STUDY GUIDE TO CONSULTATION-LIAISON PSYCHIATRY

A Companion to
The American Psychiatric Association Publishing Textbook of Psychosomatic Medicine and Consultation-Liaison Psychiatry, Third Edition

STUDY GUIDE TO CONSULTATION-LIAISON PSYCHIATRY

A Companion to
The American Psychiatric Association Publishing Textbook of Psychosomatic Medicine and Consultation-Liaison Psychiatry, Third Edition

Edited by

Philip R. Muskin, M.D., M.A.
Anna L. Dickerman, M.D.
Sara Siris Nash, M.D.

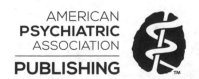

AMERICAN
PSYCHIATRIC
ASSOCIATION
PUBLISHING
™

If you wish to buy 50 or more copies of the same title, please go to www.appi.org/specialdiscounts for more information.

Copyright © 2020 American Psychiatric Association Publishing

ALL RIGHTS RESERVED

Manufactured in the United States of America on acid-free paper
23 22 21 20 19   5 4 3 2 1

ISBN 978-1-61537-261-4

First Edition

American Psychiatric Association Publishing
800 Maine Avenue SW
Suite 900
Washington, DC 20024-2812
www.appi.org

Contents

Part II: Answer Guide

Contributors

Nicole Allen, M.D.
Assistant Professor of Psychiatry, Division of Consultation-Liaison Psychiatry, Columbia University Medical Center, and Department of Psychiatry, Columbia University Vagelos College of Physicians and Surgeons, New York, New York

Rachel Anne Caravella, M.D.
Clinical Assistant Professor and Attending, Consultation-Liaison Psychiatry Service, NYU School of Medicine, New York, New York

Stephanie Cheung, M.D.
Assistant Professor of Psychiatry, Division of Consultation-Liaison Psychiatry, Columbia University Medical Center, and Department of Psychiatry, Columbia University Vagelos College of Physicians and Surgeons, New York, New York

Eric D. Collins, M.D.
Associate Clinical Professor of Psychiatry, Columbia University Vagelos College of Physicians and Surgeons; Physician-in-Chief: Silver Hill Hospital, New Canaan, Connecticut

Roberta De Oliveira, M.D., Ph.D.
Instructor in Psychiatry, Columbia University/NewYork-Presbyterian Hospital/Comprehensive Health Program, Department of Psychiatry, Columbia University Vagelos College of Physicians and Surgeons, New York, New York

Anna L. Dickerman, M.D.
Assistant Professor of Psychiatry and Chief of Consultation-Liaison Psychiatry, Weill Cornell Medical College/NewYork-Presbyterian Hospital, New York, New York

David A. Fedoronko, M.D.
Assistant Professor of Psychiatry, Division of Consultation-Liaison Psychiatry, Columbia University Medical Center, and Department of Psychiatry, Columbia University Vagelos College of Physicians and Surgeons, New York, New York

Elena Friedman, M.D.
Assistant Professor of Psychiatry, Weill Cornell Medical College/NewYork-Presbyterian Hospital, New York, New York

Liliya Gershengoren, M.D., M.P.H.
Assistant Professor of Clinical Psychiatry, Weill Cornell Medical College/NewYork-Presbyterian Hospital, New York, New York

Janna S. Gordon-Elliott, M.D.
Assistant Professor of Clinical Psychiatry, Weill Cornell Medical College/NewYork-Presbyterian Hospital, New York, New York

Mark Groves, M.D.
Assistant Clinical Professor of Psychiatry and Neurology, Icahn School of Medicine at Mount Sinai, New York, New York

Elizabeth Haase, M.D.
Associate Professor of Psychiatry, University of Nevada School of Medicine, Reno

Silvia Hafliger, M.D.
Assistant Clinical Professor of Psychiatry, UT Health, McGovern Medical School, The University of Texas/Health Science Center at Houston

Lucy A. Hutner, M.D.
Cofounder Phoebe

Alexander Kane, M.D.
Assistant Professor of Clinical Psychiatry, Weill Cornell Medical College, New York, New York

Edward T. Kenny, M.D.
Assistant Professor of Clinical Psychiatry, Department of Psychiatry, Columbia University Vagelos College of Physicians and Surgeons, New York, New York

Donald S. Kornfeld, M.D.
Professor Emeritus of Psychiatry and Special Lecturer, Columbia University Vagelos College of Physicians and Surgeons, New York, New York

Mallika Lavakumar, M.D.
Assistant Professor, Case Western Reserve University School of Medicine, Department of Psychiatry, Cleveland, Ohio

Jon A. Levenson, M.D.
Associate Professor of Psychiatry, Division of Consultation-Liaison Psychiatry, and Director, Undergraduate Medical Education in Consultation-Liaison Psychiatry, Department of Psychiatry, Columbia University Vagelos College of Physicians and Surgeons, New York, New York

Stephan J. Levitan, M.D.
Clinical Professor of Psychiatry, Columbia University Vagelos College of Physicians and Surgeons, and Training and Supervising Psychoanalyst, Columbia University Center for Psychoanalytic Training and Research, New York, New York

Vivian Liu, M.D.
PGY1 Resident in Psychiatry, Mt. Sinai Beth Israel Hospital, New York, New York

Elsa Gisella E. Mirasol, M.D.
Physician-in-Charge, Mental Health Clinic - Veterans Affairs Medical Center, Northport, New York

Adrienne D. Mishkin, M.D., M.P.H.
Assistant Professor of Psychiatry, Division of Consultation-Liaison Psychiatry, Department of Psychiatry, Columbia University Vagelos College of Physicians and Surgeons, New York, New York

Philip R. Muskin, M.D., M.A.
Professor of Psychiatry and Senior Consultant in Consultation-Liaison Psychiatry, Columbia University Medical Center, Department of Psychiatry, Columbia University Vagelos College of Physicians and Surgeons, New York, New York

Sara Siris Nash, M.D.
Assistant Professor of Psychiatry and Fellowship Director in Consultation-Liaison Psychiatry, Columbia University Medical Center, Department of Psychiatry, Columbia University Vagelos College of Physicians and Surgeons, New York, New York

Roger Nathaniel, M.D.
Assistant Clinical Professor of Psychiatry, Department of Psychiatry, Columbia University Vagelos College of Physicians and Surgeons; Assistant Attending Psychiatrist, NewYork-Presbyterian Hospital; Voluntary Faculty, New York State Psychiatric Institute; Voluntary Faculty, Columbia University Center for Psychoanalytic Teaching and Research, New York, New York

Gaddy Noy, D.O.
Postdoctoral Clinical Fellow in Consultation-Liaison Psychiatry, Department of Psychiatry, NewYork-Presbyterian Hospital and the New York State Psychiatric Institute, New York, New York

Luis F. Pereira, M.D., M.S.
Instructor in Psychiatry, Department of Psychiatry, Columbia University Vagelos College of Physicians and Surgeons, New York, New York

Shabnam Shakibaie Smith, M.D.
Assistant Professor of Psychiatry, Department of Psychiatry, Columbia University Vagelos College of Physicians and Surgeons, New York, New York

Daniel Shalev, M.D.
Postdoctoral Clinical Fellow in Consultation-Liaison Psychiatry, Department of Psychiatry, New York-Presbyterian Hospital and the New York State Psychiatric Institute, New York, New York

Akhil Shenoy, M.D.
Assistant Professor of Psychiatry and Director of Transplant Psychiatry, Department of Psychiatry, Columbia University Vagelos College of Physicians and Surgeons, New York, New York

Geoffrey Taylor, M.D.
Assistant Professor of Clinical Psychiatry, Department of Psychiatry, University of Pennsylvania, Philadelphia

Katherine E. Taylor, M.D.
Clinical Assistant Professor of Psychiatry, NYU School of Medicine; Attending Psychiatrist, NYU Langone Perlmutter Cancer Center, New York, New York

Leslie R. Vogel, M.D.
Psychiatric Consultant, Spaulding Nursing and Therapy Center Brighton, Spaulding Rehabilitation Network; Psychiatric Consultant, Nova Psychiatric Services, Quincy, Massachusetts

Rebecca Weiss, P.M.H.N.P.
Psychiatric Mental Health Nurse Practitioner, Mental Health Services, Student Health Services, Columbia University Medical Center, New York, New York

Ilona Wiener, M.D.
Assistant Professor of Psychiatry and Consultant to Kidney and Heart Transplant Services, Department of Psychiatry, Columbia University Vagelos College of Physicians and Surgeons, New York, New York

Preface

This self-examination guide is a companion to, but not a replacement for, The American Psychiatric Association Publishing Textbook of Psychosomatic Medicine and Consultation-Liaison Psychiatry, Third Edition. This self-examination guide has special meaning for the contributors and editors because we are consultation-liaison (C-L) psychiatrists. Thus, we took on this project as a "family"; that is, the contributors are all people associated with the C-L service of Columbia University Irving Medical Center, including a medical student, a nurse practitioner, residents, fellows, graduates of the fellowship program, and faculty. We hope that using this guide will prepare readers to understand the assessment and treatment of medically ill patients. As such, the guide is organized around each chapter in the textbook. As you work through this self-examination book, let it guide you to focus on chapters in the textbook as a path to your self-education. Some questions will seem obvious or easy, whereas others will be quite difficult. In the close to 400 questions in the guide, we have endeavored to use the style of question writing found in certification examinations; however, this is not a board preparation book. For each question, we provide explanations for both the correct and incorrect options. In some cases, we have gone to the primary source listed in the textbook and referenced it because there is more information in that article than is in the textbook. In a few cases, we provide an additional reference to explain why a particular option is incorrect if the textbook did not contain that information.

The contributors have graciously agreed that the proceeds from this book will be donated to charitable foundations dedicated to mental health.

Editors

Philip R. Muskin, M.D., M.A.
Anna L. Dickerman, M.D.
Sara Siris Nash, M.D.

PART I

Questions

CHAPTER 1

Psychiatric Assessment and Consultation

1.1   What is the essential element of the collaborative care model?

    A. There is consultation and appropriate sharing of information among the primary care provider, the care manager, and the consulting psychiatrist.
    B. The psychiatric specialist provides a consultation for every patient.
    C. Mental health specialists treat all patients with diagnosed mental illnesses.
    D. All interventions are performed by the same clinician.

1.2   For which of these presentations should neuroimaging be considered?

    A. A patient with a recurrent psychotic episode.
    B. A patient with established dementia when admitted to the hospital.
    C. A patient with an acute change in mental status who also has abnormal findings on neurological examination.
    D. A patient undergoing a second course of electroconvulsive therapy treatments.

1.3   Which of the following statements about the electroencephalogram (EEG) is true?

    A. The EEG is rarely available.
    B. The EEG generally indicates a specific etiology for generalized delirium.
    C. The EEG can be helpful in distinguishing between neurological and psychiatric etiologies in mute, uncommunicative patients.
    D. The EEG is useful in the screening evaluation of patients with head injury.

1.4   Which statement about screening tools for psychiatric illness is correct?

    A. Psychiatric screening tools are useful on their own in the evaluation of and treatment planning for patients.
    B. Psychiatric screening tools are unaffected by cognitive status.

C. Psychiatric screening tools have not been translated into other languages or validated cross-culturally.

D. Psychiatric screening tools may identify patients who may benefit from further psychiatric assessment.

1.5   The extensive body of research into the utility of the psychiatric consultation for medical patients has demonstrated which of the following?

A. There appears to be no link between comorbid psychopathology and increased length of hospital stay, independent of the severity of the medical illness.

B. There appears to be no link between comorbid psychopathology and increased inpatient costs, independent of the severity of the medical illness.

C. Depressed elderly patients have less frequent and shorter hospitalizations than their nondepressed cohorts.

D. Psychiatric consultation improves the medical care of complex patients.

CHAPTER 2

Legal and Ethical Issues

2.1 Which of the following, alone, would be insufficient to justify compromising patient confidentiality?

A. Suspected child abuse.
B. Suspected elder abuse.
C. Patient threatens to sign out against medical advice.
D. Patient has expressed intent to harm a specific individual.

2.2 A 72-year-old patient tells his physician he no longer wishes to be treated and wants to sign out of the hospital, despite medical advice that he remain. Which of the following is not legally required to permit the patient to leave?

A. Patient expresses a preference to leave the hospital.
B. Patient signs AMA discharge form to waive hospital liability.
C. Patient comprehends pertinent medical facts.
D. Patient rationally comprehends potential consequences.

2.3 Which of the following scenarios would not necessarily warrant a psychiatric consultation to assess a mother's ability to care for her child?

A. Maternal substance abuse.
B. Mother has a severe mental disorder.
C. Suspected child abuse or neglect.
D. Suspected intimate partner violence.

2.4 A psychiatrist is called to evaluate a patient who is a Jehovah's Witness and has refused to accept a life-saving blood transfusion. Which of the following must be present to determine that the patient has capacity to make such a decision?

A. Patient understands why the transfusion is required.
B. Patient understands refusing the transfusion will lead to his discharge from the hospital.
C. Patient's wife, who is also a Jehovah's Witness, agrees with the patient's decision.
D. Patient must consult with a psychiatrist who agrees with the patient.

2.5   A 60-year-old woman is admitted for recurrent depression that is not responsive to adequate medication trials, but four prior courses of electroconvulsive therapy (ECT) treatment were successful. She has no medical comorbidities, denies suicidal or homicidal ideation, and has no evidence of delusions or hallucinations. She lives with her husband and is independent in all activities of daily living. ECT is recommended, and the patient receives appropriate information and counseling, which she is able to repeat in her own words. She signs a consent form, although she tells staff her husband threatened divorce unless she receives ECT, and if it were up to her alone, she would not want ECT. Which of the following best describes the validity of the patient's consent?

A. Consent is valid, because the patient's decision is both knowing and voluntary.
B. Consent is valid, because the patient's husband also agrees with treatment recommendations.
C. Consent is not valid, because the patient has not received adequate information about the proposed treatment.
D. Consent is not valid even with a signed consent form, because the patient has verbally expressed reservations.

2.6   Which of the following is not a required component to meet the standard for informed consent?

A. Consent form was read to the patient.
B. Patient's spouse agrees the proposed intervention is needed.
C. Patient is presented information including the diagnosis and nature of the condition being treated; reasonably expected benefits from the proposed treatment; nature and likelihood of risks involved; inability to precisely predict results of treatment; potential irreversibility of the treatment; the expected risks, benefits, and results of alternative, or no, treatment.
D. Patient is able to repeat the information provided regarding the medical problem and proposed treatment in his own words.

2.7   A 71-year-old man presents to the emergency room with symptoms suggestive of a cerebral vascular accident. He is unable to speak and appears to have difficulty comprehending. It is determined that immediate intravascular removal of the clot causing the patient's stroke is required. Treatment may proceed without the patient's informed consent based on which of the following principles?

A. Beneficence.
B. Justice.
C. Nonmaleficence.
D. Autonomy.

2.8   Which of the following is the physician's obligation in reporting elder abuse?

A. Physicians are not mandated reporters of suspected elder abuse and neglect.
B. Reporting is mandated only when there is physical evidence of abuse.

C. Reporting suspected elder neglect should be deferred until a full assessment of cognitive decline has been performed.

D. Physicians must report suspected abuse, although elder patients may ultimately refuse intervention by protective services agencies.

2.9   A psychiatric consultation is requested to evaluate a medical patient who is irritable, agitated, and grandiose. The patient has not slept in several days. The consulting psychiatrist makes a diagnosis of bipolar disorder and recommends treatment with lithium. Three days later, lab results show the patient's serum creatinine is 1.5 mg/dL, up from a previous baseline of 1.3 mg/dL. Lithium is discontinued, and a different mood-stabilizing medication is prescribed. Which of the following is true of the consulting psychiatrist's duty to the patient regarding treatment?

A. The consulting psychiatrist has a duty directly to the patient.
B. The consulting psychiatrist assumes responsibility for monitoring the outcome of all treatment recommendations.
C. The consulting psychiatrist may assume a primary treatment role.
D. The consulting psychiatrist must enter orders for all recommendations.

2.10   Which of the following is not an element that would contribute to establishing a clear claim of malpractice against a consultation-liaison psychiatrist?

A. Proof that the consultation-liaison psychiatrist offered a general curbside opinion to a colleague.
B. Proof that the consultation-liaison psychiatrist acted intentionally to harm the patient.
C. Proof that the consultation-liaison psychiatrist directly caused a medical error.
D. Proof that the consultation-liaison psychiatrist violated the standard of care.

CHAPTER 3

Psychological Responses to Illness

3.1   What variable best accounts for interindividual differences in psychological responses to the stress of illness?

    A. Illness severity.
    B. Subjective experience of illness.
    C. Illness chronicity.
    D. Organ system involvement.

3.2   Coping is a powerful mediator of how a patient responds emotionally to a given stressor. Research by Folkman and others has demonstrated that patients tend to choose which category of coping style when the condition is appraised as out of their control?

    A. Emotion focused.
    B. Repression.
    C. Problem focused.
    D. Denial.

3.3   A middle-aged executive is threatening to sign out against medical advice after long delays in transportation to radiology for a study. A psychiatrist is consulted to assess capacity and arrives at the nursing station to hear nurses angrily complaining, "Who does she think she is?" Upon entering the room to greet the patient, the consultant spends some time inquiring about the patient's profession and achievements. The consultant says to the patient, "We aim to give you the best care and aspire to run things as efficiently as it sounds like you are able to in your business; unfortunately, emergencies frequently derail our ability to meet our ideal—please be patient with us." A dramatic de-escalation in complaints occurs, and the patient agrees to stay. What predominant personality style best describes this patient?

    A. Histrionic.
    B. Obsessional.

C. Masochistic.

D. Narcissistic.

3.4 Which attachment style is associated with consciously or unconsciously exaggerated illness behavior and high medical services use?

A. Fearful attachment style.

B. Secure attachment style.

C. Preoccupied attachment style.

D. Dismissing attachment style.

3.5 A 35-year-old woman is admitted to the hospital with orthopedic injuries sustained in a motor vehicle accident. She is found to have a growing breast mass that she has been hiding under loose clothing for many months; she is terrified that she might have cancer. A psychiatric review of systems fails to find any psychotic symptoms or any clinically significant evidence of depression. The primary medical team describes her as being in "psychotic denial." What is the best approach for the consulting psychiatrist to take in addressing her denial of cancer?

A. Direct confrontation of the denial.

B. Exploration of the underlying emotions provoking the denial.

C. Prescription of an antipsychotic medication.

D. Immediate referral to oncology.

3.6 Vaillant and others have conceptualized a hierarchy of defense mechanisms ranked in four levels of adaptivity. Defense mechanisms on which hierarchical level tend to be irritating to others, transmitting "shame, impulses, and anxiety to those around them"?

A. Psychotic defenses.

B. Mature defenses.

C. Neurotic defenses.

D. Immature defenses.

3.7 Which attachment style is predictive of worse diabetes self-care, lower adherence to hypoglycemic agents, and higher blood glucose levels in studies of diabetic patients by Ciechanowski and colleagues?

A. Preoccupied attachment style.

B. All insecure attachment styles (fearful, preoccupied, and dismissing).

C. Fearful and dismissing attachment styles.

D. Preoccupied and fearful attachment styles.

3.8   A consulting psychiatrist realizes that she dreads seeing a patient on the oncology service and has been finding excuses to see all of the other patients on her caseload first. Calls from the patient to the consultation-liaison service have begun to escalate over the past week. In noticing her countertransference response and the patient's behavior, what predominant personality style is the patient likely to have?

A. Obsessional.
B. Paranoid.
C. Dependent.
D. Narcissistic.

3.9   Adjusting to a recent diagnosis of metastatic pancreatic cancer and given a prognosis of less than 6 months to live, a patient plans to take a month vacation with family prior to medical follow-up. He tells his physician, "There is no value in my getting consumed every day in thinking about my illness if I can't do anything about it." What defense mechanism is this patient employing?

A. Repression.
B. Suppression.
C. Rationalization.
D. Denial.

3.10   The psychiatry consult service is called to assess the capacity to sign out against medical advice of a 34-year-old man who was admitted for treatment of a postsurgical infection requiring intravenous antibiotics and wound care. Nurses describe the patient as demanding and hostile, frequently calling them, and demanding to speak to the attending about discharge planning. What is the first intervention the psychiatrist should do in assessing capacity to sign out against medical advice?

A. Clarify that the patient really wants to leave the hospital.
B. Sit down and empathically listen to the patient's frustrations.
C. Assess his understanding about his medical condition.
D. Conduct a brief cognitive examination to assess orientation among other domains.

CHAPTER 4

Delirium

4.1   What is the *primary* cognitive disturbance in delirium?

    A. Attention.
    B. Short-term memory.
    C. Orientation.
    D. Visuospatial processing.

4.2   When do symptoms of a hospitalization-related delirium typically resolve in elderly patients?

    A. Before discharge in about 80% of cases.
    B. By 1 month postdischarge in about 90% of cases.
    C. By 3 months postdischarge in about 90% of cases.
    D. By 6 months postdischarge in about 80% of cases.

4.3   What physiological disturbance is associated with delirium in addition to reduced cholinergic activity?

    A. Reduced dopaminergic activity.
    B. Excess dopaminergic activity.
    C. Decreased cytokine levels.
    D. Low glucocorticoid levels.

4.4   Which strategy was found to reduce the incidence of delirium in elderly medical patients?

    A. Only pharmacological risk-reduction strategies have been shown to work.
    B. Simple interventions (e.g., consensus guidelines, educational approaches) have the greatest impact.
    C. Special medical and nursing interventions.
    D. Sleep promotion.

4.5   Studies on pharmacological prophylaxis for delirium support which statement?

A. Cholinesterase inhibitors prevent delirium.
B. Antipsychotic use in intensive care unit (ICU) patients prevents delirium.
C. Evidence so far does not support routine pharmacological prophylaxis of delirium.
D. Antipsychotic use had a positive impact on hospital length of stay and mortality.

4.6   What is the additional cost of delirium to a hospital stay?

A. An extra $5,000 to ICU costs per delirious patient.
B. An extra $5,000 to total hospital cost per delirious patient.
C. Approximately an extra $150 billion per year in the United States.
D. A 25% increase in cost of pediatric ICU stays per delirious patient.

CHAPTER 5

Dementia

5.1 Which of the following statements is true regarding the concept and epidemiology of dementia?

A. Most cases of mild cognitive impairment, including mild neurocognitive disorder, do not progress to dementia.
B. The prevalence and incidence rates of dementia remain constant as age increases.
C. The prevalence rate for all dementias in the U.S. population older than 65 years is 1%.
D. Vascular dementia is the most common neurodegenerative disorder.

5.2 Which of the following is a confirmed risk factor for dementia of the Alzheimer's type (DAT)?

A. Low education.
B. Hypertension.
C. Age.
D. Depression.

5.3 Which of the following is true regarding genes and the inheritance of Huntington's disease?

A. The amyloid precursor protein (APP) gene is a genetic locus for Huntington's disease.
B. The mutation responsible for Huntington's disease is an elongated and unstable trinucleotide (CAG) repeat.
C. A mutation in the presenilin-2 gene is responsible for Huntington's disease.
D. Mutations in the tau gene are responsible for Huntington's disease.

5.4 Which of the following is a clinical finding in patients with mild DAT?

A. Total disorientation.
B. Difficulties in planning, sequencing, and executing instrumental activities of daily living.

C. Extreme impoverishment of language; communication impossible.

D. Double incontinence (urinary and fecal).

5.5   Which of the following is true regarding the behavioral and psychological symptoms of dementia (BPSDs)?

A. BPSDs are associated with slower disease progression.

B. The course of BPSDs parallels cognitive and functional deterioration in patients with DAT.

C. BPSDs are only observed after cognitive or functional decline is apparent.

D. BPSDs may include depression, hallucinations, disinhibition, wandering, and eating disturbances.

5.6   Which of the following is a clinical characteristic of cortical dementia?

A. Late appearance of primitive reflexes.

B. Early marked apathy.

C. Early, very marked extrapyramidal signs.

D. Frequent, severe affective syndromes.

5.7   Early gait disturbance, subcortical dementia with severe apathetic features, and urinary incontinence are characteristic of which of the following dementia syndromes?

A. DAT.

B. Huntington's disease.

C. Normal-pressure hydrocephalus (NPH).

D. Wilson's disease.

5.8   Which of the following is a strength of the Mini-Mental State Examination (MMSE)?

A. It can document degree of functional impairment.

B. It tests well for executive function deficits.

C. It is sensitive to mild cognitive impairment.

D. It fares very well in different cultures.

5.9   Neuroimaging in the diagnosis of dementia is useful in which of the following situations?

A. To diagnose dementia in cases involving advanced symptoms and a long history of disease.

B. To rule out reversible conditions such as NPH, subdural hematoma, and brain tumors.

C. To identify general atrophy, which is diagnostic for DAT.

D. To demonstrate increased fluorodeoxyglucose uptake in the temporoparietal cortex on positron emission tomography (PET), which is a major biomarker of DAT.

5.10   Which of the following is a suggested guideline for psychotropic medication use
       in patients with dementia?

       A. Treat behavioral symptoms immediately with sedatives.
       B. Add an anticholinergic agent if extrapyramidal symptoms occur.
       C. Quickly up titrate dosages in order to achieve optimal symptoms control.
       D. Reassess risks and benefits of psychotropic treatment on an ongoing basis.

CHAPTER 6

Aggression and Violence

6.1 What is the relationship between violence and mental illness?

A. Mental illness does not affect an individual's risk for violence.
B. People with mental illness are two to eight times more likely to be violent than people without mental illness only by virtue of their illness.
C. People with mental illness are two to eight times more likely to be violent than people without mental illness for a variety of reasons including clinical, historical, demographic, and social factors.
D. People with mental illness are two to eight times more likely to be violent than people without mental illness, but this is simply because of the increased rate of substance use.

6.2 Which of the following is a feature of instrumental aggression?

A. It is associated with high emotional sensitivity and autonomic arousal.
B. It is often unintentional.
C. It is purposeful and premeditated.
D. It is inherently pathological in nature.

6.3 What personality disorder is most likely to be associated with habitual violence?

A. Antisocial personality disorder.
B. Borderline personality disorder.
C. Narcissistic personality disorder.
D. Paranoid personality disorder.

6.4 Lesions of what brain regions have been associated with episodes of uncontrollable rage?

A. Hypothalamus and prefrontal cortex.
B. Hypothalamus and amygdala.
C. Hypothalamus and insula.
D. Amygdala and prefrontal cortex.

6.5   What is the *most* common cause of substance-induced violent behavior?

A. Hallucinogens.
B. Cocaine and amphetamines.
C. Anticholinergic substances.
D. Alcohol.

6.6   What is the most common association between violence and ictal/postictal states in patients with epilepsy?

A. Most violent behavior in patients with epilepsy occurs during the ictal state.
B. Most violent behavior in patients with epilepsy occurs during the postictal state because of postictal psychosis.
C. Most violent behavior in patients with epilepsy is not associated with preictal, ictal, or postictal states.
D. Most violent behavior in patients with epilepsy occurs during preictal affective instability.

6.7   What is *most* characteristic of aggression among people with dementia?

A. Simple behaviors like throwing objects, pushing, kicking, pinching, biting, and scratching.
B. Destruction of property.
C. Aggressive sexual behaviors.
D. Complex, coordinated violent activity driven by a consistent goal.

6.8   Which of the following is true of routine screening for intimate partner violence?

A. The evidence suggests that all women should be routinely screened for intimate partner violence.
B. Victims prefer face-to-face questioning rather than self-completed questionnaires.
C. Computer screening in the emergency department (ED) setting is likely to be widely implemented.
D. Although the U.S. Preventive Services Task Force and many advocacy organizations advocate universal screening, there is a lack of evidence that such screening improves outcomes.

6.9   What *best* describes the role of medication in the treatment of aggression?

A. There is no evidence for any particular pharmacological intervention in either acute or chronic aggressive behavior.
B. Although antipsychotics and benzodiazepines are most frequently used for acute agitation, a broad range of medications are used for chronic aggressive behavior depending on context.

C. Only valproate has demonstrated efficacy as a treatment for acute aggression.

D. Antipsychotics are never first-line medication choices for chronic aggressive behavior.

6.10 Which of the following is characteristic of communication-based de-escalation techniques for aggressive behavior?

A. They are exclusively used in lieu of pharmacological management.

B. They should be deployed as an unstructured, instinctive intervention.

C. They are most useful in situations that involve patient-staff conflict.

D. The basic goal is to assume an authoritative stance that compels patients to acquiesce.

CHAPTER 7

Depression

7.1 Which of the following depressive diagnoses was reclassified as a trauma- and stressor-related disorder in DSM-5?

   A. Persistent depressive disorder.
   B. Bereavement.
   C. Adjustment disorder with depressed features.
   D. Depressive disorder due to another medical condition.

7.2 Which of the following illnesses has the highest prevalence of major depressive disorder (MDD)?

   A. Stroke.
   B. HIV/AIDS.
   C. Cancer.
   D. Alzheimer's disease.

7.3 Inflammatory cytokine-associated depression is most likely to present with which of the following symptoms of depression?

   A. Anhedonia.
   B. Suicidality.
   C. Guilty ruminations.
   D. Fatigue.

7.4 Which of the following is more consistent with subthreshold depression than with normal sadness?

   A. Potentially transient and self-limited, including mood episodes lasting less than 2 weeks.
   B. Belief that things will get better.
   C. Maintenance of will to live.
   D. Sense of self-worth fluctuating with thoughts of illness.

7.5   To what are the increased mortality rates among depressed patients with cardio-vascular disease most attributable?

A. Cigarette smoking.
B. Alcohol use.
C. Severity of medical illness.
D. Effects on the autonomic nervous system.

7.6   Which of the following depression self-report measures includes the fewest somatic items?

A. Center for Epidemiologic Studies–Depression Scale (CES-D).
B. Hospital Anxiety and Depression Scale (HADS).
C. Beck Depression Inventory–II (BDI-II).
D. Patient Health Questionnaire–9 (PHQ-9).

7.7   What is considered the most important clinical psychotherapeutic tool in treating depression in many medically ill patients?

A. Psychoeducation techniques.
B. Behavioral activation techniques.
C. Supportive-expressive psychotherapy.
D. Relationship with the primary medical provider.

7.8   Which of the following can lead to the overdiagnosis and treatment of depression in the medical setting?

A. Time-pressured medical visits.
B. Patients' comfort with spontaneous disclosure of psychological issues.
C. Practitioners' comfort with managing psychological issues.
D. Identification of depression as an understandable reaction to medical illness.

7.9   Which of the following statements about repetitive transcranial magnetic stimulation (rTMS) is correct?

A. rTMS treatment is associated with short-term memory impairment.
B. rTMS has a similar antidepressant effect to selective serotonin reuptake inhibitors (SSRIs) in patients with Parkinson's disease.
C. rTMS has a robust antidepressant effect for depression, but not in specific medical populations.
D. rTMS use is discouraged in patients with neurological disorders.

7.10   Which of the following antidepressants is most effective in treating hot flashes in breast cancer?

A. Milnacipran.
B. Bupropion.
C. Venlafaxine.
D. Mirtazapine.

CHAPTER 8

Suicidality

8.1   Which of the following statements is true regarding gender differences in suicide rates?

    A. Men age 75 years and older have the highest suicide rate.

    B. Suicide rates in women are high in younger ages, decline in midlife, and peak as they get older.

    C. Suicide rates in men decrease with age.

    D. Men consistently have a lower suicide rate than women.

8.2   Which of the following is *true* regarding predicting suicide risk?

    A. Chronically suicidal individuals rarely end up committing suicide.

    B. History of suicide attempts is an important predictor of future suicide risk.

    C. Active alcohol use and other substances play an insignificant role in predicting suicide risk.

    D. Opiate use disorder does not increase suicide risk.

8.3   Which of the following statements is *true* regarding the demographics of suicide attempts?

    A. Medical illness in those who attempt suicide is uncommon.

    B. Those who attempt suicide have very different predictors compared with those who complete suicide.

    C. Life-threatening illness and chronic deteriorating illness are rare in those who attempt suicide.

    D. The ratio of attempts to completed suicides narrows precipitously in old age.

8.4   What is the focus when assessing suicide risk in medically ill patients?

    A. The medical diagnosis.

    B. Understanding that comorbid psychiatric illnesses play only a limited role in suicide risk.

    C. Assessment of psychiatric conditions associated with suicide.

    D. Understanding that there is a high risk of completed suicides in inpatient units.

8.5   Suicide risk is the highest in which of the following groups of cancer patients?

A. Good prognosis group.
B. Patients with lung and bronchial cancer.
C. Patients with laryngeal cancer.
D. Patients in the later stages of cancer illness.

8.6   The suicide rates in people with HIV/AIDS have decreased but remain elevated. Which factors contribute to this elevated risk?

A. Treatment with highly active antiretroviral therapy (HAART).
B. Living with long-term AIDS.
C. Substance abuse, psychiatric illness, and intimate partner violence contribute independently to elevated suicide risk.
D. Lack of intimate partner violence does not protect against the risk of a suicide attempt.

8.7   Along with early detection and treatment of comorbid psychiatric disorders, which of the following is helpful in preventing suicide in the medically ill?

A. Always prescribing antidepressant medications for medically ill patients expressing suicidal ideation.
B. Diagnosing depression when patients are fatigued, have trouble concentrating, and are expressing disappointment.
C. Avoiding any direct questions about suicidal ideations.
D. Advocating psychotherapy.

8.8   What is the most important factor to consider for managing a patient admitted to a medical unit after a suicide attempt?

A. Psychiatrists should trust the judgment of the primary team about whether patients are medically cleared for transfer.
B. Hospital environments are generally safe.
C. Attention should be paid to items that could be used for self-strangulation.
D. One-to-one observation by sitters is not cost-effective and should be avoided.

8.9   A competent, terminally ill patient whose decision-making ability is not compromised by psychiatric illness can request hastened death or physician-assisted suicide (PAS) in which of the following states?

A. Massachusetts, New York, New Hampshire, Maryland, and Maine.
B. The majority of states because voters have passed PAS ballot measures even though the states have not put the legislation into effect.
C. Oregon, Washington, Vermont, Colorado, California, and the District of Columbia.
D. Arizona, New Mexico, Texas, Montana, and Idaho.

8.10 Within the ethos and practice of palliative care, which of the following is correct in the assessment of patients requesting PAS?

A. Depression and cognitive impairment play no role when assessing patients requesting PAS.
B. The Oregon experience has shown that offering palliative interventions results in higher PAS requests.
C. Pain, mental anguish, strained interpersonal relationships, spiritual despair, and iatrogenic anxiety about the dying process should be addressed.
D. Physical distress motivates desire for hastened death.

CHAPTER 9

Psychosis, Mania, and Catatonia

9.1 Which of the following would be considered a secondary psychosis in a medically hospitalized patient?

A. Acute exacerbation of schizophrenia.
B. A patient with schizophrenia and Grave's disease with psychosis due to thyroid abnormalities.
C. Psychosis due to epilepsy.
D. Psychosis with no Schneiderian first-rank symptoms.

9.2 How can psychosis affect care in the medical setting?

A. Need for legal intervention can result in treatment delays.
B. Staff may increase interaction and become more responsive to the patient.
C. Patients with dementia may be less likely to be admitted to a nursing home.
D. Life span of patients with schizophrenia may improve.

9.3 Which of the following considerations are *true* when making recommendations for managing psychosis in a patient with dementia who has Parkinson's disease?

A. Benzodiazepines are the treatment of choice for secondary psychosis.
B. Clozapine has few potential side effects in patients with Parkinson's disease.
C. There may be an increased risk of death in patients with dementia treated with antipsychotics.
D. No selective serotonin reuptake inhibitors (SSRIs) have shown efficacy in treating psychotic agitation.

9.4 What is the best way to distinguish delirium from secondary mania?

A. The gradual onset of delirium.
B. The waxing and waning course of delirium.
C. The sleep disturbance found in mania.
D. The presence of psychosis in mania.

9.5 Which of the following is a *rare* cause of secondary mania?

    A. Frontotemporal dementia.
    B. Epilepsy.
    C. Alzheimer's disease.
    D. Central nervous system infection.

9.6 Which of the following conditions is *most* likely to cause secondary mania?

    A. Hypothyroidism.
    B. Alzheimer's disease.
    C. Cushing's disease.
    D. Epilepsy.

9.7 In which of the following patient populations does catatonia have the *highest* incidence?

    A. Patients hospitalized with acute psychotic episodes.
    B. Patients with mood disorders.
    C. Patients with medical illness.
    D. Patients with mental retardation and autistic spectrum disorders.

9.8 What is the *most* effective treatment for catatonia?

    A. Benzodiazepines.
    B. First-generation high-potency antipsychotics.
    C. Electroconvulsive therapy (ECT).
    D. Second-generation antipsychotics.

9.9 Which of the following is a secondary catatonia?

    A. Neuroleptic malignant syndrome (NMS).
    B. Stiff person syndrome.
    C. Malignant hyperthermia.
    D. Locked-in syndrome.

9.10 Which of the following is an example of malignant catatonia?

    A. Bell's mania.
    B. Kahlbaum's syndrome.
    C. A score of at least 9/14 on the Bush-Francis Catatonia Rating Scale (BFCRS).
    D. Catatonia causing critical illness with hyperthermia or autonomic instability.

CHAPTER 10

Anxiety Disorders

10.1 What percentage of primary care patients with generalized anxiety disorder (GAD) are correctly diagnosed?

A. 14%.
B. 24%.
C. 34%.
D. 44%.

10.2 Which measure is considered the *gold standard* for diagnosis of an anxiety disorder?

A. A clinical interview using DSM-5 criteria.
B. The Generalized Anxiety Disorder–7 (GAD-7) scale.
C. The Hospital Anxiety and Depression Scale (HADS).
D. The Patient Health Questionnaire–4 (PHQ-4).

10.3 Which type of anxiety disorder is quite common but rarely comes to the attention of primary care physicians?

A. GAD.
B. Panic disorder.
C. Specific phobia.
D. Posttraumatic stress disorder.

10.4 Which of the following scenarios should prompt consideration of a medical cause for anxiety?

A. When there is a personal or family history of primary anxiety disorder.
B. When the onset of anxiety is at a younger age.
C. When psychosocial stressors are present.
D. When anxiety is accompanied by disproportionate or atypical physical symptoms.

10.5 How can one distinguish between anxiety secondary to hyperthyroidism and a primary anxiety disorder?

A. Hyperthyroidism is associated with persistent tachycardia.
B. Hyperthyroidism is associated with cold intolerance.
C. Anxiety associated with hyperthyroidism is alleviated by treatment with beta-blockers.
D. Hyperthyroidism is accompanied by adrenergic overreactivity.

10.6 How does PTSD based on the trauma of a medical experience, such as cancer or myocardial infarction, differ from more usual PTSD stressors such as rape?

A. In PTSD associated with a medical experience, the stressor is related to memory of a past event rather than fear of recurrence.
B. In PTSD associated with a medical experience, the threat arises from one's own body.
C. PTSD associated with a medical experience does not arise out of a perceived trauma.
D. Development of PTSD in medical illness is predicted by disease severity.

10.7 Which class of medication might contribute to anxiety both with therapeutic use as well as during withdrawal?

A. Antidepressants.
B. Antineoplastic agents.
C. Phenethylamines.
D. Interferons.

10.8 Which modality of psychotherapeutic treatment for anxiety involves promoting the patient's adaptive defenses and challenging only clearly maladaptive defenses?

A. Cognitive-behavioral therapy.
B. Psychodynamic therapy.
C. Supportive psychotherapy.
D. Mindfulness-based stress reduction.

10.9 Which statement best reflects the recommended treatment approach for managing death anxiety in patients confronting life-threatening or terminal illnesses such as cancer?

A. Open discussions about death should be avoided, as they increase anxiety and distress.
B. Emphasizing the importance of patients to their families can potentially increase anxiety and distress.
C. The primary goal should remain full recovery.
D. Helping patients find meaning despite their suffering is an important therapy goal.

10.10 Which benzodiazepine has the advantages of oral, intravenous, or intramuscular administration?

A. Diazepam.
B. Oxazepam.
C. Lorazepam.
D. Midazolam.

CHAPTER 11

Somatic Symptom Disorder and Illness Anxiety Disorder

11.1   Which of the following is a major change in the DSM-5 diagnostic criteria for somatic symptom disorders?

A. Positive psychobehavioral features in criterion B have been eliminated.
B. Multiple distressing bodily symptoms are a requirement for the diagnosis.
C. The diagnosis rests on the determination that the bodily symptoms be medically unexplained.
D. Illness anxiety disorder (IAD) replaces hypochondriasis in older *Diagnostic and Statistical Manual of Mental Disorders* (DSM) editions.

11.2   Which of the following is a predisposing factor for bodily distress and somatization?

A. Childhood adversity.
B. Ability to read one's own emotional states.
C. Attachment security.
D. Single gene inheritance.

11.3   What advice would be most appropriate for an internist regarding management of a patient with somatic symptom disorder?

A. Repetitive investigations should be undertaken to reassure and calm the patient.
B. Persistent physical symptoms should be equated with malingering.
C. Pay attention to patient clues indicating distress beyond the current main symptom.
D. Do not screen for anxiety and depression as it is outside your specialist field.

11.4   Which of the following is a helpful theragnostic principle for management of patients with IAD?

A. Avoid taking bodily complaints seriously when no well-defined organic pathology is demonstrated.
B. Frame context factors as amplifiers rather than causes of symptoms.
C. Symptomatic measures from complementary medicine should be strictly prohibited.
D. Wait for the patient to initiate appointments.

11.5   Which of the following is a rigorously evidence-based intervention for somatic symptom disorder (SSD)?

A. Cognitive-behavioral interventions.
B. Tricyclic antidepressants.
C. St. John's wort.
D. Training in enhanced care for primary care physicians.

11.6   What is the prevalence of health anxiety across the life span?

A. 3.4%.
B. 5.7%.
C. 7%.
D. 20%.

11.7   What is the most relevant disorder in the differential diagnosis of IAD?

A. Factitious disorder.
B. Depressive disorder.
C. Generalized anxiety disorder.
D. Personality disorder.

11.8   Which recommendation is most appropriate for the initial phase of psychotherapy in patients with SSD/IAD?

A. Establish "cure" as a treatment goal.
B. Listen attentively to bodily complaints.
C. Concentrate on psychosocial issues independently of lead complaints.
D. Avoid discussing the patient with others involved in his or her care.

CHAPTER 12

Deception Syndromes: Factitious Disorders and Malingering

12.1   Which psychiatric condition is often associated with pseudologia fantastica?

   A. Learning disability.
   B. Adult trauma.
   C. Superior intelligence.
   D. Malingering.

12.2   Which deception syndrome is *not* a psychiatric diagnosis?

   A. Factitious disorder with physical symptoms.
   B. Factitious disorder with psychological symptoms.
   C. Factitious disorder imposed on another.
   D. Malingering.

12.3   Which patient phenotype is usually associated with common factitious disorder?

   A. Single, male, age in the 40s, antisocial traits.
   B. Single, female, age in the 30s, Cluster B traits.
   C. Married, female, age in the 50s, Cluster B traits.
   D. Married, male, age in the 20s, histrionic traits.

12.4   Which feature occurs in classic Munchausen syndrome and distinguishes it from common factitious disorder?

   A. Simulation of disease.
   B. Self-induction of disease.
   C. Pseudologia fantastica.
   D. Peregrinating behavior.

12.5   Which symptoms are most commonly reported in patients with factitious disorder with psychological symptoms?

    A. Depression and suicidal ideation.
    B. Dissociative identity disorder.
    C. Substance use disorder.
    D. Posttraumatic stress disorder.

12.6   What treatment strategy is recommended for patients with factitious disorder?

    A. Direct confrontation of the patient to "let them have it."
    B. Invasive diagnostic testing to rule out "real" disease.
    C. Indirect "interpretation" and therapy focused on acting-out behaviors.
    D. Identify the patient on circulated "blacklists" for other hospitals.

12.7   When should a clinician entertain the diagnosis of factitious disorder imposed on another (FDIA)?

    A. If the illness resolves when the child is separated from the caregiver.
    B. In spite of the absence of a parental history of psychiatric treatment.
    C. When an angry parent seems very comfortable with the child staying in the hospital.
    D. When the mother adamantly denies a personal history of abuse as a child.

12.8   What is the feared outcome of FDIA?

    A. Failure to meet developmental milestones.
    B. False accusations.
    C. High cost of medical care.
    D. Death of a child.

12.9   When malingering is suspected, how should the psychiatric consultant approach the case?

    A. Direct patient confrontation.
    B. Diagnosis of antisocial personality disorder.
    C. Careful written documentation.
    D. Functional neuroimaging assessment.

12.10   Who is a typical victim in angel of death syndrome?

    A. The patient who intentionally feigns physical disease.
    B. The patient who gives approximate answers.
    C. The elderly patient resuscitated by a nurse on an evening shift.
    D. The wealthy housewife seeking to evade arrest by feigning coma.

CHAPTER 13

Eating Disorders

13.1 You evaluate a 4-year-old boy for significant weight loss who does not exhibit fear of weight gain, body image disturbance, or drive for thinness. His mother reports noticing that he avoids food with a certain bitter taste, will only eat foods that are crunchy, does not engage in recurrent regurgitation of food, and does not consume nonnutritive substances (e.g., dirt, clay, soap, paper). His day care teachers have requested an evaluation for suspected autism spectrum diagnoses. What is the most appropriate diagnosis given the aforementioned information from the evaluation?

A. Pica.
B. Avoidant/restrictive food intake disorder (ARFID).
C. Rumination disorder.
D. Anorexia nervosa (AN).

13.2 How do patients with eating disorder typically approach behavior change?

A. Ambivalence toward behavior change is the norm.
B. They exhibit overall comfort with engaging in weight-control behaviors.
C. Symptom concealment is uncommon.
D. Embarrassment and shame typically do not complicate patient engagement.

13.3 A 34-year-old woman discloses feeling depressed and guilty about weekly episodes of heavy consumption of food over a period of 6 months during a consultation regarding depression. She typically eats alone, even when not hungry, consumes food more rapidly than usual, and eats until physically full and uncomfortable. She does not vomit and experiences strong feelings of disgust. She denies any compensatory behaviors in order to lose weight and does not engage in restricting behaviors to limit caloric intake. She has metabolic syndrome and newly diagnosed hypertension. She is concerned about her obesity and has been considering weight-loss surgery. Given the aforementioned presentation, what is the most appropriate diagnosis?

A. Bulimia nervosa (BN).
B. Anorexia nervosa (AN).

C. Binge-eating disorder (BED).

D. Rumination disorder.

13.4   Which of the following treatment plans is recommended for individuals with co-morbid eating disorders and substance use disorders (SUDs)?

A. Both disorders should be addressed at the same time.

B. Patients with eating disorders do not have an elevated prevalence of SUDs and therefore SUDs are of little concern.

C. Addressing each disorder one at a time will result in symptomatic improvement of both disorders.

D. Comorbid SUDs have not been shown to increase mortality, medical complications, and psychopathology and are, therefore, of little concern.

13.5   Which of the following phenomena should raise suspicion for an underlying eating disorder in patients with type 1 diabetes mellitus?

A. Frequent requests to be weighed during medical appointments.

B. Optimal glycemic control.

C. Requests for multiple medical appointments.

D. Skipping doses of insulin.

13.6   Signs and symptoms of starvation and purging include which of the following?

A. Increase in energy.

B. Sinus tachycardia.

C. Parotid gland enlargement.

D. Elevated mood.

13.7   Which of the following factors contributes to the sustaining behavior of eating disorders?

A. Cognitive rigidity.

B. Low self-directedness.

C. Alterations in satiety and hunger signaling.

D. Excessive exercise.

13.8   Which of the electrolyte abnormalities is seen in patients with AN?

A. Hypokalemia.

B. Hyperglycemia.

C. Hyperphosphatemia.

D. Hypernatremia.

13.9   A woman with a recent diagnosis of AN is contemplating becoming pregnant. What are the gynecological and obstetric complications associated with AN?

A. Patients with AN do not respond to fertility treatment.
B. AN is associated with high estrogen levels.
C. AN is associated with primary hypogonadotropic amenorrhea.
D. AN is associated with low follicle-stimulating hormone and luteinizing hormone.

13.10 Refeeding syndrome carries which of the following risks to patients?

A. High risk of hypophosphatemia.
B. High risk of hyperglycemia.
C. Rare risk of edema or congestive heart failure.
D. Higher risk from oral feeding than parenteral feeding.

13.11 Which of the following patient populations has been shown to benefit from outpatient interventions designed for weight restoration and symptom remission in medically stable patients diagnosed with AN?

A. Acutely ill patients.
B. Chronic cases.
C. Adults rather than adolescents.
D. Only inpatient treatments are indicated for patients with AN.

13.12 What medication is approved by the U.S. Food and Drug Administration (FDA) for the treatment of BN?

A. Topiramate.
B. Fluoxetine.
C. Ondansetron.
D. Bupropion.

13.13 A consultation-liaison psychiatrist is asked to evaluate a patient hospitalized after a syncopal episode, who was found to have a low BMI. The patient is a 20-year-old woman who presents with recent significant weight loss, persistent food intake restriction, and intense fear of gaining weight. She reluctantly admits to occasional laxative use in order to maintain low weight. The patient does not believe that she has an eating disorder despite her hospitalization in the setting of a syncopal episode due to prolonged starvation. After discussing the patient's diagnosis, the psychiatrist is considering pharmacological interventions. Which of the following is correct regarding pharmacological agents approved for the treatment of a diagnosis of AN?

A. To date, no pharmacological agent is approved for the treatment of AN.
B. Fluoxetine has been FDA approved for the treatment of AN.
C. Chlorpromazine has been FDA approved for the treatment of AN.
D. Alprazolam has been FDA approved for the treatment of AN.

13.14 Which of the following eating disorders meets all the criteria for AN except for low weight?

    A. Night eating syndrome.
    B. BED.
    C. ARFID.
    D. Atypical AN.

CHAPTER 14

Sleep Disorders

14.1   What characterizes rapid eye movement (REM) sleep?

A. Three distinct stages.
B. Decreased levels of cortical activation.
C. Reduced muscle tone.
D. Spindles and K complexes.

14.2   Which of the following conditions is most likely to cause insomnia?

A. Hyperglycemia.
B. Hypothyroidism.
C. Psychostimulant withdrawal.
D. Gastrointestinal reflux.

14.3   For which sleep disorder is a portable sleep study appropriate?

A. Obstructive sleep apnea hypopnea (OSAH).
B. Central sleep apnea.
C. Restless leg syndrome.
D. Fatal familial insomnia.

14.4   What is the most important part of an evaluation for narcolepsy?

A. Decreased cerebrospinal fluid (CSF) hypocretin levels.
B. Clinical interview.
C. Presence of deep-tendon reflexes during cataplexy episode.
D. Negative wrist actigraphy.

14.5   What is the cardinal feature of hypersomnolence disorder?

A. Sleep-onset REM episodes.
B. Undetectable CSF hypocretin levels.
C. Excessive daytime sleepiness.
D. Short duration of nocturnal sleep.

14.6   Which of the following is a risk factor for REM sleep behavior disorder?

   A. Selective serotonin reuptake inhibitors (SSRIs).
   B. Female gender.
   C. Childhood age.
   D. Alzheimer's dementia.

14.7   Which of the following sleep disorders is treated with behavioral techniques, such as relaxation and exposure?

   A. Non–rapid eye movement (NREM) sleep behavior disorder.
   B. Hypersomnolence disorder.
   C. Narcolepsy.
   D. Nightmare disorder.

14.8   What is an appropriate treatment for an obese patient with OSAH unable to tolerate continuous positive airway pressure (CPAP)?

   A. Bilevel positive airway pressure.
   B. Supplemental oxygen.
   C. Tonsillectomy.
   D. A 10-pound weight loss.

14.9   How does central sleep apnea differ from OSAH?

   A. Central sleep apnea is characterized by respiratory pauses with airway collapse.
   B. Patient's airway is narrowed in central sleep apnea.
   C. Patients with central sleep apnea present with insomnia.
   D. Snoring is a typical warning sign in central sleep apnea.

14.10 What is the treatment of choice for restless leg syndrome (RLS)?

   A. Clonazepam.
   B. Gabapentin.
   C. Pramipexole.
   D. Methadone.

CHAPTER 15

Sexual Dysfunctions

15.1   What type of therapy for sexual dysfunction includes sensate focus therapy?

A. Mindfulness-based cognitive therapy.
B. Sex therapy.
C. Hypnotherapy.
D. Cognitive-behavioral therapy (CBT).

15.2   Which of the following disease categories is considered high risk and would defer sexual dysfunction treatment?

A. Moderate or severe valve disease.
B. Stable angina.
C. History of uncomplicated myocardial infarction (MI).
D. Left ventricular dysfunction/congestive heart failure (LVD/CHF) (New York Heart Association [NYHA] Class II).

15.3   Which of the following medications would be safe to use with vardenafil?

A. Cimetidine.
B. Amiodarone.
C. Nitroglycerin.
D. Sertraline.

15.4   What is a predictor of sexual dysfunction in patients with rheumatic disease?

A. Genital tissue changes.
B. Impaired mobility.
C. Comorbid anxiety disorder.
D. Pain.

15.5   The treatment of which neurological condition puts male patients at risk for hypersexuality?

A. Seizure disorder.
B. Stroke.

C. Spinal cord injury.
D. Parkinson's disease.

15.6   Erectile dysfunction (ED) in a patient with uncomplicated type 2 diabetes could be an indicator of which of the following conditions?

A. Cardiac ischemia.
B. Neuropathy.
C. Hypertension.
D. Hypoglycemia.

15.7   Which of the following anticonvulsants has the lowest profile of sexual side effects in men?

A. Lamotrigine.
B. Carbamazepine.
C. Phenytoin.
D. Barbiturates.

15.8   Which of the following factors is directly involved in sexual dysfunction associated with chronic disease?

A. Reduction of self-image.
B. Fear of sexual activity worsening medical condition.
C. Disruption of sexual desire and response because of nonhormonal medications.
D. Partnership difficulties.

15.9   Which of the following has evidence to support its use in reversing ejaculatory dysfunction?

A. Improving glycemic control.
B. Narcotics.
C. Anabolic steroids.
D. Diuretics.

15.10 Which of the following combinations are predictors of sexual dysfunction in diabetes?

A. Depression and being married, in women.
B. Depression and being married, in men.
C. Depression and poor glycemic control, in women.
D. Depression and poor glycemic control, in men.

CHAPTER 16

Substance-Related Disorders

16.1   You are called to help manage severe alcohol withdrawal in a 64-year-old patient who is extremely agitated and aggressive. Which of the following is appropriate as a single-agent treatment for moderate to severe alcohol withdrawal?

A. Propranolol.
B. Phenobarbital.
C. Carbamazepine.
D. Clonidine.

16.2   A 56-year-old diabetic man is brought to the emergency room for altered mental status and receives IV glucose. Shortly after his admission, he becomes confused and displays difficulty with coordination with an abnormal gait. Immediate treatment with which of the following IV medications is most appropriate for this patient?

A. Flumazenil.
B. Magnesium.
C. Ethanol.
D. Thiamine.

16.3   You are called to see a 35-year-old woman who takes oral naltrexone 50 mg daily for alcohol use disorder (AUD). Two days ago, she began taking a prescription medication for a newly diagnosed condition. Earlier today, she consumed several mixed drinks at a wedding reception. On presentation to the emergency room, she had palpitations, nausea, vomiting, headache, hypotension, shortness of breath, and flushing. Which of the following medications is the most likely cause of the patient's symptoms?

A. Metronidazole.
B. Meperidine.
C. Diazepam.
D. Naltrexone.

16.4 A 49-year-old man, maintained on methadone 80 mg daily, is hit by a car and suffers compound fractures of both femurs. Which of the following is the most appropriate approach to managing the patient's acute pain in the hospital?

A. Continue the methadone maintenance dosage and use only nonsteroidal analgesics because the methadone maintenance doses will produce sufficient analgesia.
B. Divide the patient's daily methadone maintenance dosage into four equal amounts to be given orally every 6 hours.
C. Continue the patient's methadone maintenance dosage once daily by the intravenous route.
D. Continue the methadone maintenance dosage and treat with additional opioid analgesics, as well as other analgesics, as needed.

16.5 A 58-year-old homeless man with AUD and opioid use disorder, maintained on methadone 100 mg daily, is treated with rifampicin for tuberculosis. His physicians should monitor for which of the following potential adverse reactions due to the antibiotic?

A. Opioid intoxication due to inhibition of cytochrome P450 3A4.
B. Opioid withdrawal due to induction of cytochrome P450 3A4.
C. Development of torsades de pointes due to prolongation of the QTc interval.
D. Emergence of hypomagnesemia and/or hypokalemia.

16.6 You are asked to help manage a 34-year-old woman at 22 weeks gestation who presents with vaginal bleeding in the setting of heroin withdrawal; the patient's Clinical Opiate Withdrawal Scale (COWS) score is 8 points. Which of the following is the most appropriate next step in management?

A. Treat symptoms with nonopioid medications only until the opioid withdrawal syndrome resolves.
B. Administer naloxone 1 mg intravenously to reduce the opioid-induced uterine bleeding.
C. Induct the patient onto buprenorphine for maintenance treatment of opioid use disorder during pregnancy.
D. Begin intramuscular naltrexone for maintenance treatment of opioid use disorder during pregnancy and to protect the fetus from the effects of opioids.

16.7 A 23-year-old man is brought to the emergency room after developing grandiosity, auditory hallucinations, paranoia, and agitation. Vitals signs are notable for blood pressure of 160/105 mmHg and heart rate of 125 beats per minute. Friends report he has been compulsively using a new drug and may have accidentally overdosed. Which of the following is the most likely causative agent of this patient's presentation?

A. Methcathinone (a synthetic cathinone compound).
B. Gamma-hydroxybutyrate (GHB).

C. NBOMe ("N-bomb").

D. Nitrous oxide ("laughing gas").

16.8 A daily marijuana smoker for many years, a 25-year-old man is hospitalized for several weeks for treatment of pneumonia. He develops the following symptoms: insomnia with strange dreams, nausea, tremor, elevated mood, decreased appetite, and marked irritability. Which of this patient's symptoms is uncharacteristic of cannabis withdrawal?

A. Nausea.

B. Irritability.

C. Tremor.

D. Elevated mood.

16.9 You are called to evaluate a patient who was admitted a week ago for abdominal pain and vomiting, for which no immediate cause is identified. Symptoms have been refractory to usual antiemetics. The patient frequently insists upon using the bathroom and takes multiple long showers each day, which, according to nursing staff, is both highly unusual and often disruptive to the patient sharing the room. Chronic use of which of the following drugs can lead to cycles of abdominal pain and vomiting, often relieved by bathing or showering with hot water?

A. Cathinone (khat).

B. Meperidine.

C. Cannabis.

D. GHB.

16.10 A 19-year-old patient with a severe daily substance use disorder presents to the emergency room with severe gastrointestinal cramping. The patient is fully oriented and remains alert, with an unremarkable mental status examination. Review of systems is notable for abdominal pain but is otherwise negative, with no nausea, diarrhea, or constipation. Use of which substance most likely caused this presentation?

A. Heroin.

B. Ketamine.

C. PCP (phencyclidine).

D. Cannabis.

CHAPTER 17

Heart Disease

17.1 Which of the following is true regarding the relationship between congenital heart disease and psychiatric illness?

A. The lifetime rates of mood and anxiety disorders in survivors of congenital heart disease may be as high as 90%.
B. Subtle neuropsychological deficits are common in persons with congenital heart disease.
C. In cyanotic conditions, the time of surgical repair does not seem to have an impact on intellectual function.
D. Low rates of posttraumatic stress disorder (PTSD) are found in parents of children with critical congenital heart disease.

17.2 Which of the following statements is true regarding coronary artery disease (CAD)–associated depression?

A. Depression is the most common psychiatric disorder in patients with CAD.
B. It is not recommended to screen for depression in patients with CAD.
C. There is no association between social support and the likelihood of persistent depression after an acute coronary event.
D. Depression is a normal reaction to illness; subsyndromal depression in CAD patients rarely evolves into major depressive disorder.

17.3 Which of the following is a proposed risk factor for PTSD in patients with cardiac disease?

A. Male gender.
B. Older age.
C. Delayed acute stress reaction following cardiac event.
D. Personality traits such as repressive coping, alexithymia, and neuroticism.

17.4 Which of the following is considered a risk factor for delirium after cardiac surgery?

A. Short time on ventilator support.
B. Preoperative atrial fibrillation.

51

C. Preoperative or postoperative blood product transfusions.

D. Absence of history of psychiatric illness.

17.5   What is the correct pairing regarding cardiac medications and their most likely neuropsychiatric side effects?

A. Beta-blockers/increased energy.

B. Digoxin/visual hallucinations.

C. Reserpine/mania.

D. Diuretics/hypernatremia resulting in weakness.

17.6   Which of the following symptoms is the best indicator of depression in a patient with advanced heart failure?

A. Anhedonia.

B. Appetite loss.

C. Cachexia.

D. Fatigue.

17.7   In the absence of CAD, which of the following characteristics of patients with chest pain is predictive of panic disorder?

A. Male sex.

B. Older age.

C. Higher education and income.

D. Atypical chest pain quality.

17.8   Which of the following drugs has the *least* potential for causing cardiac conduction side effects?

A. Sertraline.

B. Desipramine.

C. Nortriptyline.

D. Carbamazepine.

17.9   What selective serotonin reuptake inhibitor (SSRI) has a black box warning against its use at dosages greater than 40 mg/day because it causes dose-dependent QT interval prolongation?

A. Fluoxetine.

B. Sertraline.

C. Paroxetine.

D. Citalopram.

17.10 Which cytochrome P450 (CYP) isoenzyme is responsible for the caution when beta-blockers are coadministered with known inhibitors of this isoenzyme, such as haloperidol or paroxetine?

A. CYP2D6.
B. CYP3A4.
C. CYP1A2.
D. CYP2B6.

17.11 You are asked to counsel a 50-year-old man regarding resumption of sexual activity following a myocardial infarction. Which of the following statements regarding energy equivalence is true regarding the safety of resuming sexual activity?

A. The energy requirement necessary increases the chance of a recurrence five-fold following sexual activity.
B. The risk of further cardiac damage is very high following sexual activity.
C. The patient should be able to walk up one flight of stairs.
D. The patient should be able to walk up three flights of stairs.

CHAPTER 18

Lung Disease

18.1 Which of the following diagnoses is most appropriate for a patient who has a psychogenic cough consisting of single dry coughs that are suppressible, distractible, suggestible, and variable?

A. Hyperventilation syndrome.
B. Somatic cough disorder.
C. Tic cough.
D. Vocal cord dysfunction.

18.2 Which of the following is a factor predictive of vocal cord dysfunction?

A. Female sex.
B. Older age.
C. Low body mass index.
D. Absence of psychiatric illness.

18.3 What is the *most* definitively established risk factor for psychiatric side effects of corticosteroids?

A. Dose of corticosteroid.
B. Inhaled route of administration.
C. Duration of exposure to corticosteroid.
D. Recurrent treatment with corticosteroid.

18.4 A pulmonologist colleague asks you about managing the psychiatric side effects of theophylline. Which of the following is the most appropriate response?

A. Theophylline has been linked to completed suicide.
B. Theophylline is sometimes associated with anxiety.
C. There are several established treatments for psychiatric side effects of theophylline.
D. Dose reduction does not impact psychiatric side effects.

18.5   Which class of medications has *most* strongly demonstrated improved respiratory outcomes in patients with asthma as evidenced by decreased corticosteroid use?

A. Antipsychotics.
B. Benzodiazepines.
C. Opioids.
D. Antidepressants.

18.6   Which psychiatric comorbidity has been shown to be *most* common in patients with sarcoidosis?

A. Panic disorder.
B. Major depressive disorder (MDD).
C. Bipolar disorder.
D. Generalized anxiety disorder.

18.7   Which behavioral intervention for asthma patients has shown the *most* beneficial impact on quality of life and respiratory symptoms?

A. Meditation.
B. Yoga.
C. Breathing training.
D. Relaxation training.

18.8   The symptoms of which psychiatric disorder show the *greatest* relative increase in prevalence in patients with chronic obstructive pulmonary disease (COPD) compared with the general population?

A. Generalized anxiety.
B. Panic disorder.
C. Depression.
D. Alcohol use disorder.

18.9   Which individual component of rehabilitation programs for COPD has been found to yield substantial effects on physical activity levels?

A. Exercise training.
B. Smoking cessation.
C. Nutrition counseling.
D. Psychosocial support.

Gastrointestinal Disorders

19.1 What should a patient taking daily ibuprofen as well as fluoxetine be informed about regarding the risk for an upper gastrointestinal (GI) bleed?

   A. The risk is unaffected by fluoxetine.
   B. The patient should immediately stop fluoxetine and start sertraline, given the extremely high risk of upper-GI bleed.
   C. The patient's absolute risk is more than twice as high as a healthy control subject not taking fluoxetine and ibuprofen.
   D. Evidence demonstrates that venlafaxine would have a similar effect on his risk for upper-GI bleed.

19.2 What psychopharmacological intervention is best supported for treatment of poorly controlled irritable bowel syndrome (IBS)–diarrhea symptoms in a patient with comorbid depression and anxiety?

   A. Duloxetine.
   B. Desipramine.
   C. Paroxetine.
   D. Sertraline.

19.3 Which of the following is the reason for caution in the use of direct-acting antiviral agents (DAAs) for hepatitis C treatment in patients with comorbid psychiatric illness?

   A. DAAs are not effective in patients with active substance use.
   B. DAAs carry a significant risk of drug-induced depression and suicidality.
   C. Given longer duration of DAA therapy, "high-risk" patients are less likely to remain adherent to DAA versus interferon (IFN).
   D. DAA regimens containing ritonavir may have significant drug-drug interactions with psychotropic medications.

19.4   What abnormality seen in patients with liver disease necessitates cautious inter-
       pretation of therapeutic drug-monitoring results?

       A. Disruption of phase II glucuronidation metabolism.
       B. Prolongation of elimination half-life.
       C. Altered plasma protein binding.
       D. Impaired renal function and fluctuations in fluid balance.

19.5   A healthy 31-year-old man who recently started taking duloxetine develops ab-
       normal liver function test results thought to be secondary to a drug-induced liver
       injury (DILI). His alanine aminotransferase is elevated more than his alkaline
       phosphatase. Which statement about DILI in this patient is correct?

       A. The patient's liver function tests are most consistent with cholestatic DILI.
       B. The patient's liver function tests should have been monitored more closely
          during initiation of duloxetine.
       C. The patient's liver injury is likely to resolve with discontinuation of duloxetine.
       D. The risk of DILI would have been significantly reduced by maintaining dulox-
          etine at 30 mg.

19.6   Which of the following medications is the most common cause of psychotropic-
       induced pancreatitis?

       A. Valproic acid.
       B. Ziprasidone.
       C. Haloperidol.
       D. Sertraline.

19.7   Which of the following statements most accurately describes the relationship be-
       tween inflammatory bowel disease (IBD) and anxiety and depression?

       A. Patients with active IBD symptoms have similar rates of anxiety and depres-
          sion as do patients whose IBD symptoms are well controlled.
       B. Antidepressants improve both psychological well-being and IBD disease ac-
          tivity in most patients with IBD.
       C. Levels of anxiety and depression are lower among patients with IBD with co-
          morbid IBS.
       D. Evidence suggests that there is a significant relationship between the presence
          of depressive and anxiety symptoms and risk for clinical recurrence of IBD.

19.8   Which of the following is *not* a mechanism through which psychiatric medica-
       tions may contribute to gastroesophageal reflux disease (GERD) symptoms?

       A. Clonazepam may increase lower esophageal sphincter pressure.
       B. Amitriptyline may lead to decreased gastric transit or impaired GI peristalsis.

C. Sertraline may increase gastric acidity via increased vagal tone.

D. Psychotropic medications with anticholinergic effects may decrease salivary secretions.

19.9 What is the *best* treatment for dysphagia in a patient with haloperidol-induced parkinsonism and chronic complaints of difficulty swallowing?

A. Intravenous diphenhydramine.

B. Discontinuation of haloperidol.

C. Intravenous benztropine.

D. Oral clonazepam.

19.10 A 37-year-old woman recently diagnosed with peptic ulcer disease (PUD) is concerned that work-related stress and anxiety may have contributed to her condition. What should the patient be counseled regarding the relationship between stress and PUD?

A. Stress is the definitive cause of most cases of PUD.

B. *Helicobacter pylori* or nonsteroidal anti-inflammatory drug (NSAID) use are now recognized as the causes of PUD, and stress has no bearing on the development of PUD.

C. Studies suggest that high levels of stress may more than double the chances of developing an ulcer.

D. Given that her high levels of stress and anxiety are contributing to her GI illness, the patient should be started on a tricyclic antidepressant (TCA) for PUD.

CHAPTER 20

Renal Disease

20.1   What is the *most* common psychiatric diagnosis in dialysis patients?

    A. Delirium.
    B. Dementia.
    C. Depression.
    D. Substance abuse.

20.2   Withdrawal from dialysis is most common in which of the following patient groups in the United States?

    A. Younger patients.
    B. Women.
    C. African American patients.
    D. Asian patients.

20.3   Which anxiety- or stressor-related disorder has been shown to be *much* higher in end-stage renal disease (ESRD) patients than in community samples?

    A. Anxiety disorders are equally prevalent in community and ESRD samples.
    B. Phobias.
    C. Posttraumatic stress disorder (PTSD).
    D. Panic disorder.

20.4   How does a disruptive patient *most* commonly interfere with the dialysis unit and staff?

    A. Verbal aggression.
    B. Noncompliance with treatment.
    C. Coming late to appointments.
    D. Physical abuse.

20.5   Which of the following is associated with dialysis termination?

    A. Pain.
    B. Median time to death of 14 days.

C. Lethargy.

D. Increased suffering at the end of life.

20.6 Which selective serotonin reuptake inhibitor (SSRI) would be expected to have the fewest potential interactions with other medications *and* may not need dose adjustment in patients with renal insufficiency?

A. Paroxetine.

B. Fluoxetine.

C. Citalopram.

D. Escitalopram.

20.7 Which antipsychotic medication depends on renal elimination?

A. Haloperidol.

B. Paliperidone.

C. Prolixin.

D. Chlorpromazine.

20.8 Which diuretics reduce lithium excretion?

A. Carbonic anhydrase inhibitors.

B. Thiazide diuretics.

C. Potassium-sparing diuretics.

D. Loop diuretics.

20.9 Which of the following medications may cause hypernatremia due to nephrogenic diabetes insipidus?

A. Amiloride.

B. Thiazides.

C. Nonsteroidal anti-inflammatory drugs (NSAID)s.

D. Lithium.

20.10 Which of the following medications is removed during dialysis?

A. Valproate.

B. Carbamazepine.

C. Paroxetine.

D. Lorazepam.

C H A P T E R   2 1

Endocrine and Metabolic Disorders

21.1   Which of the following describes the impact of stress on patients with diabetes?

   A. Those with an active lifestyle have high levels of stress.
   B. Repeated stress leads to inhibition of the hypothalamic-pituitary-adrenal (HPA) axis.
   C. Repeated stress leads to overstimulation of the HPA axis.
   D. Glycemic control is poorer in people with diabetes who report less stress.

21.2   Which antipsychotic is the *least* likely to cause weight gain and glucose intolerance?

   A. Clozapine.
   B. Olanzapine.
   C. Aripiprazole.
   D. Quetiapine.

21.3   Which of the following is the *most* common manifesting symptom of hyperthyroidism in younger patients?

   A. Paranoia.
   B. Apathy.
   C. Confusion.
   D. Anxious dysphoria.

21.4   For a patient with rapid-cycling bipolar disorder and abnormal thyroid function tests, what is the most appropriate next step in management?

   A. Discontinue lithium and switch to a different mood stabilizer.
   B. Begin treatment with T_4 if thyroid-stimulating hormone (TSH) levels are elevated.
   C. Begin treatment with T_4 only if TSH and T_4 levels are abnormal.
   D. Begin treatment with T_4 only if patient has psychotic symptoms.

21.5 A 50-year-old man with a history of bipolar disorder, who has been stable for many years, presents with new onset of inattention, confusion, and belief that his coworker has planted a camera in his office to spy on him. He also complains of feeling thirsty, needing to urinate frequently, and pain in his joints. His wife mentions that about 1 year ago he became indifferent to events at home and work. Which of the following is the most likely explanation?

A. Valproate treatment for bipolar disorder caused hyperparathyroidism and severe hypercalcemia.
B. Lithium treatment for bipolar disorder caused hyperparathyroidism and severe hypercalcemia.
C. Lamotrigine treatment for bipolar disorder caused hyperparathyroidism and severe hypercalcemia.
D. Olanzapine treatment for bipolar disorder caused hyperparathyroidism and severe hypercalcemia.

21.6 Which of the following best characterizes the relationship between psychiatric disorders and osteoporosis?

A. Depression is a risk factor for osteoporosis in women but not men.
B. Osteoporosis in uncommon in patients with schizophrenia.
C. Depression is a risk factor for osteoporosis in both women and men.
D. Depression is a risk factor for osteoporosis in men but not women.

21.7 Which neuropsychiatric symptom is *most* prevalent in Cushing's syndrome?

A. Psychosis.
B. Mania.
C. Anxiety.
D. Depression.

21.8 Which of the following tests can be used to definitively diagnose adrenal insufficiency?

A. Morning serum cortisol level.
B. Corticotropin stimulation test.
C. Adrenocorticotropic hormone (ACTH) level.
D. Fasting plasma glucose.

21.9 Which antipsychotic can be used to treat medication-induced prolactinemia?

A. Aripiprazole.
B. Haloperidol.
C. Risperidone.
D. Paliperidone.

21.10 Polycystic ovarian syndrome (PCOS) is associated with which of the following adverse psychiatric consequences?

A. Psychosis.
B. Cognitive impairment.
C. Depression.
D. Mania.

CHAPTER 22

Oncology

22.1 Which of the following is a risk factor for the development of depression in cancer patients?

    A. Older age.
    B. Early stage of disease.
    C. Female sex.
    D. Insecure attachment style.

22.2 Which of the following events is associated with a high risk of suicide in cancer patients?

    A. Referral to palliative care.
    B. Initial cancer diagnosis.
    C. Completing chemotherapy treatment.
    D. Undergoing surgery.

22.3 Paroxetine affects which cytochrome P450 (CYP) enzyme important in the metabolism of tamoxifen?

    A. CYP2D6.
    B. CYP2C19.
    C. CYP3A4.
    D. CYP1A2.

22.4 In breast cancer patients, which of the following is associated with development of cancer-related fatigue?

    A. Having a partner.
    B. Being treated with surgery.
    C. Being treated with surgery plus radiation.
    D. Being treated with chemotherapy.

22.5 What is the *most* common motivation cited by patients for requesting physician-assisted suicide?

    A. Loss of autonomy/dignity and the ability to enjoy life's activities.
    B. Fears of increased pain and symptoms.
    C. A sense of being a burden on loved ones.
    D. Economic hardship associated with the costs of health care.

22.6 Which of the following cancer types has been linked to the development of depression prior to the cancer diagnosis?

    A. Esophageal cancer.
    B. Gastric cancer.
    C. Pancreatic cancer.
    D. Colorectal cancer.

22.7 What is the *most* common cause of hypomania or mania in cancer patients?

    A. Interferon-alpha.
    B. Methotrexate.
    C. Corticosteroids.
    D. Tamoxifen.

22.8 A 67-year-old woman is receiving chemotherapy for non-small-cell adenocarcinoma of the lung. She currently complains of low mood, hopelessness, poor appetite, and chemotherapy-induced nausea. Which of the following antidepressants may be helpful for its antiemetic and appetite-stimulating effects?

    A. Mirtazapine.
    B. Sertraline.
    C. Citalopram.
    D. Paroxetine.

CHAPTER 23

Hematology

23.1 Which of the following is most likely to be seen in patients with folate deficiency anemia?

    A. Hashimoto's thyroiditis.
    B. Vegetarian diet.
    C. Depression.
    D. Subacute combined degeneration of the spinal cord.

23.2 Which of the following is a major neuropsychiatric manifestation of sickle cell disease (SCD)?

    A. Depression and anxiety related to stigma, unpredictable pain crises, and high mortality rates.
    B. Depression and anxiety secondary to substance abuse.
    C. Central nervous system damage resulting from opiate drug overuse.
    D. Poor cognitive performance from frequent school absences.

23.3 How does opioid treatment typically impact patients with sickle cell disease?

    A. Opioids help control pain but decrease functional capacity and can lead to tolerance and addiction.
    B. Opioids help control pain but increase hospitalizations and can lead to tolerance and addiction.
    C. Opioids help control pain but consistently lead to tolerance and addiction.
    D. Opioids help control pain, improve functional capacity, and decrease hospitalizations.

23.4 Which best describes the risk of agranulocytosis with clozapine use?

    A. The highest risk is present during the first 3 weeks of treatment and then decreases significantly.
    B. A white blood cell (WBC) count lower than $1,000/mm^3$ or an absolute neutrophil count lower than $500/mm^3$ is an indication for immediate cessation of clozapine.

C. The fatality rate of clozapine-induced agranulocytosis is 4.2%–16%.

D. Stopping clozapine is not typically a sufficient intervention.

23.5   Which of the following is an indication for cessation of treatment with a selective serotonin reuptake inhibitor (SSRI)?

A. SSRIs should be discontinued before any major surgery.

B. The SSRI in use is sertraline or citalopram, and the patient needs warfarin.

C. The patient is at high risk of gastrointestinal hemorrhage.

D. The patient has other sources of bleeding risk that outweigh the benefits of antidepressant treatment.

23.6   Why is carbamazepine contraindicated in patients with a history of bone marrow depression?

A. Carbamazepine is directly toxic to bone marrow and can cause potentially fatal agranulocytosis and aplastic anemia.

B. Carbamazepine causes a transient reduction in platelet count in approximately 10% of patients during the first 4 months of treatment.

C. Carbamazepine stimulates WBC production, predominantly neutrophils.

D. Potentially fatal hematopoietic complications such as neutropenia, thrombocytopenia, and macrocytic anemia have been associated with carbamazepine.

CHAPTER 24

Rheumatology

24.1 What class of pharmacological management of rheumatoid arthritis (RA) is associated with a lower prevalence of depressive and anxiety disorders?

    A. Nonsteroidal anti-inflammatory drugs (NSAIDs).
    B. Methotrexate and antimalarials.
    C. Corticosteroids.
    D. Biological response modifiers.

24.2 What is the *strongest* proximal risk factor for depression in RA?

    A. Burden of chronic physical symptoms.
    B. Personal losses resulting from RA.
    C. Major life stressors, including interpersonal stress and social rejection.
    D. Disability.

24.3 Which cluster symptom in RA is associated with greater pain?

    A. Sleep difficulties.
    B. Depressed mood.
    C. Fatigue.
    D. Functional disability.

24.4 What is the single strongest marker of central nervous system (CNS) risk in systemic lupus erythematosus (SLE) patients?

    A. Articular manifestation or discoid rash.
    B. Antinuclear antibody (ANA)–negative.
    C. Antiphospholipid antibodies.
    D. Drug-induced SLE.

24.5 To define neuropsychiatric lupus according to the American College of Rheumatology Ad Hoc Committee on Neuropsychiatric Lupus Nomenclature (1999), which disorder is the *most* common?

A. Cognitive dysfunction.
B. Anxiety.
C. Depression.
D. Mania.

24.6 Which of the following is more likely due to a CNS lupus flare-up than a corticosteroid-induced psychiatric reaction?

A. Increases in indices of inflammation.
B. Mania or mixed states.
C. Exacerbation of symptoms in response to corticosteroids.
D. SLE symptoms preceding the onset of psychiatric symptoms.

24.7 As a wide variety of diseases can mimic neuropsychiatric SLE, which of the following may be mistaken for CNS lupus but is characterized by a negative ANA?

A. Mixed or undifferentiated connective tissue disease.
B. Hepatitis C.
C. Wegener's granulomatosis.
D. Multiple sclerosis.

24.8 CNS involvement is rare in which of the following rheumatological conditions?

A. Sjögren's syndrome.
B. Temporal arteritis.
C. Granulomatosis with polyangiitis.
D. RA.

24.9 Which rheumatological disorder is *not* likely to respond to corticosteroid treatment?

A. Systemic sclerosis (scleroderma).
B. Temporal arteritis.
C. RA.
D. SLE.

24.10 Which medication is likely to cause confusion, psychosis, mania, nightmares, and aggression?

A. Infliximab.
B. Tocilizumab.
C. Hydroxychloroquine.
D. Mycophenolate mofetil.

CHAPTER 25

Chronic Fatigue and Fibromyalgia Syndromes

25.1   Which of the following statements most accurately describes chronic fatigue syndrome (CFS) and fibromyalgia syndrome (FMS)?

A. CFS and FMS are as firmly based in disease pathology as any other medical condition.
B. CFS and FMS are symptom-defined somatic syndromes in which biological, psychological, and social factors play a role.
C. CFS and FMS are social constructions based on psychological amplification of somatic sensation.
D. CFS and FMS are syndromes in which psychological conflicts are expressed in physical symptoms.

25.2   A patient presents with 7 months of fatigue and malaise after exercising and reports that sleep is not restorative. What is an additional physical symptom that would support the diagnosis of CFS?

A. Chest pain.
B. Gastrointestinal problems.
C. Sore throat.
D. Chronic pelvic pain.

25.3   Which of the following is an accurate statement about the revised 2010 American College of Rheumatology (ACR) criteria for FMS?

A. Patient must have a minimum number of tender point sites on palpation.
B. Patient must have widespread pain of at least 6 months' duration.
C. Patient must report fatigue, waking unrefreshed, cognitive symptoms, or somatic symptoms.
D. A distinguishing diagnostic feature is the presence of distressing bodily symptoms.

25.4 Which of the following statements most accurately describes the association between CFS and FMS with psychiatric disorders?

  A. Incidence of major depressive disorder (MDD) in patients with CFS and FMS is similar.
  B. CFS, but not FMS, is associated with increased prevalence of posttraumatic stress disorder.
  C. After adjusting for hierarchical rules that subsume generalized anxiety disorder (GAD) under MDD, the prevalence of GAD in patients with CFS and FMS is similar to that in the general population.
  D. Most patients with CFS and FMS would meet criteria for somatic symptom disorder.

25.5 Which of the following is a predictor of poor outcome in CFS?

  A. Short duration of illness.
  B. Younger age.
  C. Minimal symptom severity.
  D. Belief that the illness has a physical cause.

25.6 Which of the following statements regarding predisposing and precipitating factors for CFS is most supported by currently available evidence?

  A. There is a strong heritable component to CFS and FMS, including likely candidate genes.
  B. Certain personality types are predictive of developing CFS and FMS.
  C. Patients with CFS and FMS often had highly active lives prior to onset of illness.
  D. Chronic back pain is known to precipitate the onset of FMS and may of CFS also.

25.7 A 35-year-old man presents with symptoms suggestive of CFS, which he reports began a few months ago when he was offered a lucrative and exciting job promotion that would require frequent travel, but he felt pressured by family to decline when they learned he was the best human leukocyte antigen match for his critically ill brother who was awaiting renal transplantation. What type of stress does this patient demonstrate that may be relevant to the etiology of CFS?

  A. Denial.
  B. Fear.
  C. Dilemma.
  D. Altruism.

25.8 In a patient with severe fatigue, which of the findings below would be most supportive of a diagnosis of CFS or FMS?

  A. Elevated interleukin-6 (IL-6).
  B. Low cortisol.

C. Myoglobinuria.

D. Positive Epstein-Barr virus test.

25.9 What measures should a therapist recommend that might improve the recovery of a patient with CFS/FMS?

A. Graded exercise therapy.

B. Avoiding activities that might lead to an increase in symptoms.

C. Keeping a daily symptom record.

D. Active involvement in a CFS/FMS patient support group.

25.10 What is the most appropriate initial approach to evaluate CFS or FMS for a new patient presenting with 3 weeks of fatigue and generalized pain?

A. Follow-up visit at 1 month.

B. Viral and immunological studies for CFS.

C. Discontinuing statin medication.

D. Sleep study.

25.11 What would be the most effective medication to prescribe to a 30-year-old otherwise healthy depressed patient with FMS and widespread pain?

A. Nonsteroidal anti-inflammatory drugs (NSAIDs).

B. Nortriptyline.

C. Fluoxetine.

D. Citalopram.

CHAPTER 26

Infectious Diseases

26.1   After returning from a summer trip to North Carolina where he was bitten by a tick, an otherwise healthy young man developed fever and a rash with erythematous macules that eventually progressed to maculopapular lesions with central petechiae. What organism is most likely responsible for this clinical presentation?

   A. *Borrelia burgdorferi.*
   B. *Treponema pallidum.*
   C. *Tropheryma whipplei.*
   D. *Rickettsia rickettsii.*

26.2   Which microorganism classically causes muscle stiffness signs, such as "lockjaw" and *risus sardonicus*?

   A. *Salmonella typhi.*
   B. *Clostridium tetani.*
   C. Group A beta-hemolytic streptococci.
   D. *Leptospira interrogans.*

26.3   Which of the following serological tests can be used to confirm a diagnosis of syphilis after a positive screening test?

   A. Microhemagglutination assay of *T. pallidum* (MHA-TP).
   B. Rapid plasma reagin test.
   C. Venereal Disease Research Laboratory test.
   D. Monospot test.

26.4   Which stage of syphilis infection is characterized by tabes dorsalis?

   A. Primary syphilis.
   B. Secondary syphilis.
   C. Tertiary syphilis.
   D. Acute syphilitic infection.

26.5   What AIDS-associated opportunistic infection characteristically causes nerve demyelination and manifests with multiple focal neurological deficits?

   A. Progressive multifocal leukoencephalopathy.
   B. Cryptococcal meningitis.

C. Central nervous system (CNS) lymphoma.

D. Toxoplasmosis.

26.6 Which of the following is a risk factor for HIV-associated neurocognitive disorder (HAND)?

A. Younger age.

B. Absence of cerebrovascular disease.

C. Higher CD4 nadir.

D. Co-infection with hepatitis C.

26.7 Which of the following is true regarding HIV infection and depression?

A. Depression has no effect on adherence to HIV treatment.

B. Major depressive disorder is not a risk factor for HIV infection.

C. HAND and other HIV-related CNS conditions can produce a flat, apathetic state that is often misdiagnosed as depression.

D. Fatigue has been found to be more associated with HIV disease progression than with depression.

26.8 Which of the following best describes the relationship between bipolar disorder and HIV infection?

A. Patients with bipolar disorder are less likely to engage in behaviors that place them at risk for HIV infection.

B. Irritable mood is a prominent feature of "AIDS mania."

C. The prevalence of mania is about the same in patients with AIDS as in the general population.

D. Mania remains a common manifestation of AIDS.

26.9 What potential drug-drug interaction can occur when erythromycin is coadministered with the following medications?

A. Antipsychotics and tricyclic antidepressants—prolongation of QT interval.

B. Alprazolam—decrease in alprazolam levels.

C. Buspirone—decrease in buspirone levels.

D. Carbamazepine—decrease in carbamazepine levels.

26.10 Which of the following antiretroviral drugs is known to cause vivid dreams and nightmares?

A. Maraviroc.

B. Atazanavir.

C. Zidovudine.

D. Efavirenz.

CHAPTER 27

Dermatology

27.1 Studies of patients with psychogenic purpura suggest which of the following to be a likely etiologic process?

A. Autoimmune.
B. Factitious.
C. Psychotic.
D. Infectious.

27.2 Which of the following findings is most consistent with somatoform pruritus?

A. The lesions on the skin are in areas where it is difficult for patients to reach with their hands.
B. The pruritus wakes patients from sleep.
C. The pruritus is associated with a starvation state.
D. The pruritus first started after a traumatic experience.

27.3 In which dermatological disorder do a predominance of those affected experience onset of symptoms during childhood, onset frequently occurring after a stressful event, higher rates of attention-deficit/hyperactivity disorder (ADHD) and depression and suicidality, and blunted cortisol responsiveness to a stressor?

A. Psoriasis.
B. Atopic dermatitis.
C. Acne.
D. Chronic urticaria.

27.4 Patients with body dysmorphic disorder (BDD) are overrepresented in dermatological treatment settings, with dermatological concerns being the most common reason for seeking nonpsychiatric treatment. Which of the following patterns of treatment-seeking behavior is most likely among patients with BDD?

A. The interventions most commonly requested by patients with BDD in dermatological practice are systemic acne treatments.
B. Patients with BDD are likely to report satisfaction with their treatment outcome.

C. Patients with BDD are more likely to agree to a trial of isotretinoin than the general acne population.

D. Patients seeking dermatological care for more severe acne have higher rates of having a diagnosis of BDD.

27.5   Which of the following psychotropic medications is approved by the U.S. Food and Drug Administration (FDA) for management of a condition with both dermatological and psychiatric manifestations?

A. Pimozide (for delusional infestation).
B. Doxepin topical cream (for atopic dermatitis [AD]).
C. Lamotrigine (for skin-picking disorder).
D. Venlafaxine (for the mucocutaneous dysesthesias).

27.6   Which of the following disorders that manifest in the skin and in psychological ways is best categorized as a somatic symptom disorder?

A. Excoriation (skin-picking) disorder.
B. Body dysmorphic disorder.
C. Dermatitis artefacta.
D. Morgellon's disease.

27.7   Which of the following is a known dermatological manifestation of binge-eating disorder?

A. Acne.
B. Russell's sign.
C. Pruritus.
D. Subconjunctival hemorrhage.

27.8   In which scenario should the clinician be most concerned for Stevens-Johnson syndrome/toxic epidermal necrolysis (SJS/TEN) for a patient taking carbamazepine for bipolar disorder?

A. New addition of lithium.
B. Use of carbamazepine for more than 1 year.
C. Recent ketoconazole treatment of a fungal infection.
D. A patient of Caucasian ancestry.

27.9   A dermatologist consults a psychiatrist for help with a patient who has diffuse pruritus and repetitive scratching that is causing lesions, leading to more scratching. What recommendation might the psychiatrist suggest as part of the evaluation and management?

A. Initiation of olanzapine.
B. Review of the patient's sleep patterns.
C. Discontinuation of the patient's benzodiazepines.
D. Referral for meaning-centered psychotherapy.

CHAPTER 28

Surgery

28.1   In patients with which psychiatric illness is postoperative pain most likely to be underrecognized?

A. Depression.
B. Schizophrenia.
C. Body dysmorphic disorder (BDD).
D. Bipolar disorder.

28.2   What is the most common theme in preoperative fears of anesthesia across multiple studies?

A. Fear of postoperative pain.
B. Fear of not waking up after surgery.
C. Fear of being nauseous or vomiting.
D. Fear of intraoperative awareness.

28.3   Which sedative used in postoperative intensive care unit (ICU) patients is associated with the lowest incidence of delirium?

A. Midazolam.
B. Dexmedetomidine.
C. Lorazepam.
D. Propofol.

28.4   Which common type of bariatric surgery is most effective at promoting weight loss?

A. Sleeve gastrectomy.
B. Biliopancreatic bypass with duodenal switch.
C. Laparoscopic adjustable gastric banding.
D. Laparoscopic Roux-en-Y gastric bypass.

28.5   BDD is *most* common in patients seeking which type of surgery?

   A. Cosmetic.
   B. Bariatric.
   C. Healthy limb amputation.
   D. Strabismus correction.

28.6   Which type of drug forms the pharmacological basis of burn pain management?

   A. Nonsteroidal anti-inflammatory agents.
   B. Benzodiazepines.
   C. Acetaminophen.
   D. Opioids.

28.7   Concerns about bodily noises occur commonly after what type of surgery?

   A. Bariatric.
   B. Limb amputation.
   C. Ostomies.
   D. Prostatectomy.

28.8   Which of the following is a risk factor for intraoperative awareness during surgery?

   A. Male gender.
   B. Inpatient surgery.
   C. Cardiac surgery.
   D. Absence of serious systemic illness.

28.9   Which sensation associated with limb amputation may patients with body integrity identity disorder (BIID) experience?

   A. Phantom limb.
   B. Stump pain.
   C. Overcompleteness.
   D. Residual pain.

28.10   Which is most likely to be the best predictor of postoperative posttraumatic stress disorder (PTSD)?

   A. Quality of prior emotional adjustment.
   B. Severity of condition requiring surgery.
   C. Alcohol use.
   D. Presence of acute stress disorder during acute ICU hospitalization.

CHAPTER 29

Organ Transplantation

29.1   For which organ is the U.S. transplant wait list the largest?

A. Heart.
B. Lung.
C. Liver.
D. Kidney.

29.2   Which group of patients has the best 10-year survival rate?

A. Living-donor liver transplant.
B. Deceased-donor liver transplant.
C. Deceased-donor kidney transplant.
D. Heart transplant.

29.3   Which pretransplant psychiatric condition has consistently been shown to be associated with early graft loss and patient death?

A. Schizophrenia.
B. Bipolar.
C. Depression.
D. Anxiety.

29.4   Which is the correct list of organs according to psychosocial stringency of clearance?

A. Heart, liver, kidney.
B. Heart, kidney, liver.
C. Liver, kidney, heart.
D. Lung, kidney, liver.

29.5   Which strategy has demonstrated its ability to improve adherence to medical regimes posttransplantation?

A. Excluding patients with severe personality disorders from transplant.
B. Allowing occasional missed doses to improve alliance with the patient.

C. Implementing mobile phone apps.

D. Reviewing standard deviation of tacrolimus blood levels.

29.6 Nicotine replacement, despite dose adjustment, is relatively contraindicated in which of these potential organ transplant patients?

A. Kidney.

B. Liver.

C. Heart.

D. Lung.

29.7 Which is a standard treatment for hepatic or portosystemic encephalopathy?

A. Benztropine.

B. Shunting to relieve portal hypertension.

C. Osmotic laxatives.

D. High-protein diets.

29.8 Which of the following has become an increasing concern for solid organ donors in the United States?

A. Regret after poor recipient outcomes.

B. Financial hardship.

C. Coercion to donate.

D. Postdonation decrease in general well-being.

29.9 A 55-year-old male with bipolar disorder, alcohol use disorder, in full sustained remission, and hepatic encephalopathy receives a liver transplant complicated by acute cellular rejection. He remains in the surgical intensive care unit and develops mania on postoperative day 7. Which medication is most likely contributing to the secondary mania?

A. Tacrolimus.

B. Mycophenolate mofetil.

C. Methylprednisolone.

D. Cyclosporine.

29.10 A 25-year-old female with borderline personality disorder receives a liver transplant after fulminant hepatic failure from an acetaminophen overdose. She is transferred to inpatient psychiatry on daily tacrolimus, prednisone, and oxycodone as needed. Which psychotropic should be used with the most caution given the risk of posterior reversible encephalopathy syndrome?

A. Venlafaxine.

B. Fluoxetine.

C. Paroxetine.

D. Sertraline.

CHAPTER 30

Neurology and Neurosurgery

30.1   Of the following common and observable poststroke changes in brain function, which should be specifically tested for because it is easily overlooked?

    A. Dementia.
    B. Delirium.
    C. Vascular cognitive impairment.
    D. Strategic infarction.

30.2   In which of the following poststroke behavioral changes does recognition of the deficit remain intact?

    A. Affective dysprosody.
    B. Anosognosia.
    C. Somatoparaphrenia.
    D. Wernicke's aphasia.

30.3   Which of the following statements about poststroke depression is *most* supported by current research consensus?

    A. Poststroke depression affects fewer than 5% of stroke patients.
    B. Left frontal lesions are associated with an increased rate of depressive illness.
    C. SSRIs (selective serotonin reuptake inhibitors) are ineffective in treating depression after stroke.
    D. Silent infarcts are a risk factor for poststroke depression.

30.4   Which of the following is relatively rare poststroke?

    A. Anxiety.
    B. Hyposexuality.
    C. Self-directed anger or frustration.
    D. Impairment of executive function.

30.5 What medication is *best* supported in the literature for the treatment of psychosis in the setting of Parkinson's disease (PD)?

A. Quetiapine.
B. Clozapine.
C. Pimavanserin.
D. Cholinesterase inhibitors.

30.6 Which of the following symptoms is *most* useful in diagnosing depression in patients with PD?

A. Preoccupation with health.
B. Sleep disturbance.
C. Anhedonia.
D. Attention deficit.

30.7 Which of the following statements about symptoms that commonly occur with multiple sclerosis (MS) is correct?

A. Fatigue is the most common single symptom in MS.
B. Cognitive impairment is uncommon with MS.
C. Mood symptoms comorbid with MS are a depressive psychological reaction to the illness.
D. There is no increased risk of psychosis with MS.

30.8 Which of the following is *most* helpful in differentiating epileptic seizures from psychogenic nonepileptic seizures?

A. Frequent occurrence of seizures in public spaces.
B. Tremulous movements of varying frequency.
C. Resistance to attempted eye opening.
D. Acceptance that psychological factors contribute to the illness.

30.9 Which of the following is *true* regarding the relationship between depression and epilepsy?

A. Depression is an independent risk factor for unprovoked seizures.
B. The prevalence of depression is similar in people with or without epilepsy.
C. Antidepressant medication should be avoided in people with epilepsy.
D. Anticonvulsant medication has no association with increased risk for suicide.

30.10 Which of the following signs or symptoms occurs with equal frequency in both functional neurological symptom disorders and organic neurological disorders?

A. Fixed dystonia.
B. *La belle indifférence.*

C. Depersonalization or derealization at the time of onset.

D. Tremor with variable frequency and entrainment.

30.11 Which of the following psychotropic medications appears to be *most* effective in treating fatigue associated with MS?

A. Amantadine.

B. Psychostimulants.

C. Modafinil.

D. Bupropion.

30.12 Which of the following cognitive impairments is typical of MS?

A. Procedural and implicit memory functions are impaired.

B. Aphasia and apraxia are common.

C. Cognitive impairment in MS is rare.

D. Impairment is usually a subcortical dementia.

30.13 Which of the following psychiatric conditions is rarely associated with Wilson's disease?

A. Depression.

B. Dementia.

C. Schizophreniform psychosis.

D. Personality change.

30.14 Which of the following findings of cognitive function is *most* likely to be observed in a patient with Wernicke-Korsakoff syndrome?

A. Severely impaired executive function.

B. Retrograde amnesia with relative sparing of anterograde memory.

C. Flattened affect with normal levels of motivation and interest.

D. Minimal difficulty on standard tasks of attention and working memory.

30.15 Which of the following is the *most* likely initial presentation of an autoimmune encephalitis?

A. Episodic impairment of working memory without focal neurologic deficits.

B. Acute onset of autonomic dysfunction, preceding psychiatric symptoms.

C. Numerous metastatic tumors on magnetic resonance imaging.

D. Subacute onset of psychiatric symptoms, with no identifiable tumor.

CHAPTER 31

Obstetrics and Gynecology

31.1 Which psychiatric disorder is *more* common among women with infertility?

A. Posttraumatic stress disorder.
B. Psychosis.
C. Major depressive disorder (MDD).
D. Anxiety disorder.

31.2 Which psychiatric medication is most likely to be associated with infertility due to hyperprolactinemia?

A. Escitalopram.
B. Haloperidol.
C. Valproic acid.
D. Fluoxetine.

31.3 How does infertility most commonly impact a couple's mental health?

A. Duration of infertility does not affect the couple's mental health.
B. Fertility treatments themselves may have adverse effects on mental health.
C. Men show the same distress and guilt whether the infertility is attributed to male-factor etiology or female-factor etiology.
D. The rate of anxiety and depression is higher among men with infertility than women with infertility.

31.4 Which of the following psychotropic medications reduces the efficacy of hormonal contraception?

A. Phenobarbital.
B. Valproate.
C. Lamotrigine.
D. Amitriptyline.

31.5   Electroconvulsive therapy (ECT) is generally regarded as a safe and effective treatment for which one of the following conditions in pregnancy?

   A. Hyperemesis.
   B. All forms of MDD.
   C. A patient with schizophrenia who is stable on medications.
   D. Affective psychosis.

31.6   Which of the following atypical antipsychotics is most likely to impair fertility?

   A. Quetiapine.
   B. Ziprasidone.
   C. Risperidone.
   D. Lurasidone.

31.7   Which of the following is considered to be a risk factor for poor outcome after hysterectomy?

   A. Preoperative pain.
   B. Lack of psychiatric history.
   C. Clear indications for hysterectomy.
   D. Use of laparoscopic rather than robotic surgery.

31.8   How does spontaneous abortion typically impact mental health?

   A. Spontaneous abortion does not precipitate psychiatric consequences, as it is not associated with serious medical or obstetric complications.
   B. Only women with repeated miscarriages are at risk of psychological sequelae.
   C. Increased attention from health care providers exacerbates the emotional effect of spontaneous abortion.
   D. The end of pregnancy through miscarriage or stillbirth is associated with an increase in anxiety and depression during a subsequent pregnancy.

31.9   Which one of the following pieces of a patient's history would indicate a risk for depression in pregnancy?

   A. No prior psychiatric history.
   B. Higher-powered, high-stress employment.
   C. Intimate partner violence.
   D. Fair social support.

31.10   Which of the following conditions is potentially increased, in either mother or fetus, with a selective serotonin reuptake inhibitor (SSRI) antidepressant use in pregnancy?

   A. Cardiac malformation in fetus.
   B. Persistent pulmonary hypertension of the newborn.

C. Risk of preeclampsia.

D. Renal hypoplasia in fetus.

31.11 Which of the following is associated with untreated depression during pregnancy or the postpartum period?

A. No change in risk of morbidity in the mother and her offspring.

B. Increased risk of preterm birth.

C. No change in infant birth weight.

D. No change in risk related to substance use during pregnancy.

31.12 Which one of the following medications is associated with the greatest risk of teratogenicity in the fetus?

A. Lorazepam.

B. Quetiapine.

C. Valproic acid.

D. Lithium.

31.13 Which one of the following strategies should be implemented in the care of a pregnant woman being treated with lithium?

A. Divided dosing.

B. Keeping the daily dose of lithium the same throughout the pregnancy.

C. Checking lithium levels only at the beginning and at the end of the pregnancy.

D. Maintain the dose used during the pregnancy after delivery.

31.14 The levels of which of the following psychotropic medications can be increased by oral contraceptives?

A. Modafinil.

B. Oxcarbazepine.

C. Lamotrigine.

D. Phenobarbital.

CHAPTER 32

Pediatrics

32.1 A 9-year-old child has which of the following cognitive understandings of their body?

A. Ability to apply logic to his or her understanding of physical illness and is eager for factual information about the body.
B. Lack of capacity to create a narrative about his or her experience.
C. Ability to use abstract reasoning and can discuss body systems and not just individual organs.
D. Ability to understand basic concepts of cause and effect and is most aware of body parts he or she can directly sense, like the heart.

32.2 Which of the following statements is *true* about parents and their children in a medical system?

A. Parents may not be involved in significant aspects of their children's medical care.
B. Children do not let their parents' reactions to an illness determine how they should respond.
C. Parents (or legal guardian equivalents) are the legal decision makers for the child and thus are deeply involved in the child's care.
D. Heightened parental stress plays no role in how the child adjusts psychologically to illness.

32.3 Which of the following risk factors is *not* linked to illness- or treatment-related posttraumatic stress symptoms in children?

A. Premorbid psychopathology.
B. Female gender.
C. Maternal negative life events.
D. Older age.

32.4 Which of the following factors does *not* increase the risk of suicide in medically ill adolescents?

A. Suicidal intent and plan.
B. Recent improvement in depressive symptoms.
C. Family history of suicide.
D. Hypersomnia.

32.5 Which of the following selective serotonin reuptake inhibitor (SSRI) medications is *not* considered first-line in the treatment of depression in medically ill youth?

A. Escitalopram.
B. Sertraline.
C. Citalopram.
D. Fluoxetine.

32.6 According to the chronic illness literature, which percentage is the most accurate estimate of nonadherence to prescribed treatment in pediatric patients?

A. 50%.
B. 10%.
C. 75%.
D. 90%.

32.7 Which of the following features is *not* considered more specific to pediatric delirium compared with delirium in adults?

A. Psychosis.
B. Inconsolability.
C. Autonomic dysregulation.
D. Purposeless actions.

32.8 Which of the following is *not* a common psychiatric reason for consultation for patients with autism who have medical illness?

A. Difficulty coping with hospitalization/illness.
B. Nonadherence to treatment plan.
C. Substance abuse.
D. Homicidal ideation.

32.9 Which statistic correctly represents the risk of posttraumatic stress disorder (PTSD) in childhood cancer survivors compared with their siblings?

A. PTSD occurs less frequently in childhood cancer survivors compared with their siblings.
B. PTSD is found in roughly the same proportion in childhood cancer survivors compared with their siblings.

C. There is roughly twice the risk of PTSD in childhood cancer survivors compared with their siblings.

D. There is roughly four times the risk of PTSD in childhood cancer survivors compared with their siblings.

32.10 Which explanation is most accurate in terms of the link between asthma and panic symptoms?

A. Panic symptoms are not common in patients with asthma because the physiologic reactions to strong emotions do not trigger wheezing.

B. Panic can act like an "asphyxia alarm system" triggered by central chemoreceptors in response to changes in partial pressure of carbon dioxide.

C. Panic symptoms are uncommon because asthma medications such as steroids and beta-agonists are not associated with psychiatric side effects.

D. Periodic increases in partial pressure of carbon dioxide from asthma exacerbations are unrelated to panic attacks in patients with a genetic vulnerability to panic disorder.

CHAPTER 33

Physical Medicine and Rehabilitation

33.1 What is expected in terms of cognitive recovery after a traumatic brain injury (TBI)?

    A. TBI is associated with an acute decrement in cognitive function, which routinely improves within 2 years.

    B. Individuals with severe brain injury can be expected to have made all of their cognitive gains by the first year after the injury.

    C. The severity of the TBI correlates with the severity of the neurocognitive disorder (NCD).

    D. In patients who have lost consciousness for 30 minutes or less, 80%–85% are expected to recover within 3–6 months without permanent deficits.

33.2 Which criterion for major depressive disorder does not overlap with the ICD-10 criteria for postconcussive syndrome?

    A. Insomnia.

    B. Decreased concentration.

    C. Depressed mood.

    D. Psychomotor changes.

33.3 Which of the following does the research indicate as the *strongest* predictive factor for postconcussive symptoms at 6 months?

    A. Postinjury posttraumatic stress.

    B. Years of education.

    C. Anxiety.

    D. Successful outcome of litigation.

33.4 Which of the following defines a moderate traumatic brain injury?

    A. Loss of consciousness less than half an hour.

    B. Posttraumatic amnesia of 1–7 days.

C. Glasgow Coma Scale of 13–15 at 30 minutes postinjury.

D. Loss of consciousness greater than 24 hours.

33.5 A 27-year-old man with a history of cannabis use disorder is admitted with a TBI after a motor vehicle accident. His family gets information from the internet that some people diagnosed with a TBI behave aggressively. They want to know if their loved one is likely to act aggressively once he returns home. How should this family be counseled?

A. Approximately 95% of patients with moderate-severe TBI demonstrate aggression.

B. Aggression in most patients with a TBI is not premeditated, does not achieve a particular goal for the individual, is triggered by an out of proportion reaction to a stimulus, does not have a prodromal buildup, and causes them distress.

C. His preinjury history of substance abuse does not predispose him to aggression after a TBI.

D. The most significant predictors of later aggression after TBI are worse depressive symptoms and older age.

33.6 When patients are depressed after spinal cord injury (SCI), which of these factors is *most* predictive of suicide?

A. Lower functional independence.

B. Poorer social integration.

C. Shame and apathy.

D. High use of paid personal care and higher medical expenses.

33.7 After an SCI, a woman is told that she has suffered an incomplete lower motor neuron lesion affecting the sacral segments. How is this injury expected to impact her sexual functioning?

A. As in 25% of cases, she is expected to achieve psychogenic lubrication but will have no reflex lubrication.

B. She is likely to have vaginal lubrication from reflexive but not psychogenic mechanisms.

C. After SCI, she may, like 25% of women, achieve orgasm.

D. She will only retain psychogenic lubrication if she has intact light touch sensation in the T11–L2 thoracic and lumbar dermatomes.

33.8 According to the Consortium for Spinal Cord Medicine (2010), what is the first-line treatment for erectile dysfunction in patients with SCI?

A. Sildenafil.

B. Pharmacological penile injections.

C. Penile implants.

D. Vacuum erection devices.

33.9   On the basis of multiple randomized controlled trials (RCTs), which of the follow-
       ing has been recommended by the international team of experts in cognitive re-
       habilitation (INCOG) to manage inattention after a traumatic brain injury?

       A. Methylphenidate.
       B. Metacognitive strategies and dual tasking.
       C. Self-cueing.
       D. Structured problem solving.

33.10 A 35-year-old woman who suffered a complete SCI in a motor vehicle accident
       has been learning to move around with a wheelchair as well as performing self-
       catheterization. When discussing treatment goals with her medical team, she in-
       sists that she will be able to walk again. Psychiatry is consulted to assess the patient
       and to deal with her denial. On assessment, the patient does not display any signs
       of major depression, psychosis, or cognitive dysfunction. According to the dual-
       process model of grief, what would be the *most* appropriate response to this pa-
       tient's insistence that she will walk again?

       A. Continue to educate her on the nature of her injury.
       B. Review the prognosis for recovery.
       C. Discuss the limitations of current research seeking a cure for SCI.
       D. Refrain from confronting her denial.

33.11 Which of the following psychological interventions is effective in improving pain
       and sleep in patients with a spinal cord injury?

       A. Motivational interviewing plus self-management.
       B. Telephone-delivered cognitive-behavioral counseling.
       C. Peer-led brief action planning.
       D. Telephone-delivered problem-solving therapy.

C H A P T E R   3 4

Pain

34.1 What is the term for pain that results from a stimulus that does not normally pro-voke pain?

    A. Hyperalgesia.
    B. Nociception.
    C. Allodynia.
    D. Sensitization.

34.2 Which of the following statements describes the relationship between depression and pain?

    A. Baseline depressive symptoms more accurately predict future pain and dis-ability than do initial ratings of the actual pain.
    B. Chronic pain conditions have not been found to increase suicide risk.
    C. Patients with depression have twice the prevalence of pain conditions.
    D. Pain intensity is a better prediction of disability than depression.

34.3 In which of the following neuropathic conditions has lamotrigine demonstrated efficacy in treatment?

    A. Fibromyalgia.
    B. Postamputation phantom limb pain.
    C. Central neuropathic pain.
    D. HIV-related neuropathy.

34.4 A positive placebo response to a treatment would indicate which of the following?

    A. The patient has not had a biological response to the treatment.
    B. The patient would not benefit from active treatment.
    C. Expectation has played a role in the patient's response.
    D. The patient's pain is psychogenic.

34.5 Which opioid, because of its delayed central nervous system absorption and on-set of action, has a prolonged analgesic effect relative to its plasma half-life and therefore reduced potential for accumulation and toxicity with repeated dosing?

A. Morphine.
B. Oxycodone.
C. Fentanyl.
D. Hydrocodone.

34.6 Which medication is the most effective choice for neuropathic pain?

A. Nortriptyline.
B. Fluoxetine.
C. Vortioxetine.
D. Venlafaxine.

34.7 Which of the following is *not* an element of the fear-avoidance model of musculo-skeletal pain?

A. Pain severity.
B. Pain catastrophizing.
C. Avoidance behavior.
D. Internal locus of control.

CHAPTER 35

Medical Toxicology

35.1 What pharmacokinetic property of a drug increases the risks of toxicity?

A. Acute exposure.
B. Narrow therapeutic window.
C. Short half-life.
D. Abrupt absorption.

35.2 What is an advantage of using standard urine drug screening over other toxin assays?

A. It allows for a comprehensive detection of potentially dangerous substances.
B. It has a low rate of false negatives.
C. It is frequently updated to include novel substances of abuse.
D. It provides rapid results, which expedites intervention.

35.3 What is a *main* goal in the acute phase of toxicological treatment?

A. Hastening the elimination of an absorbed toxin.
B. Rapid tranquilization with benzodiazepines or antipsychotics.
C. Preventing seizures, which can cause additional injury.
D. Use of physical restraint to prevent physical injury.

35.4 What is the antidote to overdose with propranolol?

A. Flumazenil.
B. Glucagon.
C. *N*-acetylcysteine.
D. Physostigmine.

35.5 A patient makes a suicide attempt by overdose of lithium and presents with a high lithium level. What is the most appropriate treatment?

A. Activated charcoal.
B. Gastric lavage.

C. Chelation therapy.

D. Hemodialysis.

35.6 In acetaminophen overdose, what is the *most* important predictor of poor prognosis?

A. Alcohol co-ingestion at the time of overdose.

B. Presenting for medical care later than 24 hours after overdose.

C. Eating disorder.

D. Adolescent age.

35.7 A patient was recently discharged from your hospital's addiction unit. His wife brings him into your outpatient practice visibly altered, which she cannot under-stand because she disposed of all of the alcohol in their house. She did notice that he had windshield wiper fluid in the bathroom. While your colleague calls 911, you quickly administer what substance to protect him from permanent damage?

A. Ethanol.

B. Water.

C. 100% oxygen.

D. Diazepam.

35.8 A patient is concerned about neurotoxicity from radiation coming from her micro-wave. What do you tell her?

A. Microwaves produce non-ionizing radiation, so people should not stand in front of the microwave when it's on.

B. Microwaves produce ionizing radiation, so people should not stand in front of the microwave when it's on.

C. Microwaves produce non-ionizing radiation, which does not have toxic potential.

D. Microwaves produce ionizing radiation, which does not have toxic potential.

35.9 A patient tests positive for lead level of 20 µg/dL. Which symptom would make you suspect the exposure was *chronic*?

A. Peripheral motor neuropathy.

B. Coma.

C. Convulsions.

D. Clumsiness.

35.10 Which of the following is helpful in treating patients with "medication sensitivity"?

A. Extensive diagnostic and toxicological testing.

B. Treatment assuming the primary issue is psychiatric.

C. Using a disease model that anticipates identification of specific etiological agents.

D. Encouraging patients to seek relief from nonpharmacological therapies.

CHAPTER 36

Psychopharmacology

36.1 Which of the following antidepressant side effects is long term and may not abate unless the medication is discontinued?

A. Anxiety.
B. Sexual dysfunction.
C. Vomiting.
D. Headache.

36.2 Which of the following statements most accurately describes the treatment principle for patients with comorbid mood disorder and migraine headaches?

A. Coadministration of triptans and serotonergic antidepressants is not contraindicated.
B. Coadministration of triptans and serotonergic medications is safe because there have never been case reports of serotonin syndrome.
C. All triptans should be avoided when coadministered with a monoamine oxidase inhibitor (MAOI).
D. Antidepressants have no role in the treatment of migraine headache.

36.3 Which of the following medications requires no dosage adjustment or caution in patients with renal insufficiency?

A. Venlafaxine.
B. Pregabalin.
C. Olanzapine.
D. Gabapentin.

36.4 Which of the following natural medicines is thought to have clinically significant cytochrome interactions?

A. Ginkgo biloba.
B. Ginseng.
C. Kava.
D. Valerian.

36.5 Which antipsychotic carries the lowest risk of affecting a patient's seizure threshold?

A. Olanzapine.
B. Clozapine.
C. Fluphenazine.
D. Quetiapine.

36.6 Which of the following psychostimulants is preferred in the treatment of patients for whom weight loss and appetite suppression are a concern?

A. Methylphenidate.
B. Dexmethylphenidate.
C. Atomoxetine.
D. Modafinil.

36.7 Which of the following injectable benzodiazepines is preferred in behavioral emergencies?

A. Lorazepam, because it is readily absorbed and has no active metabolites.
B. Clonazepam, because of its onset of action.
C. Diazepam, because it is readily absorbed and has no active metabolites.
D. Diazepam, because of its onset of action.

36.8 Which medication is contraindicated in patients who have had a recent myocardial infarction?

A. Nortriptyline.
B. Ziprasidone.
C. Lorazepam.
D. Memantine.

36.9 Which of the following statements is true regarding psychotropic medications and syndrome of inappropriate antidiuretic hormone secretion (SIADH)?

A. Only antidepressant medications carry a risk of precipitating SIADH.
B. SSRIs and venlafaxine carry a higher risk of precipitating SIADH than other antidepressants.
C. Second-generation antipsychotics (SGAs), but not first-generation antipsychotics (FGAs), carry a risk of precipitating SIADH.
D. SIADH is not a dose-dependent phenomenon and therefore dosage adjustment has no place in the treatment of SIADH.

36.10 When considering the impact of antipsychotic medication on metabolic and endocrinologic indices of glucose tolerance, lipid levels, prolactin levels, and weight gain, which of the following medications has the lowest overall risk?

A. Clozapine.
B. Risperidone.
C. Ziprasidone.
D. Quetiapine.

36.11 What is the definition of pharmacodynamics?

A. Determines the relationship between drug concentration and response for both therapeutic and adverse effects.
B. Characterizes the rate and extent of drug absorption, distribution, metabolism, and excretion, thus determining the rate of drug delivery to, and concentration at, its sites of action.
C. Describes the rate and extent to which the drug ingredient is absorbed from the drug product and available for drug action.
D. Is an active drug.

36.12 A patient who has been stable on aripiprazole for the alleviation of psychotic symptoms has been experiencing worsened depression. His psychiatrist starts him on fluoxetine to target his depressive symptoms. What is the possible effect of adding fluoxetine?

A. Fluoxetine will increase the activity of the metabolic enzyme, causing increased metabolism of aripiprazole.
B. Fluoxetine will increase the activity of the metabolic enzyme, causing increased metabolism of fluoxetine.
C. Fluoxetine will decrease the activity of the metabolic enzyme, causing decreased metabolism of aripiprazole.
D. Fluoxetine will decrease the activity of the metabolic enzyme, causing increased metabolism of fluoxetine.

36.13 Which antidepressant should be avoided in patients with comorbid depression and hypertension?

A. Fluoxetine.
B. Venlafaxine.
C. Trazodone.
D. Mirtazapine.

36.14 A patient with a long history of bipolar disorder, stabilized on lithium, has a new diagnosis of diabetes insipidus. His primary doctor consults you for management recommendations. What is the treatment of choice for his patient?

A. Immediately stop his lithium as his nephrogenic diabetes insipidus will continue to progress/worsen.
B. Change his dosing from single-day to double-day dosing.
C. Increase his dose of lithium to cause his kidneys to respond to antidiuretic hormone.
D. Add amiloride to patient's medication regimen.

36.15 What is the correct procedure in prescribing a psychotropic drug that is primarily hepatically metabolized to a patient with impaired hepatic function?

A. Increase the initial dosage.
B. Titrate more slowly.
C. Monitor for clinical response as they would for any other patient.
D. Choose drugs with a narrow therapeutic index.

36.16 Which of the following medications has minimal effect on lithium levels?

A. Caffeine.
B. Nonsteroidal anti-inflammatory drugs (NSAIDs).
C. Loop diuretics.
D. Potassium-sparing diuretics.

36.17 Among the various antipsychotic agents, which of the following medications is associated with the greatest mean QTc interval prolongation?

A. Olanzapine.
B. Aripiprazole.
C. Ziprasidone.
D. Thioridazine.

36.18 Which SGA has been demonstrated to be *most* effective against psychosis without worsening a patient's underlying Parkinson's disease?

A. Clozapine.
B. Quetiapine.
C. Olanzapine.
D. Ziprasidone.

36.19 A patient with a history of chronic obstructive pulmonary disease (COPD) presents for treatment of anxiety. Which of the following best describes the approach to using benzodiazepines in this patient?

A. There is no concern about using benzodiazepines in this patient.
B. Benzodiazepines can significantly reduce the ventilatory response to hypoxia, so benzodiazepines should be used with caution.
C. Long-acting benzodiazepines are preferred over intermediate-acting benzodiazepines.
D. Benzodiazepines are contraindicated in patients with a diagnosis of COPD.

36.20 Which one of the following is a clinical feature of neuroleptic malignant syndrome (NMS)?

A. Hypothermia.
B. Generalized muscle flaccidity.
C. Autonomic instability.
D. Low white blood cell count, "leukopenia."

CHAPTER 37

Psychotherapy

37.1   Hypnotherapy has the best evidence in treating which of the following conditions?

   A. Irritable bowel syndrome.
   B. Cancer.
   C. Chronic obstructive pulmonary disease (COPD).
   D. Diabetes.

37.2   Which of the following should be offered first in the stepped-care model to deliver psychological treatment?

   A. Guided self-help.
   B. Watchful waiting.
   C. Cognitive-behavioral therapy (CBT).
   D. Inpatient treatment.

37.3   Homework is often assigned to patients in what type of therapy modality?

   A. Supportive and problem-solving approaches.
   B. Person-centered counseling.
   C. Structured therapies.
   D. Psychodynamic interpersonal therapy (PIT).

37.4   On the basis of findings from systematic reviews, which of the following psycho-social interventions has the *greatest* evidence to support recommending it to cancer patients?

   A. Involving families in the treatment process.
   B. Pharmacotherapy.
   C. Liaison activities with staff.
   D. Counseling.

37.5   Women attending clinics for breast cancer were found to express which of the following preferences?

   A. A more active, authoritative role in decision making by their doctors.
   B. Emotional space to voice their fears and uncertainties.

C. Pharmacotherapy.

D. Hypnotherapy

37.6 Which of the following is *least* supported by findings from published studies of patients with cancer?

A. Breast cancer patients may want doctors to play an authoritative role in decision making.

B. Supportive group therapies reduce distress and prolong survival in cancer patients.

C. Collaborative care models have shown benefit in depressed patients with cancer.

D. Psychosocial treatments for cancer have positive effects on mood and well-being.

37.7 Which type of therapy is best described as using a treatment strategy to facilitate discussion of topics uppermost in the minds of patients with terminal illness, with an existential orientation based on the rationale that living with a terminal illness amplifies existential concerns of death, meaning, freedom, and isolation?

A. Interpersonal therapy.

B. Supportive-expressive group therapy.

C. CBT.

D. Mindfulness-based cognitive therapy (MBCT).

37.8 For which condition does the existing evidence base show comparable effects of internet-based and face-to-face psychological treatments?

A. Diabetes.

B. Tinnitus.

C. Pain.

D. Breast cancer.

37.9 Which therapies are based on the premise that feelings, thoughts, and relationships are intimately tied up with each other?

A. Stepped care.

B. PIT.

C. Collaborative care.

D. Relational therapies.

37.10 Which of the following is specific to PIT as compared with interpersonal therapy?

A. The creation of an interpersonal inventory.

B. The use of role play to modify problematic interactions.

C. The focus on strategies to prevent recurrent depression.

D. The use of the therapeutic relationship to address problems in the "here and now."

CHAPTER 38

Electroconvulsive Therapy and Other Brain Stimulation Therapies

38.1 Whose responsibility is it to ensure that information obtained from previous electroconvulsive therapy (ECT) treatments is passed on before starting a new course of ECT?

A. The anesthesiologist.
B. The internist.
C. Other specialist consultants.
D. The psychiatrist.

38.2 What is the initial autonomic response to the electrical stimulus during ECT?

A. Bradycardia.
B. Tachycardia.
C. Hypotension.
D. Atrial fibrillation.

38.3 What cardioprotective agent is administered during ECT for patients with congestive heart failure (CHF)?

A. An antimuscarinic is administered.
B. All cardiac medications should be held on the morning of the ECT.
C. A beta-blocker is administered.
D. CHF is an absolute contraindication to ECT.

38.4 Which is the most common dysrhythmia among patients presenting for ECT?

A. Atrial fibrillation.
B. Sinus arrhythmia.
C. Premature ventricular contractions.
D. Premature atrial contractions.

38.5 Following ECT, which of the following conditions in neurological disorders have been shown to improve?

A. Treatment-emergent dyskinesias.
B. Core motor deficits.
C. Cognitive impairment.
D. Symptoms of recent stroke.

38.6 Transcranial magnetic stimulation (TMS) is U.S. Food and Drug Administration (FDA)–approved for which of the following disorders?

A. Treatment-resistant depression.
B. Cognitive impairment.
C. Parkinson's disease.
D. Migraine.

38.7 Contraindications regarding vagal nerve stimulation (VNS) occur in which of the following situations?

A. Patients with epilepsy.
B. Patients with treatment-resistant depression.
C. Patients with left vagotomy.
D. Patients requiring diagnostic ultrasound.

38.8 For which of the following conditions does deep brain stimulation have FDA approval?

A. Cerebrovascular disease.
B. Increased bleeding risk.
C. Treatment-resistant obsessive-compulsive disorder.
D. Immunodeficiency.

38.9 For which of the following conditions may ECT be lifesaving?

A. Patients with a recent stroke.
B. Intracerebral aneurysm.
C. Intracranial masses.
D. Neuroleptic-induced malignant catatonia.

C H A P T E R   3 9

Palliative Care

39.1 Which of the following statements best describes the *primary* role of the consultation-liaison psychiatrist in the palliative care setting?

A. Address bereavement issues with the patient and family.
B. Encourage discussion of end-of-life ethical issues regarding provision or nonprovision of treatment.
C. Assist clinicians in how to deliver bad news and discuss treatment preferences.
D. Diagnose and treat comorbid psychiatric disorders in the palliative care setting.

39.2 A 60-year-old woman with advanced chronic obstructive pulmonary disease and current tobacco use disorder is admitted for workup and care of a newly diagnosed left lung adenocarcinoma. She and her family report that she does not drink alcohol and has been using e-cigarettes for the past year. On the third hospital day, her nurses report that she is highly anxious. The psychiatric consultant notes that she is irritable, anxious, and complains of confusion; however, she is not delirious. What is the single best first approach to patient engagement and management in this case?

A. Start citalopram 20 mg daily.
B. Offer counseling only because e-cigarette use does not cause withdrawal.
C. Initiate nicotine replacement therapy with a transdermal nicotine patch.
D. Instruct house staff to give a stat dose of intramuscular lorazepam 1 mg.

39.3 You are consulting in hospital on a 66-year-old man with advanced metastatic prostate cancer. He has multiple painful bony metastases to spine and femur and is expected to live for only a few weeks. Parenteral hydromorphone is effective at controlling his pain, radiation therapy is started, and a discussion regarding home hospice is held with the patient and family. The patient becomes acutely depressed, hopeless, and feels guilty about his illness. The symptoms are distressing and persist over the next week. What is the best initial medical approach to managing depression in this patient?

A. Start fluoxetine at 20 mg daily.
B. Start methylphenidate 2.5 mg at 8 A.M. and 1 P.M.

C. Reduce hydromorphone dosage.

D. Start sertraline at 50 mg daily.

39.4 Which of the following statements is *most* accurate regarding models of delivery of palliative care?

A. Palliative care is synonymous with end-of-life care.

B. Bereavement programs are carved out of traditional models of palliative care delivery.

C. Model palliative care programs are hospital based in setting.

D. Model programs typically include both research and education as core components.

39.5 You are consulting in an inpatient hospice setting on an 82-year-old man with advanced lung cancer with recent progression of disease who is actively dying; he is both anxious and dyspneic. Which medicine would be the most appropriate to palliate these distressing symptoms?

A. Buspirone.

B. Morphine.

C. Trazodone.

D. Mirtazapine.

39.6 A 66-year-old woman has end-stage refractory leukemia with impaired quality of life (pain, fatigue). She begins a palliative psychotherapy intervention, which combines didactics and personal exploration with assigned writing to promote self-reflection outside of sessions. Which of the following palliative psychotherapies is consistent with this specific intervention?

A. Dignity therapy.

B. Cognitive-behavioral therapy.

C. Meaning-centered psychotherapy.

D. Life review.

39.7 A 36-year-old woman with breast cancer is receiving cyclic systemic chemotherapy and develops severe, refractory nausea, and vomiting. First-line antiemetics have been ineffective or intolerable because of extrapyramidal side effects. Which of the following would be the most appropriate next treatment to initiate?

A. Metoclopramide.

B. Prochlorperazine.

C. Dronabinol.

D. Haloperidol.

39.8 A 52-year-old man is confronting the death of his husband due to amyotrophic lateral sclerosis (ALS) 3 months earlier. He is successfully integrating this loss without significant detriment in self-care, and he has maintained social interactions. Which of the following terms *best* describes his current coping with this loss?

A. Mourning.
B. Bereavement.
C. Uncomplicated grief.
D. Complicated grief.

PART II

Answer Guide

CHAPTER 1

Psychiatric Assessment and Consultation

1.1   What is the essential element of the collaborative care model?

A. There is consultation and appropriate sharing of information among the primary care provider, the care manager, and the consulting psychiatrist.
B. The psychiatric specialist provides a consultation for every patient.
C. Mental health specialists treat all patients with diagnosed mental illnesses.
D. All interventions are performed by the same clinician.

The correct response is option A: There is consultation and appropriate sharing of information among the primary care provider, the care manager, and the consulting psychiatrist.

Collaborative care refers to the joining together of mental health care providers with primary care physicians and their teams to deliver specialized care within the outpatient primary care setting. Consultation psychiatrists are uniquely positioned for this role, given the focus of psychosomatic medicine at the interface of medicine and psychiatry. Although specific models of collaborative care vary, effective programs generally share certain key components. The first is systematic care management (often by a trained nurse, social worker, or psychologist). The care manager helps identify patients in need, coordinates an initial treatment plan, educates patients, provides follow-up, monitors progress, and helps change the treatment course as needed. These tasks may be performed in person (e.g., in the primary care clinic) or by telephone (Worth and Stern 2003). The next essential piece is consultation and appropriate sharing of information among the primary care provider, the care manager, and the consulting psychiatrist (Unützer et al. 2006) (option A is correct). This does not necessarily mean that the psychiatric specialist provides a consultation for every patient (option B is incorrect); in fact, research has shown that the most efficient and cost-effective measures often involve a stepwise approach, in which progressively more intensive interventions are applied until a successful outcome is achieved (option C is incorrect) (Katon et al. 2005, 2008; Richards et al. 2008). Thus, stepped care for a patient with depression might involve an initial intervention of prescription of an antidepressant by the primary care provider along with care management either by phone or in person, as detailed above. If the patient remains symptomatic, the next step would be referral for brief psychotherapy or other behavioral interventions and/or a switch to another medication. Although much of this process takes place under the supervision of a consulting psychiatrist, referral to mental health care specialists is generally reserved for treatment nonresponders. For example, in the IMPACT (Improving Mood—Promoting Access to Collaborative Treatment) randomized trial for depressed elderly patients in primary care, consulting psychiatrists saw only about 10% of patients, but they served as key members of the collaborative team by providing consultation and education to care managers and primary care providers (Hunkeler et al. 2006; Unützer et al. 2002) (option D is incorrect). Collaborative care models have been shown to improve outcomes and enhance patient function and quality of life as well as to be cost-effective (Rossom et al. 2017). **Chapter 1 (p. 18)**

1.2   For which of these presentations should neuroimaging be considered?

A. A patient with a recurrent psychotic episode.
B. A patient with established dementia when admitted to the hospital.
C. A patient with an acute change in mental status who also has abnormal findings on neurological examination.
D. A patient undergoing a second course of electroconvulsive therapy treatments.

The correct response is option C: A patient with an acute change in mental status who also has abnormal findings on neurological examination.

Dougherty and Rauch (2004) suggest that the following conditions and situations merit consideration of neuroimaging: new-onset psychosis (option A is incorrect), new-onset dementia (option B is incorrect) , delirium of unknown cause prior to an initial course of electroconvulsive therapy (option D is incorrect), and an acute mental status change with an abnormal neurological examination in a patient with either a history of head trauma or an age of 50 years or older (option C is correct). Regardless of the modality, the consultant should read the radiologist's report because other physicians tend to dismiss all but acute focal findings and, as a result, misleadingly record the results of the study as normal in the chart. Psychiatrists recognize, however, that even small abnormalities (e.g., periventricular white matter changes) or chronic changes (e.g., cortical atrophy) have diagnostic and therapeutic implications. **Chapter 1 (p. 14)**

1.3   Which of the following statements about the electroencephalogram (EEG) is true?

A. The EEG is rarely available.
B. The EEG generally indicates a specific etiology for generalized delirium.

C. The EEG can be helpful in distinguishing between neurological and psychiatric etiologies in mute, uncommunicative patients.
D. The EEG is useful in the screening evaluation of patients with head injury.

The correct response is option C: The EEG can be helpful in distinguishing between neurological and psychiatric etiologies in mute, uncommunicative patients.

The EEG is the most widely available test that can assess brain activity (option A is incorrect). The EEG is most often indicated in patients with paroxysmal or other symptoms suggestive of a seizure disorder, especially complex partial seizures or pseudoseizures (see Chapter 30, "Neurology and Neurosurgery"). An EEG may also be helpful in distinguishing between neurological and psychiatric etiologies for a mute, uncommunicative patient (option C is correct). An EEG may be helpful in documenting the presence of generalized slowing in a delirious patient, but it rarely indicates a specific etiology of delirium, and an EEG is not indicated in every delirious patient (option B is incorrect). However, when the diagnosis of delirium is uncertain, EEG evidence of dysrhythmia may prove useful. For example, when the primary treatment team insists that a patient should be transferred to a psychiatric inpatient service because of a mistaken belief that the symptoms of delirium represent schizophrenia or depression, an EEG can provide concrete data to support the correct diagnosis. EEGs may also facilitate the evaluation of rapidly progressive dementia or profound coma; but because findings are neither sensitive nor specific, they are not often helpful in the evaluation of space-occupying lesions, cerebral infarctions, or head injury (Bostwick and Philbrick 2002) (option D is incorrect). Continuous EEG recordings with video monitoring or ambulatory EEG monitoring may be necessary in order to document abnormal electrical activity in cases of complex partial seizures or when psychogenic seizures are suspected. As with neuroimaging reports, the psychiatric consultant must read the EEG report because nonpsychiatrists often misinterpret the absence of dramatic focal abnormalities (e.g., spikes) as indicative of normality, even though psychiatrically significant brain dysfunction may be associated with focal or generalized slowing or with sharp waves. Other electrophysiological tests may be helpful in specific situations, for example, sensory evoked potentials testing to distinguish multiple sclerosis from conversion disorder or electromyography with nerve conduction velocities to differentiate neuropathy from malingering. **Chapter 1 (pp. 14–15)**

1.4   Which statement about screening tools for psychiatric illness is correct?

A. Psychiatric screening tools are useful on their own in the evaluation of and treatment planning for patients.
B. Psychiatric screening tools are unaffected by cognitive status.
C. Psychiatric screening tools have not been translated into other languages or validated cross-culturally.
D. Psychiatric screening tools may identify patients who may benefit from further psychiatric assessment.

The correct response is option D: Psychiatric screening tools may identify patients who may benefit from further psychiatric assessment.

The use of screening tools may be helpful in specific situations. For example, even though a comprehensive assessment of cognitive function is not required for every patient, even a slim suspicion of the possibility of a cognitive deficit should prompt performance of cognitive screening. Although individualized mental status examinations performed as part of a psychiatrist's clinical interview are much preferred to standardized tests, screening tests may be particularly useful in case finding (e.g., in primary care settings as part of a collaborative care approach) and in research (option D is correct). The same has been proposed for a variety of other psychiatric disorders, including depressive, anxiety, and substance use disorders. An important note in this regard, however, is that screening is unlikely to be helpful without a systematic approach to treatment and may even have negative effects (option A is incorrect) (Thombs et al. 2012).

A formal neuropsychological battery may be useful if these bedside tests produce abnormal results. In a patient with an altered level of awareness or attention, formal cognitive tests should be deferred until the sensorium clears because clouding of consciousness will produce uninterpretable results (option B is incorrect).

Other screening instruments may also help to identify patients in medical settings who could benefit from a comprehensive psychiatric interview. The Patient Health Questionnaire (PHQ), an abbreviated form of the Primary Care Evaluation of Mental Disorders (PRIME-MD), is a three-page questionnaire that can be entirely self-administered by the patient (Spitzer et al. 1999). In addition to the assessment of mood, anxiety, eating, alcohol use, and somatization disorders, the PHQ screens for posttraumatic stress disorder and common psychosocial stressors and also elicits a pregnancy history. The PHQ is valid and reliable and has improved the diagnosis of psychiatric conditions in primary care and other ambulatory medical settings (Spitzer et al. 1999); it may also have a role at the bedside. Subsets of the PHQ's items have been validated for specific screening purposes. For example, the nine-item PHQ-9, a self-administered depression-specific questionnaire that can be completed by the patient in roughly 2 minutes (Gilbody et al. 2007a; Kroenke et al. 2001) has been shown to perform as well (in a range of countries, populations, and clinical settings) as longer clinician-administered instruments that screen for depression in medical settings (Gilbody et al. 2007b); it can also be used to monitor the severity of depression (option C is incorrect). The PHQ-2 for depression, which includes just the items for mood and anhedonia, is sensitive and specific for both major depressive disorder and other depressive disorders, performing almost as well as the PHQ-9 (Löwe et al. 2005). **Chapter 1 (pp. 18–20)**

1.5 The extensive body of research into the utility of the psychiatric consultation for medical patients has demonstrated which of the following?

A. There appears to be no link between comorbid psychopathology and increased length of hospital stay, independent of the severity of the medical illness.
B. There appears to be no link between comorbid psychopathology and increased inpatient costs, independent of the severity of the medical illness.
C. Depressed elderly patients have less frequent and shorter hospitalizations than their nondepressed cohorts.
D. Psychiatric consultation improves the medical care of complex patients.

The correct response is option D: Psychiatric consultation improves the medical care of complex patients.

The benefits of psychiatric services in health care delivery are significant. An extensive body of evidence has demonstrated a link between comorbid psychopathology and increased length of hospital stay and, consequently, increased inpatient costs (options A and B are incorrect). Levenson et al. (1990) described a longer median length of hospital stay (a 40% increase) and hospital costs that were 35% higher in medical inpatients with depression, anxiety, cognitive dysfunction, or high levels of pain (independent of severity of medical illness). Depressed elderly patients in another sample had more hospitalizations and longer hospital stays (Koenig and Kuchibhatla 1998) (option C is incorrect). Although it was hoped that psychiatric consultation might decrease lengths of stay and inpatient costs, it has been difficult to prove, and this is not where its primary value lies. Patients benefit from the reductions in mental suffering and improvements in psychological well-being that result from more accurate diagnosis and more appropriate treatment. Providers of health care profit from the added diagnostic and therapeutic expertise of the psychiatric consultant as well as from a better understanding of health behaviors. The hospital milieu also benefits from having readily available medically knowledgeable psychiatrists, whose assistance improves the care of the complex patients (option D is correct). **Chapter 1 (p. 21)**

References

Bostwick JM, Philbrick KL: The use of electroencephalography in psychiatry of the medically ill. Psychiatr Clin North Am 25(1):17–25, 2002 11912938

Dougherty DD, Rauch SL: Neuroimaging in psychiatry, in Massachusetts General Hospital Psychiatry Update and Board Preparation, 2nd Edition. Edited by Stern TA, Herman JB. New York, McGraw-Hill, 2004, pp 227–232

Gilbody S, Richards D, Barkham M: Diagnosing depression in primary care using self-completed instruments: UK validation of PHQ-9 and CORE-OM. Br J Gen Pract 57(541):650–652, 2007a 17688760

Gilbody S, Richards D, Brealey S, Hewitt C: Screening for depression in medical settings with the Patient Health Questionnaire (PHQ): a diagnostic meta-analysis. J Gen Intern Med 22(11):1596–1602, 2007b 17874169

Hunkeler EM, Katon W, Tang L, et al: Long term outcomes from the IMPACT randomised trial for depressed elderly patients in primary care. BMJ 332(7536):259–263, 2006 16428253

Katon WJ, Schoenbaum M, Fan MY, et al: Cost-effectiveness of improving primary care treatment of late-life depression. Arch Gen Psychiatry 62(12):1313–1320, 2005 16330719

Katon WJ, Russo JE, Von Korff M, et al: Long-term effects on medical costs of improving depression outcomes in patients with depression and diabetes. Diabetes Care 31(6):1155–1159, 2008 18332158

Koenig HG, Kuchibhatla M: Use of health services by hospitalized medically ill depressed elderly patients. Am J Psychiatry 155(7):871–877, 1998 9659849

Kroenke K, Spitzer RL, Williams JB: The PHQ-9: validity of a brief depression severity measure. J Gen Intern Med 16(9):606–613, 2001 11556941

Levenson JL, Hamer RM, Rossiter LF: Relation of psychopathology in general medical inpatients to use and cost of services. Am J Psychiatry 147(11):1498–1503, 1990 2121054

Löwe B, Kroenke K, Gräfe K: Detecting and monitoring depression with a two-item questionnaire (PHQ-2). J Psychosom Res 58(2):163–171, 2005 15820844

Richards DA, Lovell K, Gilbody S, et al: Collaborative care for depression in UK primary care: a randomized controlled trial. Psychol Med 38(2):279–287, 2008 17803837

Rossom RC, Solberg LI, Magnan S, et al: Impact of a national collaborative care initiative for patients with depression and diabetes or cardiovascular disease. Gen Hosp Psychiatry 44:77–85, 2017 27558106

Spitzer RL, Kroenke K, Williams JB: Validation and utility of a self-report version of PRIME-MD: the PHQ primary care study. Primary Care Evaluation of Mental Disorders. Patient Health Questionnaire. JAMA 282(18):1737–1744, 1999 10568646

Thombs BD, Coyne JC, Cuijpers P, et al: Rethinking recommendations for screening for depression in primary care. CMAJ 184(4):413–418, 2012 21930744

Unützer J, Katon W, Callahan CM, et al; IMPACT Investigators. Improving Mood-Promoting Access to Collaborative Treatment: Collaborative care management of late-life depression in the primary care setting: a randomized controlled trial. JAMA 288(22):2836–2845, 2002 12472325

Unützer J, Schoenbaum M, Druss BG, Katon WJ: Transforming mental health care at the interface with general medicine: report for the presidents commission. Psychiatr Serv 57(1):37–47, 2006 16399961

Worth JL, Stern TA: Benefits of an outpatient Psychiatric TeleConsultation Unit (PTCU): results of a one-year pilot. Prim Care Companion J Clin Psychiatry 5(2):80–84, 2003 15156235

CHAPTER 2

Legal and Ethical Issues

2.1   Which of the following, alone, would be insufficient to justify compromising patient confidentiality?

A. Suspected child abuse.
B. Suspected elder abuse.
C. Patient threatens to sign out against medical advice.
D. Patient has expressed intent to harm a specific individual.

The correct response is option C: Patient threatens to sign out against medical advice.

Medical patients are admitted voluntarily to a general hospital; therefore, discharges against medical advice (AMA) are akin to a withdrawal of the original consent to hospitalization. Decisions about AMA discharges generally follow the decisional capacity–based model of medical treatment refusal (option C is correct). Doctor-patient confidentiality is a professional, legal, and ethical requirement. However, confidentiality is not an absolute mandate, and it must give way when another ethical principle or legal requirement takes precedence. One such example is child or elder abuse and neglect; every jurisdiction in the United States mandates that physicians report suspected child or elder abuse and neglect (Brendel 2005; Milosavljevic et al. 2012, 2016) (options A and B are incorrect). Because the landmark California Supreme Court Decision in *Tarasoff v. Board of Regents of the University of California* in 1976, the concept of a duty to warn third parties or protect them from physical harm from patients has emerged as a well-known exception to doctor-patient confidentiality (Schouten and Brendel 2004) (option D is incorrect). **Chapter 2 (pp. 28–31, 43–44)**

2.2   A 72-year-old patient tells his physician he no longer wishes to be treated and wants to sign out of the hospital, despite medical advice that he remain. Which of the following is not legally required to permit the patient to leave?

A. Patient expresses a preference to leave the hospital.
B. Patient signs AMA discharge form to waive hospital liability.

C. Patient comprehends pertinent medical facts.

D. Patient rationally comprehends potential consequences.

The correct response is option B: Patient signs AMA discharge form to waive hospital liability.

Too often, hospital personnel are intent on getting a patient to sign an AMA discharge form, but the form is neither necessary nor sufficient to avoid legal liability (option B is correct). Decisions about discharges that are AMA generally follow the decisional capacity–based model of medical treatment refusal. Therefore, one role of the consulting psychiatrist is to perform a capacity assessment to determine whether the patient has the requisite capacity to decide to leave the hospital AMA. Under the model developed by Appelbaum and Grisso (Appelbaum 2007; Appelbaum and Grisso 1988), the four factors for consideration in determining decisional capacity are preference (option A is incorrect), factual understanding (option C is incorrect), appreciation of the facts presented (i.e., an understanding of how information relates to oneself and one's specific situation) (option D is incorrect), and rational manipulation of information. All four elements must be met for the individual to demonstrate decisional capacity. In addition, the psychiatrist can explore why the patient wants to leave the hospital and, when possible, help effect a solution leading to willingness of the patient to remain. A patient with decisional capacity to leave the hospital AMA should be told that he is welcome to return to the hospital if he changes his mind or his symptoms get worse, and robust efforts should be made to secure and convince the patient to accept follow-up care. **Chapter 2 (pp. 36–37, 43–44)**

2.3   Which of the following scenarios would not necessarily warrant a psychiatric consultation to assess a mother's ability to care for her child?

A. Maternal substance abuse.

B. Mother has a severe mental disorder.

C. Suspected child abuse or neglect.

D. Suspected intimate partner violence.

The correct response is option D: Suspected intimate partner violence.

Intimate partner violence denotes battery (McHugh and Frieze 2006); in some states, the physician is required by law to make a report. However, intimate partner violence may not necessarily impair a mother's ability to safely care for her child (option D is correct). Psychiatric consultations are sometimes requested to evaluate maternal competency (i.e., capacity to care for a child) when it is thought that a vulnerable infant or child will be at risk if the parent is allowed to take the child home from the hospital (Nair and Morrison 2000); this occurs most commonly in situations of maternal substance abuse (option A is incorrect), severe mental disorder (option B is incorrect), or child abuse or neglect (option C is incorrect). **Chapter 2 (p. 45); Chapter 6 (pp. 179–180)**

2.4   A psychiatrist is called to evaluate a patient who is a Jehovah's Witness and has refused to accept a life-saving blood transfusion. Which of the following must be present to determine that the patient has capacity to make such a decision?

A. Patient understands why the transfusion is required.
B. Patient understands refusing the transfusion will lead to his discharge from the hospital.
C. Patient's wife, who is also a Jehovah's Witness, agrees with the patient's decision.
D. Patient must consult with a psychiatrist who agrees with the patient.

The correct response is option A: Patient understands why the transfusion is required.

Rational manipulation of information is one of four elements that must be met in order to demonstrate decisional capacity under the model developed by Appelbaum and Grisso (1988). A patient must demonstrate that his or her decision-making process is a rational one, taking into account the individual's past preferences, values, and decisions. An often-used example is that of a Jehovah's Witness deciding whether to accept or refuse a life-saving blood transfusion. In this case, the adult individual's decision to refuse the transfusion and face certain death might seem irrational on the surface, but in the context of this individual's faith-based life decisions and belief that accepting the transfusion would be contrary to religious doctrine, the decision could meet the rationality requirement (option A is correct). Refusing a blood transfusion would not necessarily lead to discharge (option B is incorrect). A patient with decisional capacity does not require the agreement of a spouse for treatment decisions (option C is incorrect). Ethical psychiatrists may struggle when a patient's choices are inconsistent with their own personal values; however, awareness of this discomfort is critical to ensure that psychiatrists are respecting their patients by giving full credence to patients' capacitated wishes (option D is incorrect). **Chapter 2 (pp. 36–37)**

2.5   A 60-year-old woman is admitted for recurrent depression that is not responsive to adequate medication trials, but four prior courses of electroconvulsive therapy (ECT) treatment were successful. She has no medical comorbidities, denies suicidal or homicidal ideation, and has no evidence of delusions or hallucinations. She lives with her husband and is independent in all activities of daily living. ECT is recommended, and the patient receives appropriate information and counseling, which she is able to repeat in her own words. She signs a consent form, although she tells staff her husband threatened divorce unless she receives ECT, and if it were up to her alone, she would not want ECT. Which of the following best describes the validity of the patient's consent?

A. Consent is valid, because the patient's decision is both knowing and voluntary.
B. Consent is valid, because the patient's husband also agrees with treatment recommendations.

C. Consent is not valid, because the patient has not received adequate information about the proposed treatment.

D. Consent is not valid even with a signed consent form, because the patient has verbally expressed reservations.

The correct response is option A: Consent is valid, because the patient's decision is both knowing and voluntary.

In addition to requiring decisional capacity, the ethical and legal standard for informed consent requires that consent must be knowing and voluntary (Appelbaum et al. 1987; *Salgo v. Leland Stanford Jr. University Board of Trustees* 1957; *Schloendorff v. Society of New York Hospital* 1914). For informed consent to be knowing, the patient must possess the requisite information about the proposed intervention; pragmatically, to demonstrate true informed consent, the patient should be able to repeat the information in his or her own words (option C is incorrect). The second core element of informed consent is that it must be *voluntary*. Patients may be under pressure from family members to make certain treatment decisions, and in these situations, patients are generally determined to have acted voluntarily from both ethical and legal perspectives (Grisso and Appelbaum 1998; Mallary et al. 1986) (options B and D are incorrect). Nonetheless, distinguishing between voluntary and coerced choices requires a complex and nuanced inquiry (Roberts 2002). Individuals who are totally dependent on others for their care are generally deemed unable to give voluntary consent to treatment or research because of the inherent inequality between the patient and the institution; examples include nursing home residents and prisoners (Gold 1974; Moser et al. 2004; National Commission for the Protection of Human Subjects of Biomedical and Behavioral Research 1976, 1978). In the scenario here, the patient has given informed consent that is both knowing and voluntary (option A is correct). **Chapter 2 (pp. 38–39)**

2.6   Which of the following is not a required component to meet the standard for informed consent?

A. Consent form was read to the patient.

B. Patient's spouse agrees the proposed intervention is needed.

C. Patient is presented information including the diagnosis and nature of the condition being treated; reasonably expected benefits from the proposed treatment; nature and likelihood of risks involved; inability to precisely predict results of treatment; potential irreversibility of the treatment; the expected risks, benefits, and results of alternative, or no, treatment.

D. Patient is able to repeat the information provided regarding the medical problem and proposed treatment in his own words.

The correct response is option B: Patient's spouse agrees the proposed intervention is needed.

Agreement from a patient's spouse is not a required component of informed consent (option B is correct). In hospital settings, informed consent may be equated with having a signed consent form on file; however, clinicians should be aware that informed consent involves not just a reading of or signing of a form but also engaging in a process characterized by exchange of information, communication, and an active decision by the patient to accept or refuse the treatment (option A is incorrect). In addition to requiring decisional capacity, the ethical and legal standard for informed consent requires that consent must be knowing and voluntary (Appelbaum et al. 1987; *Salgo v. Leland Stanford Jr. University Board of Trustees* 1957; *Schloendorff v. Society of New York Hospital* 1914). There are six broad categories of information that, if presented to the patient, are generally accepted as meeting the standard of how much information needs to be presented, regardless of the particular jurisdictional standard (King and Moulton 2006): 1) the diagnosis and the nature of the condition being treated; 2) the reasonably expected benefits from the proposed treatment; 3) the nature and likelihood of the risks involved; 4) the inability to precisely predict results of the treatment; 5) the potential irreversibility of the treatment; and 6) the expected risks, benefits, and results of alternative, or no, treatment (option C is incorrect). Pragmatically, to demonstrate true informed consent, patients should be able to repeat the information in their own words (option D is incorrect). The second core element of informed consent is that it must be voluntary; the patient must give consent freely and unencumbered by external coercive forces. **Chapter 2 (pp. 38–39)**

2.7   A 71-year-old man presents to the emergency room with symptoms suggestive of a cerebral vascular accident. He is unable to speak and appears to have difficulty comprehending. It is determined that immediate intravascular removal of the clot causing the patient's stroke is required. Treatment may proceed without the patient's informed consent based on which of the following principles?

A. Beneficence.
B. Justice.
C. Nonmaleficence.
D. Autonomy.

The correct response is option A: Beneficence.

The most common and well-known exception to the informed consent requirement is an emergency situation in which failure to treat would result in serious and potentially irreversible deterioration of the patient's condition; therefore, invocation of the emergency exception is ethically permissible in recognition of the principle of beneficence (option A is correct). However, the presence of an emergency is not enough to authorize treatment if the physician has knowledge that the patient would have refused the emergency treatment if he or she were able to express his or her wishes; the patient's prior expressed wishes cannot be overridden by an emergency (Annas 1999; *Shine v. Vega* 1999) (option D is incorrect). In this scenario, the principles of justice and nonmaleficence do not apply in the decision to proceed with treatment (options B and C are incorrect). **Chapter 2 (pp. 39–40)**

2.8   Which of the following is the physician's obligation in reporting elder abuse?

A. Physicians are not mandated reporters of suspected elder abuse and neglect.
B. Reporting is mandated only when there is physical evidence of abuse.
C. Reporting suspected elder neglect should be deferred until a full assessment of cognitive decline has been performed.
D. Physicians must report suspected abuse, although elder patients may ultimately refuse intervention by protective services agencies.

The correct response is option D: Physicians must report suspected abuse, although elder patients may ultimately refuse intervention by protective services agencies.

Physicians are mandated reporters of suspected elder abuse and neglect in every U.S. jurisdiction (Milosavljevic et al. 2016) (option A is incorrect). The definition of elder abuse and neglect varies by state, although most states use a standard incorporating five common elements: infliction of pain or injury, infliction of emotional or psychological harm, sexual assault, material or financial exploitation, and neglect (Milosavljevic et al. 2016). Elder abuse standards may also include self-neglect, in recognition of the frequency of waning self-care abilities that accompany age-related physical and cognitive decline (Abrams et al. 2002) (option B is incorrect). Physicians are more likely to face legal liability for failure to report elder abuse and neglect than for good-faith reporting of suspected abuse and/or neglect, even when reports are "screened out" or found to be unsubstantiated following investigation by elder protective services (option C is incorrect). Unlike laws pertaining to the reporting of suspected child abuse, elder protection laws may recognize the ability of a competent elder to refuse investigation or prevention by protective services agencies (option D is correct). **Chapter 2 (p. 30)**

2.9   A psychiatric consultation is requested to evaluate a medical patient who is irritable, agitated, and grandiose. The patient has not slept in several days. The consulting psychiatrist makes a diagnosis of bipolar disorder and recommends treatment with lithium. Three days later, lab results show the patient's serum creatinine is 1.5 mg/dL, up from a previous baseline of 1.3 mg/dL. Lithium is discontinued, and a different mood-stabilizing medication is prescribed. Which of the following is true of the consulting psychiatrist's duty to the patient regarding treatment?

A. The consulting psychiatrist has a duty directly to the patient.
B. The consulting psychiatrist assumes responsibility for monitoring the outcome of all treatment recommendations.
C. The consulting psychiatrist may assume a primary treatment role.
D. The consulting psychiatrist must enter orders for all recommendations.

The correct response is option C: The consulting psychiatrist may assume a primary treatment role.

A consultation-liaison psychiatrist's primary duty is to the consultee, or the physician who requests the consult; the responsibility of the treating clinician is directly to the patient (option A is incorrect). Consultants should be careful to maintain boundaries between the role of consultant and the role of treating clinician. For example, when a psychiatrist (consultant) is requested by a treating physician (consultee) to recommend an appropriate medication to prescribe a patient, the consultant's duty is to provide appropriate recommendations and information to the consultee. But if the consultant directly enters an order for the medication to be given to the patient, the consultant will generally be held to have assumed a direct treatment role and assumed a direct responsibility to the patient (option D is incorrect). If the consultant does assume a primary treatment role (and there may be good reasons for the consultant to do so) (option C is correct), it is important that the consultant be cognizant that he or she thereby assumes all responsibilities of treating psychiatrist, including the responsibility to either monitor or follow up on the patient's progress or arrange for another clinician to do so (option B is incorrect). **Chapter 2 (pp. 45–46)**

2.10   Which of the following is not an element that would contribute to establishing a clear claim of malpractice against a consultation-liaison psychiatrist?

A. Proof that the consultation-liaison psychiatrist offered a general curbside opinion to a colleague.
B. Proof that the consultation-liaison psychiatrist acted intentionally to harm the patient.
C. Proof that the consultation-liaison psychiatrist directly caused a medical error.
D. Proof that the consultation-liaison psychiatrist violated the standard of care.

The correct response is option A: Proof that the consultation-liaison psychiatrist offered a general curbside opinion to a colleague.

Malpractice covers personal injuries resulting from medical interventions (Brendel and Schouten 2007; Schouten and Brendel 2004; Schouten et al. 2008). For a claim of malpractice to be established, four elements must be met. First, a *duty* must be established, by the existence of either a direct doctor-patient relationship or a consultant-consultee relationship (option A is correct). In some cases, even limited or cursory interactions may be considered by the court to have constituted a doctor-patient relationship. Second, a *breach* of that duty must have occurred (i.e., a violation of the standard of care). Third, this breach must have *directly* caused harm to a patient that resulted in the fourth element, *damage* to the patient. The legal requirement for malpractice is often summarized as "the four D's": duty, dereliction of duty, direct causation, and damage. Malpractice does not require that the physician acted intentionally in causing harm to the patient (option B is incorrect). Rather, malpractice is an unintentional tort, a tort of negligence, which means that deviation from the accepted standard of care caused damage to the patient (option D is incorrect). As a final note, studies of malpractice lawsuits have shown that only a small number of cases involving injury to patients due to medical errors actually lead to malpractice claims or litigation and that defendants prevail in the majority of cases that lead to litigation (Localio et al. 1991; Schouten et al. 2008) (option C is incorrect). Notwithstanding, in a study of paid claims, no medical error was found in up to one-third of claims (Brennan et al. 1996), highlighting the fact that even error-free practice does not insulate against malpractice liability (Schouten et al. 2008). **Chapter 2 (pp. 45–46)**

References

Abrams RC, Lachs M, McAvay G, et al: Predictors of self-neglect in community-dwelling elders. Am J Psychiatry 159(10):1724–1730, 2002 12359679

Annas GJ: The last resort—the use of physical restraints in medical emergencies. N Engl J Med 341(18):1408–1412, 1999 10536135

Appelbaum PS: Clinical practice. Assessment of patients' competence to consent to treatment. N Engl J Med 357(18):1834–1840, 2007 17978292

Appelbaum PS, Grisso T: Assessing patients' capacities to consent to treatment. N Engl J Med 319(25):1635–1638, 1988 3200278

Appelbaum PS, Lidz CW, Meisel A: Informed Consent: Legal Theory and Clinical Practice. New York, Oxford University Press, 1987

Brendel RW: An approach to forensic issues, in The Ten-Minute Guide to Psychiatric Diagnosis and Treatment. Edited by Stern TA. New York, Professional Publishing Group, 2005, pp 399–412

Brendel RW, Schouten R: Legal concerns in psychosomatic medicine. Psychiatr Clin North Am 30(4):663–676, 2007 17938039

Brennan TA, Sox CM, Burstin HR: Relation between negligent adverse events and the outcomes of medical-malpractice litigation. N Engl J Med 335(26):1963–1967, 1996 8960477

Gold JA: Kaimowitz v Department of Mental Health: involuntary mental patient cannot give informed consent to experimental psychosurgery. Rev Law Soc Change 4(2):207–227, 1974 11664643

Grisso T, Appelbaum PS: Assessing Competence to Consent to Treatment: A Guide for Physicians and Other Health Professionals. New York, Oxford University Press, 1998

King JS, Moulton BW: Rethinking informed consent: the case for shared medical decision-making. Am J Law Med 32(4):429–501, 2006 17240730

Localio AR, Lawthers AG, Brennan TA, et al: Relation between malpractice claims and adverse events due to negligence: results of the Harvard Medical Practice Study III. N Engl J Med 325(4):245–251, 1991 2057025

Mallary SD, Gert B, Culver CM: Family coercion and valid consent. Theor Med 7(2):123–126, 1986 3738841

McHugh MC, Frieze IH: Intimate partner violence: new directions. Ann NY Acad Sci 1087:121–141, 2006 17189502

Milosavljevic N, Green A, Brendel RW: Abuse and neglect, in Massachusetts General Hospital Psychiatry Update and Board Preparation, 3rd Edition. Edited by Stern TA, Herman JB, Gorrindo T. Boston, MA, MGH Psychiatry Academy Publishing, 2012, pp 543–545

Milosavljevic N, Taylor JB, Brendel RW: Psychiatric correlates and consequences of abuse and neglect, in Comprehensive Clinical Psychiatry, 2nd Edition. Edited by Stern TA, Rosenbaum JF, Fava M, et al. New York, Elsevier, 2016, pp 904–911

Moser DJ, Arndt S, Kanz JE, et al: Coercion and informed consent in research involving prisoners. Compr Psychiatry 45(1):1–9, 2004 14671730

Nair S, Morrison MF: The evaluation of maternal competency. Psychosomatics 41(6):523–530, 2000 11110117

National Commission for the Protection of Human Subjects of Biomedical and Behavioral Research: Report and Recommendations: Research Involving Prisoners. Washington, DC, U.S. Government Printing Office, 1976

National Commission for the Protection of Human Subjects of Biomedical and Behavioral Research: Research Involving Those Institutionalized as Mentally Infirm: Report and Recommendations. Washington, DC, U.S. Government Printing Office, 1978

Roberts LW: Informed consent and the capacity for voluntarism. Am J Psychiatry 159(5):705–712, 2002 11986120

Salgo v Leland Stanford Jr. University Board of Trustees, 154 Cal App 2d 560, 317 P2d 170 (1957)

Schloendorff v Society of New York Hospital, 105 NE 92 (NY 1914)

Schouten R, Brendel RW: Legal aspects of consultation, in The Massachusetts General Hospital Handbook of General Hospital Psychiatry, 5th Edition. Edited by Stern TA, Fricchione GL, Cassem EH, et al. Philadelphia, PA, CV Mosby, 2004, pp 349–364

Schouten R, Brendel RW, Edersheim JG: Malpractice and boundary violations, in Massachusetts General Hospital Comprehensive Clinical Psychiatry. Edited by Stern TA, Rosenbaum JF, Fava M, et al. Philadelphia, PA, Mosby/Elsevier, 2008, pp 1165–1175

Shine v Vega, 429 Mass 456, 709 NE2d 58 (Mass 1999)

Tarasoff v Board of Regents of the University of California, 17 Cal3d 425 (1976)

CHAPTER 3

Psychological Responses to Illness

3.1 What variable best accounts for interindividual differences in psychological responses to the stress of illness?

A. Illness severity.
B. Subjective experience of illness.
C. Illness chronicity.
D. Organ system involvement.

The correct response is option B: Subjective experience of illness.

Clinical experience and research indicate that illness variables such as severity (option A is incorrect), chronicity (option C is incorrect), or organ system involvement (option D is incorrect) cannot predict an individual's response to any given medical illness. It is in the realm of the individual's subjective experience of an illness that one can begin to understand his or her emotional and behavioral responses (Lipowski 1970) (option B is correct). **Chapter 3 (pp. 53–54)**

3.2 Coping is a powerful mediator of how a patient responds emotionally to a given stressor. Research by Folkman and others has demonstrated that patients tend to choose which category of coping style when the condition is appraised as out of their control?

A. Emotion focused.
B. Repression.
C. Problem focused.
D. Denial.

The correct response is option A: Emotion focused.

Research has shown that patients will tend to choose problem-focused coping strategies when they appraise the situation as being changeable or within their control (Folkman et al. 1993; Richardson et al. 2017) (option C is incorrect). In conditions considered out of their control, patients may choose emotion-focused coping styles (Folkman et al. 1993; Richardson et al. 2017) (option A is correct). Repression and denial are *defense mechanisms* (automatic psychological processes by which the mind confronts a psychological threat or conflict between a wish and the demands of reality or the dictates of conscience), not coping styles (options B and D are incorrect). Although there is some overlap of the concept of coping with that of defenses, the psychological concept of coping is more behavioral; it involves action and is generally a conscious experience. Defenses are usually conceptualized as intrapsychic processes that are largely out of the individual's awareness. **Chapter 3 (pp. 63–66)**

3.3   A middle-aged executive is threatening to sign out against medical advice after long delays in transportation to radiology for a study. A psychiatrist is consulted to assess capacity and arrives at the nursing station to hear nurses angrily complaining, "Who does she think she is?" Upon entering the room to greet the patient, the consultant spends some time inquiring about the patient's profession and achievements. The consultant says to the patient, "We aim to give you the best care and aspire to run things as efficiently as it sounds like you are able to in your business; unfortunately, emergencies frequently derail our ability to meet our ideal—please be patient with us." A dramatic de-escalation in complaints occurs, and the patient agrees to stay. What predominant personality style best describes this patient?

A. Histrionic.
B. Obsessional.
C. Masochistic.
D. Narcissistic.

The correct response is option D: Narcissistic.

Arrogant, devaluing, and demanding are common descriptors of individuals with a predominant narcissistic personality style (Table 3–1). Threats to self-concept of perfection and invulnerability inevitable in the setting of medical illness and hospitalization are likely to particularly evoke feelings of shame in individuals with a predominant narcissistic personality style. Tips on management include reframing entitlement to foster treatment adherence, taking a humble stance, and providing opportunities for the patient to show off (option D is correct). Histrionic individuals are often entertaining, melodramatic, and seductive (option A is incorrect). Those with obsessional personality styles are meticulous and orderly, they like to feel in control, and they are very concerned with right/wrong (option B is incorrect). Masochistic personality styles are typically characterized by behaving as if they are the perpetual victim; they see themselves as self-sacrificing martyrs (option C is incorrect). **Chapter 3 (Table 3–1, pp. 60–61)**

TABLE 3–1. Personality types

Type	Characteristics	Meaning of illness	Countertransference responses	Tips on management
Dependent	Needy, demanding, clingy Unable to reassure self Seeks reassurance from others	Threat of abandonment	Positive: doctor feels powerful and needed Negative: doctor feels overwhelmed and annoyed; may try to avoid patient	Reassure within limits Schedule visits Mobilize other supports Reward efforts toward independence Avoid tendency to withdraw from patient
Obsessional	Meticulous, orderly Likes to feel in control Very concerned with right/wrong	Loss of control over body/emotions/impulses	May admire When extreme: anger—a "battle of wills"	Try to set routine Give patient choices to increase sense of control Provide detailed information and "homework" Foster collaborative approach/avoid "battle of wills"
Histrionic	Entertaining Melodramatic Seductive, flirtatious	Loss of love or loss of attractiveness	Anxiety, impatience, off-putting Erotic, finds patient attractive	Strike a balance between warmth and formality Maintain clear boundaries Encourage patient to discuss fears Do not confront head-on
Masochistic	"Perpetual victim" Self-sacrificing martyr	Ego-syntonic Conscious or unconscious punishment	Anger, hate, frustration Helplessness, self-doubt	Avoid excessive encouragement Share patient's pessimism Deemphasize connection between symptoms and frequent visits Suggest that patient consider treatment as another burden to endure, or emphasize treatment's positive effect on loved ones

TABLE 3–1. Personality types *(continued)*

Type	Characteristics	Meaning of illness	Countertransference responses	Tips on management
Paranoid	Guarded, distrustful Quick to blame or counterattack Sensitive to slights	Proof that world is against patient Medical care is invasive and exploitative	Anger, feeling attacked or accused May become defensive	Avoid defensive stance Acknowledge patient's feelings without disputing them Maintain interpersonal distance; avoid excessive warmth Do not confront irrational fears
Narcissistic	Arrogant, devaluing Vain, demanding	Threat to self-concept of perfection and invulnerability Shame evoking	Anger, desire to counterattack Activation of feelings of inferiority, or enjoyment of feeling of status of working with an important patient	Resist the desire to challenge patient's entitlement Reframe entitlement to foster treatment adherence Take a humble stance, provide opportunities for patient to show off, offer consultations if appropriate
Schizoid	Aloof, remote Socially awkward Inhibited	Fear of intrusion	Little connection to patient Difficult to engage	Respect patient's privacy Prevent patient from completely withdrawing Maintain gentle, quiet interest in patient Encourage routine and regularity

Source. Derived in large part from Geringer and Stone 1986; Kahana and Bibring 1964; Perry and Viederman 1981.

3.4   Which attachment style is associated with consciously or unconsciously exaggerated illness behavior and high medical services use?

A. Fearful attachment style.
B. Secure attachment style.
C. Preoccupied attachment style.
D. Dismissing attachment style.

The correct response is option C: Preoccupied attachment style.

Attachment theory is a productive way of examining patients' interactions with the health care setting and their physicians. Inconsistently responsive caregiving is proposed as the environmental antecedent to a preoccupied attachment style, characterized by increased effort on the part of the individual to elicit caregiving and a positive expectation of others, with a negative view of self. These individuals may be particularly vulnerable to consciously or unconsciously exaggerated illness behavior and high medical services use (Ciechanowski et al. 2002) (option C is correct). Hostile, rejecting, or abusive caregiving early in life is thought to result in a fearful attachment style, characterized by negative views of self and others and a desire for support with simultaneous fears of rejection and difficulty trusting others. These individuals often alternate between help-seeking and help-rejecting behaviors and frequently demand care but are often nonadherent and miss appointments (option A is incorrect). The dismissing attachment style is thought to derive from early experiences with consistently unresponsive caregivers. As an adaptation to such an environment, these individuals come to dismiss their need for others, value extreme self-reliance, and have difficulty trusting others. Individuals with dismissing attachment styles are therefore averse to reaching out to others (Fonagy et al. 1996) (option D is incorrect). The individual with a secure attachment style is hypothesized to have experienced consistently responsive caregiving in early life and therefore has positive expectations and is comfortable depending on others for care (Ciechanowski et al. 2002) (option B is incorrect). **Chapter 3 (p. 58)**

3.5   A 35-year-old woman is admitted to the hospital with orthopedic injuries sustained in a motor vehicle accident. She is found to have a growing breast mass that she has been hiding under loose clothing for many months; she is terrified that she might have cancer. A psychiatric review of systems fails to find any psychotic symptoms or any clinically significant evidence of depression. The primary medical team describes her as being in "psychotic denial." What is the best approach for the consulting psychiatrist to take in addressing her denial of cancer?

A. Direct confrontation of the denial.
B. Exploration of the underlying emotions provoking the denial.
C. Prescription of an antipsychotic medication.
D. Immediate referral to oncology.

The correct response is option B: Exploration of the underlying emotions provoking the denial.

Direct confrontation of denial generally should be avoided because it is counterproductive (Ness and Ende 1994; Perry and Viederman 1981) (option A is incorrect). When denial is present and assessed as maladaptive, interventions usually should be directed toward the underlying emotions provoking the denial (e.g., fear) (option B is correct). Immediate referral to oncology is likely to increase the underlying emotions if exploration of underlying emotions is not done first (option D is incorrect). Most patients with pervasive denial of illness are not psychotic (option C is incorrect). Psychotic denial occurs in chronic mental illness like schizophrenia. Such patients may pay no attention to signs or symptoms of illness or may incorporate them into somatic delusions. Psychotic patients who deny illness usually do not conceal its signs. In contrast, nonpsychotic patients with pervasive denial often conceal signs of their illness from themselves and others. Diminishing the intensity of negative affects such as anxiety through psychopharmacological or psychotherapeutic interventions can be helpful. **Chapter 3 (pp. 66–69)**

3.6   Vaillant and others have conceptualized a hierarchy of defense mechanisms ranked in four levels of adaptivity. Defense mechanisms on which hierarchical level tend to be irritating to others, transmitting "shame, impulses, and anxiety to those around them"?

A. Psychotic defenses.
B. Mature defenses.
C. Neurotic defenses.
D. Immature defenses.

The correct response is option D: Immature defenses.

Vaillant (1993) proposed a hierarchy of defense mechanisms ranked in four levels of adaptivity: psychotic, immature (or borderline), neurotic, and mature. The *immature defenses* are characteristic of patients with personality disorders, especially antisocial, borderline, histrionic, and narcissistic personality disorders. Vaillant (1993) emphasized how many of these defense mechanisms are irritating to others and get under other people's skin. "Those afflicted with immature defenses often transmit their shame, impulses, and anxiety to those around them" (Vaillant 1993, p. 58) (option D is correct). *Psychotic defenses* are characterized by the extreme degree to which they distort external reality. Patients in psychotic states usually employ these defenses (option A is incorrect). The use of *mature defenses* such as humor or altruism in the confrontation of a stressor such as medical illness often earns admiration from others and can be inspirational. These defenses maximize expression of drives or wishes without negative consequences or distortion of reality (option B is incorrect). *Neurotic defenses* do not typically irritate others and are more privately experienced—they are less interpersonal and often involve mental inhibitions. They distort reality less than do immature or psychotic defenses and may go unnoticed by the observer (option C is incorrect). **Chapter 3 (p. 64)**

3.7　Which attachment style is predictive of worse diabetes self-care, lower adherence to hypoglycemic agents, and higher blood glucose levels in studies of diabetic patients by Ciechanowski and colleagues?

A. Preoccupied attachment style.
B. All insecure attachment styles (fearful, preoccupied, and dismissing).
C. Fearful and dismissing attachment styles.
D. Preoccupied and fearful attachment styles.

The correct response is option C: Fearful and dismissing attachment styles.

Ciechanowski and colleagues found that dismissive and fearful attachment styles are associated with worse diabetes self-care, lower adherence to hypoglycemic agents, and higher blood glucose levels. They describe the difficulty such patients have in trusting and depending on others, which affects their interactions with physicians (Ciechanowski and Katon 2006; Ciechanowski et al. 2001) (option C is correct). The preoccupied attachment style, characterized by increased effort on the part of the individual to elicit caregiving and a positive expectation of others, was not predictive of worse diabetes care in these studies (Ciechanowski et al. 2002) (options A, B, and D are incorrect). **Chapter 3 (pp. 58–59)**

3.8　A consulting psychiatrist realizes that she dreads seeing a patient on the oncology service and has been finding excuses to see all of the other patients on her caseload first. Calls from the patient to the consultation-liaison service have begun to escalate over the past week. In noticing her countertransference response and the patient's behavior, what predominant personality style is the patient likely to have?

A. Obsessional.
B. Paranoid.
C. Dependent.
D. Narcissistic.

The correct response is option C: Dependent.

A patient with a predominant dependent personality style is characterized as needy, demanding, clingy, and seeking reassurance from others. The threat of abandonment is a key meaning of illness to individuals with this style. Commonly, physicians working with patients with dependent personality styles will have countertransference responses of feeling overwhelmed and annoyed and may try to avoid the patient, which only can escalate the threat to the patient (option C is correct). Tips on management include regularly scheduling visits, mobilizing other supports, and avoiding the tendency to withdraw from the patient. Patients with predominant obsessional, paranoid, and narcissistic personality styles typically evoke different countertransference responses and exhibit different behaviors in the health care setting as outlined in Table 3–1 (options A, B, and D are incorrect). **Chapter 3 (pp. 59–61)**

3.9   Adjusting to a recent diagnosis of metastatic pancreatic cancer and given a prognosis of less than 6 months to live, a patient plans to take a month vacation with family prior to medical follow-up. He tells his physician, "There is no value in my getting consumed every day in thinking about my illness if I can't do anything about it." What defense mechanism is this patient employing?

A. Repression.
B. Suppression.
C. Rationalization.
D. Denial.

The correct response is option B: Suppression.

Suppression, a mature defense, is characterized by consciously putting a disturbing experience out of mind (option B is correct). In contrast, *repression* is involuntary forgetting of a painful feeling or experience (option A is incorrect). The patient in this example is not denying the seriousness of illness (option D is incorrect) nor involuntarily forgetting the situation. Patients who use the mature defense of suppression in confronting an illness are not truly in denial. *Rationalization* is a neurotic defense characterized as inventing a convincing, but usually false, reason why one is not bothered (option C is incorrect). **Chapter 3 (pp. 64–66; Table 3–2)**

TABLE 3–2. Defense mechanisms

Mature defenses

Suppression	Consciously putting a disturbing experience out of mind
Altruism	Vicarious but instinctively gratifying service to others
Humor	Overt expression of normally unacceptable feelings without unpleasant effect
Sublimation	Attenuated expression of drives in alternative fields without adverse consequences
Anticipation	Realistic planning for inevitable discomfort

Neurotic defenses

Repression	Involuntary forgetting of a painful feeling or experience
Control	Manipulation of external events to avoid unconscious anxiety
Displacement	Transfer of an experienced feeling from one person to another or to something else
Reaction formation	Expression of unacceptable impulses as directly opposite attitudes and behaviors
Intellectualization	Replacing of feelings with facts/details
Rationalization	Inventing a convincing, but usually false, reason why one is not bothered
Isolation of affect	Separating a painful idea or event from feelings associated with it
Undoing	Ritualistic "removal" of an offensive act, sometimes by atoning for it

Immature defenses

Splitting	Experiencing oneself and others as all good or all bad
Idealization	Seeing oneself or others as all-powerful, ideal, or godlike
Devaluation	Depreciating others
Projection	Attributing unacceptable impulses or ideas to others
Projective identification	Causing others to experience one's unacceptable feelings; one then fears or tries to control the unacceptable behavior in the other person
Acting out	Direct expression of an unconscious wish or impulse to avoid being conscious of the affect, and thoughts that accompany it
Passive aggression	Expressing anger indirectly and passively
Intermediate: denial	Refusal to acknowledge painful realities

Psychotic defenses

Psychotic denial	Obliteration of external reality
Delusional projection	Externalization of inner conflicts and giving them tangible reality—minimal reality testing
Schizoid fantasy	Withdrawal from conflict into social isolation and fantasizing

Source.   Carlat 1999; Muskin and Haase 2001; Vaillant 1993.

3.10   The psychiatry consult service is called to assess the capacity to sign out against medical advice of a 34-year-old man who was admitted for treatment of a post-surgical infection requiring intravenous antibiotics and wound care. Nurses describe the patient as demanding and hostile, frequently calling them, and demanding to speak to the attending about discharge planning. What is the first intervention the psychiatrist should do in assessing capacity to sign out against medical advice?

A. Clarify that the patient really wants to leave the hospital.
B. Sit down and empathically listen to the patient's frustrations.
C. Assess his understanding about his medical condition.
D. Conduct a brief cognitive examination to assess orientation among other domains.

The correct response is option B: Sit down and empathically listen to the patient's frustrations.

The patient's threat to sign out is usually not truly motivated by a primary desire to leave, but it more often reflects another agenda, intense emotion, or interpersonal friction with physicians or nursing staff (Albert and Kornfeld 1973) (option A is incorrect). In a classic study of patients threatening to sign out against medical advice, the most common underlying motivations were overwhelming fear, anger, and psychosis or confusion (Albert and Kornfeld 1973). In most cases, there had been a progressive increase in the patient's distress that had not been recognized or addressed adequately for days before the threat to sign out (Albert and Kornfeld 1973). Among interventions, empathic listening to the patient's frustrations is critical; it provides an opportunity for the patient to ventilate frustrations and to feel understood. Empathic listening will often have a dramatic de-escalating effect, enabling the team to re-engage the patient in treatment (option B is correct). The 30-day readmission rate and overall mortality of patients who sign out against medical advice is higher compared with conventionally discharged patients (Alfandre 2013). Immediate questioning about the patient's understanding of his medical condition or first conducting a cognitive examination are less likely to build rapport and may be made unnecessary were the consultant to first sit down and empathically listen to the patient's frustrations before assessing capacity (options C and D are incorrect). **Chapter 3 (pp. 76–77)**

References

Albert HD, Kornfeld DS: The threat to sign out against medical advice. Ann Intern Med 79(6):888–891, 1973 4761912
Alfandre D: Reconsidering against medical advice discharges: embracing patient-centeredness to promote high quality care and a renewed research agenda. J Gen Intern Med 28(12):1657–1662, 2013 23818160
Carlat DJ: The Psychiatric Interview: A Practical Guide. Philadelphia, PA, Lippincott Williams & Wilkins, 1999

Ciechanowski P, Katon WJ: The interpersonal experience of health care through the eyes of patients with diabetes. Soc Sci Med 63(12):3067–3079, 2006 16997440

Ciechanowski PS, Katon WJ, Russo JE, Walker EA: The patient-provider relationship: attachment theory and adherence to treatment in diabetes. Am J Psychiatry 158(1):29–35, 2001 11136630

Ciechanowski PS, Walker EA, Katon WJ, Russo JE: Attachment theory: a model for health care utilization and somatization. Psychosom Med 64(4):660–667, 2002 12140356

Folkman S, Chesney M, Pollack L, Coates T: Stress, control, coping, and depressive mood in human immunodeficiency virus-positive and -negative gay men in San Francisco. J Nerv Ment Dis 181(7):409–416, 1993 8320542

Fonagy P, Leigh T, Steele M, et al: The relation of attachment status, psychiatric classification, and response to psychotherapy. J Consult Clin Psychol 64(1):22–31, 1996 8907081

Geringer ES, Stone TA: Coping with medical illness: the impact of personality types. Psychosomatics 27(4):251–261, 1986 3704101

Kahana RJ, Bibring G: Personality types in medical management, in Psychiatry and Medical Practice in a General Hospital. Edited by Zinberg NE. New York, International Universities Press, 1964, pp 108–123

Lipowski ZJ: Physical illness, the individual and the coping processes. Psychiatry Med 1(2):91–102, 1970 4257952

Muskin PR, Haase EK: Difficult patients and patients with personality disorders, in Textbook of Primary Care Medicine, 3rd Edition (Noble J, Editor in Chief). St Louis, MO, CV Mosby, 2001, pp 458–464

Ness DE, Ende J: Denial in the medical interview. Recognition and management. JAMA 272(22):1777–1781, 1994 7966927

Perry S, Viederman M: Management of emotional reactions to acute medical illness. Med Clin North Am 65(1):3–14, 1981 7206897

Richardson EM, Schüz N, Sanderson K, et al: Illness representations, coping, and illness outcomes in people with cancer: a systematic review and meta-analysis. Psychooncology 26(6):724–737, 2017 27412423

Vaillant GE: The Wisdom of the Ego. Cambridge, MA, Harvard University Press, 1993

CHAPTER 4

Delirium

4.1   What is the *primary* cognitive disturbance in delirium?

A. Attention.
B. Short-term memory.
C. Orientation.
D. Visuospatial processing.

The correct response is option A: Attention.

The primary cognitive disturbance in delirium is in the ability to focus, sustain, and shift attention, as evidenced by difficulty in orienting to salient stimuli, poor concentration, reduced vigilance, distractibility, and impaired awareness of the immediate environment (option A is correct). Attentional abilities are disproportionately affected, but typically there are disturbances in other cognitive abilities, including orientation (option C is incorrect), visuospatial processing (option D is incorrect), executive function, and short-term memory (option B is incorrect), which can usually be demonstrated with simple bedside tests. **Chapter 4 (p. 87)**

4.2   When do symptoms of a hospitalization-related delirium typically resolve in elderly patients?

A. Before discharge in about 80% of cases.
B. By 1 month postdischarge in about 90% of cases.
C. By 3 months postdischarge in about 90% of cases.
D. By 6 months postdischarge in about 80% of cases.

The correct response is option D: By 6 months postdischarge in about 80% of cases.

DSM-5 (American Psychiatric Association 2013) notes that in hospital settings, delirium usually lasts about 1 week, but it may sometimes persist for longer periods of time and may even still be evident at the time the patient is discharged from the hospital to home or to long-term care. A subtype of chronic delirium is now recognized in DSM-5. However, persistent delirium is not rare. Especially in elderly

149

individuals and those with dementia, delirium may develop gradually and follow a chronic course. In a systematic review by Cole et al. (2009), delirious symptoms persisted in 45% of elderly hospitalized patients at discharge (option A is incorrect), and symptoms were still present in 33% of elderly patients after 1 month (option B is incorrect), in 26% after 3 months (option C is incorrect), and in 21% after 6 months (option D is correct). **Chapter 4 (p. 88)**

4.3   What physiological disturbance is associated with delirium in addition to reduced cholinergic activity?

A. Reduced dopaminergic activity.
B. Excess dopaminergic activity.
C. Decreased cytokine levels.
D. Low glucocorticoid levels.

The correct response is option B: Excess dopaminergic activity.

The delirious state is characterized by elevated cortisol levels; exogenous glucocorticoids are also known to precipitate delirium. Higher and more sustained elevations of cortisol occur in older patients when they are confronted with acute stressors such as infection. Elevated glucocorticoids are thought to be linked to delirium through their interactions with monoaminergic neurotransmission, whereas the longer-term disturbances that are noted in many patients experiencing delirium may reflect the neurotoxic effects of sustained activation of the stress axis, which can cause or accelerate neurodegeneration (Maclullich et al. 2008) (option D is incorrect). Altered central nervous system immunoreactivity is also thought to be linked to delirium pathogenesis, whereby the combination of high levels or persistence of proinflammatory cytokines and reduced cerebral reserve is associated with delirium proneness (Androsova et al. 2015) (option C is incorrect). Corroboration of this hypothesis is provided by the finding that delirium in children and older adults commonly occurs in response to relatively minor precipitating illnesses. Delirium often occurs in infectious states in which elevated cytokines are present, and therapeutic use of cytokines can also cause delirium. A further hypothesis is that cytokines exert their effects indirectly through activation of the hypothalamic-pituitary-adrenal axis, resulting in the release of glucocorticoids, occupation of the low-affinity glucocorticoid receptor, and downregulation of inflammatory responses (Maclullich et al. 2008). From a neurochemical perspective, the principal disturbances that are linked to delirium involve reduced cholinergic function and an absolute or relative excess of dopaminergic activity (option A is incorrect; option B is correct). Intoxication with dopaminergic drugs can cause delirium; elevated levels of plasma homovanillic acid (a dopaminergic metabolite) have been found during the delirious state (Ramirez-Bermudez et al. 2008). Dopamine-blocking antipsychotics are the most commonly used pharmacological intervention for delirium (Meagher et al. 2013). Similarly, in terms of cholinergic function, medications with anticholinergic effects are among the most common drug-related causes of delirium (Clegg and Young 2011), whereas delirium can sometimes be reversed by treatment with physostigmine (Dawson and Buckley 2016). Cholinergic function is reduced in states of hypoxia and hypoglycemia, which are recognized causes of delirium. Age-associated reductions in cholinergic function may underpin the increased delirium incidence with advanced age; dementia is characterized by reduced brain cholinergic activity. Dopaminergic and cholinergic mechanisms also interact, whereby D_2 receptor activation can inhibit cholinergic activity. There is also evidence for involvement of a variety of other neurochemical systems (e.g., γ-aminobutyric acid [GABA]ergic, glutamatergic, adrenergic) in delirium (Egberts et al. 2015; Fitzgerald et al. 2013), such that simple explanations are unlikely to provide a comprehensive account of the neurochemical mechanisms that underpin delirium. **Chapter 4 (pp. 100, 102)**

4.4   Which strategy was found to reduce the incidence of delirium in elderly medical patients?

    A. Only pharmacological risk-reduction strategies have been shown to work.
    B. Simple interventions (e.g., consensus guidelines, educational approaches) have the greatest impact.
    C. Special medical and nursing interventions.
    D. Sleep promotion.

The correct response is option D: Sleep promotion.

Primary prevention of delirium using nonpharmacological risk-reduction strategies has been demonstrated in elderly medical and surgical populations (Siddiqi et al. 2016) (option A is incorrect). Moreover, when delirium occurs despite these efforts, it tends to be less severe and of shorter duration. Because a complex range of factors are involved in delirium causation, simple interventions (e.g., consensus guidelines, educational approaches) have limited impact compared with multifaceted interventions (option B is incorrect). A recent meta-analysis of 14 studies of multicomponent nonpharmacological interventions found that these strategies reduced delirium incidence by 44%, with significant reductions in falls and with a trend toward decreased lengths of hospital stay and reduced need for institutionalization (Hshieh et al. 2015). These interventions typically include efforts to assist in orientation, enhance sensory efficacy (e.g., encouraging patient to use their glasses or hearing aids), promote sleep (option D is correct), minimize pain, optimize physiological parameters (e.g., electrolytes, hydration), and foster physical therapy/mobilization. Many of these components are elements that should ideally be addressed as part of standard medical and nursing care; however, given the many competing pressures in modern health care, protocolization of these elements can enhance the quality of routine care provided in real-world settings (option C is incorrect). **Chapter 4 (p. 105)**

4.5 Studies on pharmacological prophylaxis for delirium support which statement?

A. Cholinesterase inhibitors prevent delirium.
B. Antipsychotic use in intensive care unit (ICU) patients prevents delirium.
C. Evidence so far does not support routine pharmacological prophylaxis of delirium.
D. Antipsychotic use had a positive impact on hospital length of stay and mortality.

The correct response is option C: Evidence so far does not support routine pharmacological prophylaxis of delirium.

A series of studies have explored the impact of antipsychotic/antidopaminergic and procholinergic agents in prevention of delirium in high-risk populations. Some prospective work indicates that prophylactic use of low-dose typical or atypical antipsychotics may reduce delirium incidence, may reduce transition from subsyndromal delirium to full delirium, and/or may result in significantly shorter and less severe episodes when delirium does occur (Fok et al. 2015). However, the National Institute for Health and Care Excellence clinical guideline concluded that evidence for pharmacological prevention was lacking (National Institute for Health and Care Excellence 2010). A recent review (Inouye et al. 2014) likewise concluded that evidence for a positive impact of antipsychotic treatment on longer-term outcomes, such as duration of hospital stay and mortality rate, was lacking (option D is incorrect). Moreover, recent studies of prophylactic use of antipsychotics in ICU patients have not demonstrated a preventive effect on delirium (Al-Qadheeb et al. 2016; Page et al. 2013) (option B is incorrect). Studies of cholinesterase inhibitors in delirium prevention trials also have not demonstrated benefit (option A is incorrect). Preliminary evidence supports the use of the α_2-adrenergic agonist dexmedetomidine as a less deliriogenic means of sedation, as well as the use of melatonin in elderly inpatients with medical illness; both strategies have been linked with reduced delirium incidence (Djaiani et al. 2016). Careful management of analgesia and/or sedation using protocolized care can also reduce delirium incidence (Dale et al. 2014; Skrobik et al. 2010). Overall, the potential of pharmacological prophylaxis is appealing, but evidence to date does not yet support routine use because of uncertainties in usefulness across patient populations, including high-risk elderly medical inpatients and patients with comorbid dementia (option C is correct). **Chapter 4 (pp. 105–106)**

4.6 What is the additional cost of delirium to a hospital stay?

A. An extra $5,000 to ICU costs per delirious patient.
B. An extra $5,000 to total hospital cost per delirious patient.
C. Approximately an extra $150 billion per year in the United States.
D. A 25% increase in cost of pediatric ICU stays per delirious patient.

The correct response is option C: An extra $150 billion per year in the United States.

Delirium is responsible for increased health care costs. Milbrandt et al. (2004) compared ICU costs incurred by 183 mechanically ventilated medical ICU patients with at least one delirium episode against costs incurred by nondelirious control patients. The median ICU costs for delirious patients were significantly higher than those for nondelirious patients: $22,346 versus $13,332, respectively (option A is incorrect). Total hospital costs were also higher for delirious patients than for nondelirious patients: $41,836 versus $27,106, respectively (option B is incorrect). Inouye (1999) calculated the total direct 1-year health care costs in the United States attributable to delirium as somewhere between $143 billion and $152 billion (option C is correct). Implementing a multicomponent delirium prevention program can substantially reduce health care costs. The Hospital Elder Life Program saved an average of $831 per patient in annual acute hospital costs and $9,446 per patient in long-term nursing home costs (Leslie et al. 2005; Rizzo et al. 2001). In a study of children admitted to a pediatric ICU (PICU), delirium was associated with an 85% increase in PICU costs after controlling for patient age, gender, severity of illness, and PICU length of stay (Traube et al. 2016) (option D is incorrect). (Delirium in children is discussed in detail in Chapter 32, "Pediatrics.") Implementation of adequate care for hospitalized patients with delirium may lead to better outcomes for these patients as well as large cost savings. For these reasons, it has been advocated that delirium care be considered an indicator of hospital care quality (Schofield 2008; Young et al. 2008). **Chapter 4 (p. 86)**

References

Al-Qadheeb NS, Skrobik Y, Schumaker G, et al: Preventing ICU subsyndromal delirium conversion to delirium with low-dose IV haloperidol: a double-blind, placebo-controlled pilot study. Crit Care Med 44(3):583–591, 2016 26540397

American Psychiatric Association: Diagnostic and Statistical Manual of Mental Disorders, 5th Edition. Arlington, VA, American Psychiatric Association, 2013

Androsova G, Krause R, Winterer G, Schneider R: Biomarkers of postoperative delirium and cognitive dysfunction. Front Aging Neurosci 7:112, 2015 26106326

Clegg A, Young JB: Which medications to avoid in people at risk of delirium: a systematic review. Age Ageing 40(1):23–29, 2011 21068014

Cole MG, Ciampi A, Belzile E, Zhong L: Persistent delirium in older hospital patients: a systematic review of frequency and prognosis. Age Ageing 38(1):19–26, 2009 19017678

Dale CR, Kannas DA, Fan VS, et al: Improved analgesia, sedation, and delirium protocol associated with decreased duration of delirium and mechanical ventilation. Ann Am Thorac Soc 11(3):367–374, 2014 24597599

Dawson AH, Buckley NA: Pharmacological management of anticholinergic delirium - theory, evidence and practice. Br J Clin Pharmacol 81(3):516–524, 2016 26589572

Djaiani G, Silverton N, Fedorko L, et al: Dexmedetomidine versus propofol sedation reduces delirium after cardiac surgery: a randomized controlled trial. Anesthesiology 124(2):362–368, 2016 26575144

Egberts A, Fekkes D, Wijnbeld EH, et al: Disturbed serotonergic neurotransmission and oxidative stress in elderly patients with delirium. Dement Geriatr Cogn Disord Extra 5(3):450–458, 2015 26955379

Fitzgerald JM, Adamis D, Trzepacz PT, et al: Delirium: a disturbance of circadian integrity? Med Hypotheses 81(4):568–576, 2013 23916192

Fok MC, Sepehry AA, Frisch L, et al: Do antipsychotics prevent postoperative delirium? A systematic review and meta-analysis. Int J Geriatr Psychiatry 30(4):333–344, 2015 25639958

Hshieh TT, Yue J, Oh E, et al: Effectiveness of multicomponent nonpharmacological delirium interventions: a meta-analysis. JAMA Intern Med 175(4):512–520, 2015 25643002

Inouye SK: Predisposing and precipitating factors for delirium in hospitalized older patients. Dement Geriatr Cogn Disord 10(5):393–400, 1999 10473946

Inouye SK, Marcantonio ER, Metzger ED: Doing damage in delirium: the hazards of antipsychotic treatment in elderly persons. Lancet Psychiatry 1(4):312–315, 2014 25285270

Leslie DL, Zhang Y, Bogardus ST, et al: Consequences of preventing delirium in hospitalized older adults on nursing home costs. J Am Geriatr Soc 53(3):405–409, 2005 15743281

Maclullich AM, Ferguson KJ, Miller T, et al: Unravelling the pathophysiology of delirium: a focus on the role of aberrant stress responses. J Psychosom Res 65(3):229–238, 2008 18707945

Meagher DJ, McLoughlin L, Leonard M, et al: What do we really know about the treatment of delirium with antipsychotics? Ten key issues for delirium pharmacotherapy. Am J Geriatr Psychiatry 21(12):1223–1238, 2013 23567421

Milbrandt EB, Deppen S, Harrison PL, et al: Costs associated with delirium in mechanically ventilated patients. Crit Care Med 32(4):955–962, 2004 15071384

National Institute for Health and Care Excellence: Delirium: Prevention, Diagnosis and Management. NICE Clinical Guideline 103. London, National Institute for Health and Care Excellence, 2010. Available at: https://www.nice.org.uk/guidance/cg103/evidence/fullguideline-pdf-134653069. Accessed November 10, 2017.

Page VJ, Ely EW, Gates S, et al: Effect of intravenous haloperidol on the duration of delirium and coma in critically ill patients (Hope-ICU): a randomised, double-blind, placebo-controlled trial. Lancet Respir Med 1(7):515–523, 2013 24461612

Ramirez-Bermudez J, Ruiz-Chow A, Perez-Neri I, et al: Cerebrospinal fluid homovanillic acid is correlated to psychotic features in neurological patients with delirium. Gen Hosp Psychiatry 30(4):337–343, 2008 18585537

Rizzo JA, Bogardus ST Jr, Leo-Summers L, et al: Multicomponent targeted intervention to prevent delirium in hospitalized older patients: what is the economic value? Med Care 39(7):740–752, 2001 11458138

Schofield I: Delirium: challenges for clinical governance. J Nurs Manag 16(2):127–133, 2008 18269542

Siddiqi N, Harrison JK, Clegg A, et al: Interventions for preventing delirium in hospitalised non-ICU patients. Cochrane Database Syst Rev (3):CD005563, 2016 26967259

Skrobik Y, Ahern S, Leblanc M, et al: Protocolized intensive care unit management of analgesia, sedation, and delirium improves analgesia and subsyndromal delirium rates. Anesth Analg 111(2):451–463, 2010 20375300

Traube C, Mauer EA, Gerber LM, et al: Cost associated with pediatric delirium in the ICU. Crit Care Med 44(12):e1175–e1179, 2016 27518377

Young J, Leentjens AFG, George J, et al: Systematic approaches to the prevention and management of patients with delirium. J Psychosom Res 65(3):267–272, 2008 18707950

CHAPTER 5

Dementia

5.1   Which of the following statements is true regarding the concept and epidemiology of dementia?

A. Most cases of mild cognitive impairment, including mild neurocognitive disorder, do not progress to dementia.
B. The prevalence and incidence rates of dementia remain constant as age increases.
C. The prevalence rate for all dementias in the U.S. population older than 65 years is 1%.
D. Vascular dementia is the most common neurodegenerative disorder.

The correct response is option A: Most cases of mild cognitive impairment, including mild neurocognitive disorder, do not progress to dementia.

Most cases of mild cognitive impairment, including mild neurocognitive disorder cases, do not progress to dementia, even after a follow-up period of 5 years (Marcos et al. 2016) (option A is correct). Both the prevalence and the incidence rates of dementia, and of dementia of the Alzheimer's type (DAT) in particular, increase dramatically with age, doubling approximately every 5 years (option B is incorrect). The adjusted prevalence has been estimated at 8.2% for all dementias in the U.S. population older than 65 years (Koller and Bynum 2015) (option C is incorrect). DAT is the most common neurodegenerative disorder, accounting for 43.5% of dementia cases (Goodman et al. 2017) (option D is incorrect). **Chapter 5 (pp. 122–123)**

5.2   Which of the following is a confirmed risk factor for dementia of the Alzheimer's type (DAT)?

A. Low education.
B. Hypertension.
C. Age.
D. Depression.

The correct response is option C: Age.

Low education level, hypertension, and depression are probable risk factors for DAT (Gottesman et al. 2017; Medina et al. 2017; Reitz and Mayeux 2014) (options A, B, and D are incorrect). Confirmed risk factors for DAT are scarce and are limited to age, unalterable genetic factors (the apolipoprotein E epsilon4 [APOE ε4] allele), and mild cognitive impairment (option C is correct). **Chapter 5 (pp. 124, 126; Table 5–3, p. 126)**

TABLE 5–1.   Risk factors in dementias

	Strength of association[a]
Risk factors for dementia of the Alzheimer's type	
Older age	++
Female sex	+
Low education	+
First-degree relative with Alzheimer's	+
Down syndrome	+
Head trauma	+
Apolipoprotein ε4 allele	++
High aluminum levels	+/−
Cigarette smoking	+
Hypertension	+
Hyperhomocysteinemia	+/−
Depression	+
Mild cognitive impairment	++
Social isolation	+
Risk factors for vascular dementia	
Age >60 years	+
Male sex	+
Previous stroke	++
Stroke risk factors	
Hypertension	++
Heart disease/atrial fibrillation	+
Cigarette smoking	++
Diabetes mellitus	++
Excessive alcohol consumption (>3 drinks/day)	+
Hyperlipidemia	+
Hyperhomocysteinemia, low serum folate levels	+
Previous mental decline	+/−

[a]Strength of association: ++=confirmed; +=probable; +/−=controversial.
Source.   Gottesman et al. 2017; Medina et al. 2017; Reitz and Mayeux 2014.

5.3   Which of the following is true regarding genes and the inheritance of Huntington's disease?

A. The amyloid precursor protein (APP) gene is a genetic locus for Huntington's
disease.
B. The mutation responsible for Huntington's disease is an elongated and unsta-
ble trinucleotide (CAG) repeat.
C. A mutation in the presenilin-2 gene is responsible for Huntington's disease.
D. Mutations in the tau gene are responsible for Huntington's disease.

**The correct response is option B: The mutation responsible for Huntington's
disease is an elongated and unstable trinucleotide (CAG) repeat.**

Genetic loci for familial DAT were documented in chromosomes 21 (the amyloid
precursor protein [APP] gene), 14 (the presenilin-1 gene), and 1 (the presenilin-2
gene) (Medina et al. 2017) (options A and C are incorrect). Huntington's disease
is inherited as an autosomal dominant trait with complete penetrance, the mutation responsible being an elongated and unstable trinucleotide (CAG) repeat on
the short arm of chromosome 4 (Haskins and Harrison 2000) (option B is correct).
Advances in the genetics of other dementias include identification of tau gene
mutations on chromosome 17 in some familial cases of frontotemporal dementia
(option D is incorrect). **Chapter 5 (p. 125)**

5.4   Which of the following is a clinical finding in patients with mild DAT?

A. Total disorientation.
B. Difficulties in planning, sequencing, and executing instrumental activities of
daily living.
C. Extreme impoverishment of language; communication impossible.
D. Double incontinence (urinary and fecal).

**The correct response is option B: Difficulties in planning, sequencing, and ex-
ecuting instrumental activities of daily living.**

Total disorientation; extreme impoverishment of language, communication impossible; and double incontinence (urinary and fecal) are clinical findings in patients with severe DAT (options A, C, and D are incorrect). Difficulties in planning,
sequencing, and executing instrumental activities of daily living are clinical findings in patients with mild DAT (option B is correct). **Chapter 5 (Table 5–4, p. 127)**

5.5   Which of the following is true regarding the behavioral and psychological symptoms of dementia (BPSDs)?

A. BPSDs are associated with slower disease progression.
B. The course of BPSDs parallels cognitive and functional deterioration in patients with DAT.

C. BPSDs are only observed after cognitive or functional decline is apparent.

D. BPSDs may include depression, hallucinations, disinhibition, wandering, and eating disturbances.

The correct response is option D: BPSDs may include depression, hallucinations, disinhibition, wandering, and eating disturbances.

BPSDs are associated with faster disease progression (Kales et al. 2015) (option A is incorrect). The course of BPSDs does not always parallel cognitive and functional deterioration in patients with DAT (option B is incorrect). BPSDs have been observed in the prodromal stage of dementia, before any cognitive or functional decline is apparent (Stella 2014) (option C is incorrect). BPSDs occur in clusters or syndromes identified as psychosis (delusions and hallucinations), agitation (e.g., arguing, pacing, crying out), aggression (physical or verbal); depression (or dysphoria); anxiety, apathy, disinhibition (socially and sexually inappropriate behaviors), motor disturbance (wandering, rummaging), nighttime behaviors (getting up at night), and appetite and eating disturbances (option D is correct). **Chapter 5 (p. 128)**

5.6   Which of the following is a clinical characteristic of cortical dementia?

A. Late appearance of primitive reflexes.

B. Early marked apathy.

C. Early, very marked extrapyramidal signs.

D. Frequent, severe affective syndromes.

The correct response is option A: Late appearance of primitive reflexes.

The appearance of primitive reflexes (e.g., grasp, snout, suck) is a clinical characteristic of cortical dementia syndromes late in the disease but is rare in subcortical dementia (option A is correct). Marked apathy is a clinical characteristic of subcortical dementia syndromes early in the disease (option B is incorrect). Very marked extrapyramidal signs are a clinical characteristic of subcortical dementia syndromes early in the disease (option C is incorrect). Frequent, severe affective syndromes are a clinical characteristic of subcortical dementia syndromes (option D is incorrect). **Chapter 5 (pp. 128–129; Table 5–5, p. 129)**

5.7   Early gait disturbance, subcortical dementia with severe apathetic features, and urinary incontinence are characteristic of which of the following dementia syndromes?

A. DAT.

B. Huntington's disease.

C. Normal-pressure hydrocephalus (NPH).

D. Wilson's disease.

The correct response is option C: Normal-pressure hydrocephalus (NPH).

Patients with DAT typically present with prominent impairment in memory and learning. Other characteristic clinical signs and symptoms include language difficulties, and agnosia for faces (option A is incorrect). Huntington's disease has the three main characteristics of the subcortical dementia syndrome (Folstein and McHugh 1983), together with the classic choreoathetoid movement disorder and a positive family history. Psychiatric symptoms are commonly present in the early stage of the disease, with depression the most frequent symptom (option B is incorrect). NPH is a very characteristic neuropsychiatric syndrome, presenting as a triad of clinical symptoms combining motoric and psychopathological features (Folstein and McHugh 1983; McHugh 1966): 1) an early gait disturbance resembling the stiff steps of spastic paraparesis, 2) subcortical dementia with particularly severe apathetic features, and 3) urinary incontinence that may not appear until late in the disease course (option C is correct). The onset of Wilson's disease is usually during adolescence or early adulthood and is heralded by dystonia, parkinsonism, or cerebellar ataxia. Cognitive impairment is relatively mild in the early stages; however, depression, irritability, disinhibition, personality changes, and poor impulse control are common, with severity paralleling the severity of the neurological signs (Shanmugiah et al. 2008) (option D is incorrect). **Chapter 5 (pp. 129–132)**

5.8   Which of the following is a strength of the Mini-Mental State Examination (MMSE)?

A. It can document degree of functional impairment.
B. It tests well for executive function deficits.
C. It is sensitive to mild cognitive impairment.
D. It fares very well in different cultures.

The correct response is option D: It fares very well in different cultures.

The MMSE is a useful instrument for screening purposes. A variety of assessments are available for documenting functional deficits, such as the classic instruments of Lawton and Brody (1969), the Katz Index (Katz et al. 1970), and the Functional Assessment Staging Test (FAST) (option A is incorrect). Executive functions are not well covered in the MMSE (option B is incorrect). The Modified Mini-Mental State (Teng and Chui 1987) and the Montreal Cognitive Assessment (MoCA; Nasreddine et al. 2005) are more sensitive to mild cognitive impairment (option C is incorrect). The MMSE fares very well in different cultures if the standardization has been adequate (Lobo et al. 1999) (option D is correct). **Chapter 5 (p. 139)**

5.9   Neuroimaging in the diagnosis of dementia is useful in which of the following situations?

A. To diagnose dementia in cases involving advanced symptoms and a long history of disease.
B. To rule out reversible conditions such as NPH, subdural hematoma, and brain tumors.

C. To identify general atrophy, which is diagnostic for DAT.

D. To demonstrate increased fluorodeoxyglucose uptake in the temporoparietal cortex on positron emission tomography (PET), which is a major biomarker of DAT.

The correct response is option B: To rule out reversible conditions such as NPH, subdural hematoma, and brain tumors.

Neuroimaging may be unnecessary in cases involving advanced symptoms and a long history of disease (option A is incorrect). Computed tomography and magnetic resonance imaging are very useful in ruling out reversible conditions such as NPH, subdural hematoma, and brain tumors (option B is correct). General atrophy may be found in elderly patients without dementia (option C is incorrect). Decreased fluorodeoxyglucose uptake on PET in the temporoparietal cortex and positive PET amyloid imaging have been accepted as major biomarkers of DAT (option D is incorrect). **Chapter 5 (pp. 142, 143)**

5.10   Which of the following is a suggested guideline for psychotropic medication use in patients with dementia?

A. Treat behavioral symptoms immediately with sedatives.

B. Add an anticholinergic agent if extrapyramidal symptoms occur.

C. Quickly up titrate dosages in order to achieve optimal symptoms control.

D. Reassess risks and benefits of psychotropic treatment on an ongoing basis.

The correct response is option D: Reassess risks and benefits of psychotropic treatment on an ongoing basis.

The physician should use strategies to minimize the total amount of medication required; mild symptoms or limited risk often may resolve with support, reassurance, and distraction (option A is incorrect). If extrapyramidal symptoms occur, reduce the dosage or switch to another drug rather than adding anticholinergic drugs (option B is incorrect). Physicians should use low initial dosages (one-quarter to one-third of usual initial dosage); dosage increments should be smaller and between-dose intervals longer. Seek the lowest effective dosage (option C is incorrect). Physicians should reassess risks and benefits of psychotropic treatment on an ongoing basis (option D is correct). **Chapter 5 (Table 5–10, p. 148)**

TABLE 5–2.   Suggested guidelines for psychotropic medication use

Consider whether agitation and/or behavioral disturbances might be caused by:

A medical condition, pain, other psychiatric condition, or sleep loss, which could resolve with treatment of the primary condition.

Hunger, constipation, stressful atmosphere, change in living conditions, or interpersonal difficulties.

Use strategies to minimize the total amount of medication required.

Instruct caregivers to appropriately administer sedatives when warranted.

Mild symptoms or limited risk often may resolve with support, reassurance, and distraction.

Remember that dementia patients are often physically frail and have decreased renal clearance and slowed hepatic metabolism.

Be specific in selecting target symptoms.

Use low initial dosages (one-quarter to one-third of usual initial dosage); dosage increments should be smaller and between-dose intervals longer. Seek the lowest effective dosage.

Avoid polypharmacy.

Keep especially alert to:

Medical conditions and drug interactions.

Frequent and worrying side effects (orthostatic hypotension and central nervous system sedation, which may worsen cognition and cause falls; susceptibility to extrapyramidal side effects).

Idiosyncratic drug effects (mental confusion; restlessness; increased sedation; vulnerability to anticholinergic effects of psychotropic medication).

If extrapyramidal effects occur, reduce the dosage or switch to another drug rather than adding anticholinergic drugs.

Reassess risks and benefits of psychotropic treatment on an ongoing basis.

References

Folstein MF, McHugh PR: The neuropsychiatry of some specific brain disorders, in Handbook of Psychiatry 2, Mental Disorders and Somatic Illness. Edited by Lader MH. London, Cambridge University Press, 1983, pp 107–118

Goodman RA, Lochner KA, Thambisetty M, et al: Prevalence of dementia subtypes in United States Medicare fee-for-service beneficiaries, 2011-2013. Alzheimers Dement 13(1):28–37, 2017 27172148

Gottesman RF, Albert MS, Alonso A, et al: Associations between midlife vascular risk factors and 25-year incident dementia in the Atherosclerosis Risk in Communities (ARIC) cohort. JAMA Neurol 74(10):1246–1254, 2017 28783817

Haskins BA, Harrison MB: Huntington's Disease. Curr Treat Options Neurol 2(3):243–262, 2000 11096752

Kales HC, Gitlin LN, Lyketsos CG: Assessment and management of behavioral and psychological symptoms of dementia. BMJ 350:h369, 2015 25731881

Katz S, Downs TD, Cash HR, Grotz RC: Progress in development of the index of ADL. Gerontologist 10(1):20–30, 1970 5420677

Koller D, Bynum JP: Dementia in the USA: state variation in prevalence. J Public Health (Oxf) 37(4):597–604, 2015 25330771

Lawton MP, Brody EM: Assessment of older people: self-maintaining and instrumental activities of daily living. Gerontologist 9(3):179–186, 1969 5349366

Lobo A, Saz P, Marcos G, et al: Revalidation and standardization of the cognition mini-exam (first Spanish version of the Mini-Mental Status Examination) in the general geriatric population [in Spanish]. Med Clin (Barc) 112(20):767–774, 1999 10422057

Marcos G, Santabárbara J, Lopez-Anton R, et al; ZARADEMP Workgroup: Conversion to dementia in mild cognitive impairment diagnosed with DSM-5 criteria and with Petersen's criteria. Acta Psychiatr Scand 133(5):378–385, 2016 26685927

McHugh PR: Hydrocephalic dementia. Bull N Y Acad Med 42(10):907–917, 1966 5231976

Medina M, Khachaturian ZS, Rossor M, et al: Toward common mechanisms for risk factors in Alzheimer's syndrome. Alzheimers Dement (N Y) 3(4):571–578, 2017 29124116

Nasreddine ZS, Phillips NA, Bédirian V, et al: The Montreal Cognitive Assessment, MoCA: a brief screening tool for mild cognitive impairment. J Am Geriatr Soc 53(4):695–699, 2005 15817019

Reitz C, Mayeux R: Alzheimer disease: epidemiology, diagnostic criteria, risk factors and biomarkers. Biochem Pharmacol 88(4):640–651, 2014 24398425

Shanmugiah A, Sinha S, Taly AB, et al: Psychiatric manifestations in Wilson's disease: a cross-sectional analysis. J Neuropsychiatry Clin Neurosci 20(1):81–85, 2008 18305288

Stella F: Neuropsychiatric symptoms in Alzheimer's disease patients: improving the diagnosis. J Alzheimers Dis Parkinsonism 4(3):146, 2014

Teng EL, Chui HC: The Modified Mini-Mental State (3MS) examination. J Clin Psychiatry 48(8):314–318, 1987 3611032

CHAPTER 6

Aggression and Violence

6.1   What is the relationship between violence and mental illness?

A. Mental illness does not affect an individual's risk for violence.
B. People with mental illness are two to eight times more likely to be violent than people without mental illness only by virtue of their illness.
C. People with mental illness are two to eight times more likely to be violent than people without mental illness for a variety of reasons including clinical, historical, demographic, and social factors.
D. People with mental illness are two to eight times more likely to be violent than people without mental illness, but this is simply because of the increased rate of substance use.

The correct response is option C: People with mental illness are two to eight times more likely to be violent than people without mental illness for a variety of reasons including clinical, historical, demographic, and social factors.

Data from the National Comorbidity Survey show that rates of violence in adults with psychiatric illness are two to eight times higher than rates in the general population (Corrigan and Watson 2005) (option A is incorrect). These observations should not be taken to mean that violence is the inevitable outcome of mental illness. Longitudinal data from the National Epidemiologic Survey on Alcohol and Related Conditions showed that mental illness alone did not predict violent behavior (Elbogen and Johnson 2009) (option B is incorrect). Violence (measured by self-report) was instead associated with various clinical factors (e.g., substance use, perceived threats), demographic factors (e.g., age, sex, income), historical factors (e.g., past violence, juvenile detention, physical abuse, parental arrests), and social factors (e.g., recent divorce, unemployment, history of victimization) (option D is incorrect). It appears that violence among individuals with mental illness is not merely a product of the illness and that causal relationships are "complex, indirect, and embedded in a web" of pertinent personal and contextual factors (Elbogen and Johnson 2009) (option C is correct). **Chapter 6 (pp. 166–167)**

6.2   Which of the following is a feature of instrumental aggression?

   A. It is associated with high emotional sensitivity and autonomic arousal.
   B. It is often unintentional.
   C. It is purposeful and premeditated.
   D. It is inherently pathological in nature.

The correct response is option C: It is purposeful and premeditated.

Aggression and violence can be categorized as impulsive or instrumental. *Impulsive* aggression is spontaneous behavior that is typically reactive, emotion laden, and sometimes explosive, whereas *instrumental* (or *premeditated*) aggression is purposeful, controlled behavior that may be predatory (i.e., committed for material or strategic advantage) or pathological (i.e., a deliberated response to misperceptions or delusions) (option C is correct; options B and D are incorrect). In general, clinical aggression is either predominantly impulsive or predominantly instrumental. Impulsive aggression may be associated with cognitive deficits, psychotic states, and high emotional sensitivity and is usually accompanied by autonomic arousal (Nelson and Trainor 2007; Siever 2008). Instrumental aggression, on the other hand, may be associated with low sensitivity and low autonomic arousal, as in antisocial personality disorder (Nelson and Trainor 2007) (option A is incorrect). Impulsive aggression is not necessarily unintentional; rather, it occurs on a *continuum of intention,* depending on the coalescence of individual susceptibility and context, ranging from entirely unintentional reflexive behaviors (e.g., ill-directed shoving and swinging in a patient with postictal confusion) to vigorous resistance (e.g., thrashing and biting during placement of lines or tubes by an agitated patient with delirium) and spur-of-the-moment intentional behaviors (e.g., throwing of a telephone at a scolding nurse by a patient with borderline personality disorder). **Chapter 6 (p. 169)**

6.3   What personality disorder is most likely to be associated with habitual violence?

   A. Antisocial personality disorder.
   B. Borderline personality disorder.
   C. Narcissistic personality disorder.
   D. Paranoid personality disorder.

The correct response is option A: Antisocial personality disorder.

Antisocial personality disorder is the personality disorder most likely to be associated with habitual aggression (option A is correct). Patients with antisocial personality disorder often present to the Emergency Department (ED) with injuries resulting from violence (e.g., stab and gunshot wounds) and with medical complications of substance use (e.g., intoxication, wound infection, head injury, hepatitis). Borderline personality disorder is characterized by intense emotionality, intense relationships, rejection sensitivity, manipulative behaviors, impulsive-ness, low self-regard, irritability, and a tendency toward extreme reactions. The violent acts of borderline patients usually are impulsive and typically occur during interpersonal conflict (option B is incorrect). These individuals also have a high potential for self-injury and suicidal acts, for which they are often seen in the ED. Other personality disorders are less frequently associated with violent behavior, although narcissistic individuals may lash out in retaliation for perceived slights or to satiate their sense of entitlement, and individuals with paranoid personality disorder may become aggressive in response to perceived mistreatment (options C and D are incorrect). **Chapter 6 (pp. 173–174)**

6.4   Lesions of what brain regions have been associated with episodes of uncontrollable rage?

A. Hypothalamus and prefrontal cortex.
B. Hypothalamus and amygdala.
C. Hypothalamus and insula.
D. Amygdala and prefrontal cortex.

The correct response is option B: Hypothalamus and amygdala.

Although rare, rage attacks in association with neoplastic and surgical lesions of the hypothalamus and amygdala have been described (Demaree and Harrison 1996; Tonkonogy and Geller 1992). These attacks, which have been reproduced in experimental animals, have been termed *hypothalamic rage attacks or hypothalamic-limbic rage syndrome* (option B is correct). These syndromes involve provoked and unprovoked episodes of uncontrollable rage and may represent an acquired form of intermittent explosive disorder. In addition to rage attacks, patients may have symptoms such as hyperphagia, polydipsia, excessive weight gain, or obesity; clinical findings suggesting thyroid, adrenal, or pituitary disease; a history of recently diagnosed pituitary, midbrain, or temporal lobe tumor; or recent brain surgery. Treatment involves correction of the underlying condition (including surgical resection of tumors) and use of behavioral and pharmacological interventions targeted at aggression.

   Acquired antisocial behavior and aggressive behavior have also been observed in adults who sustained injuries of the prefrontal cortex in childhood (Siever 2008). Abnormalities in working memory, abstract thinking, moral reasoning, affective regulation, and behavioral inhibition have been noted in impulsively aggressive patients with antisocial personality disorder or frontal lobe injuries (Brower and Price 2001; Coccaro and Siever 2002; Davidson et al. 2000) (options A and D are incorrect). Neuroimaging studies in patients with DSM-IV pain disorder showed significant decreases in gray matter density in prefrontal, cingulate, and insular cortexes (option C is incorrect), regions that are known to modulate the subjective experience of pain (Valet et al. 2009). **Chapter 6 (pp. 170, 174–175), Chapter 34 (p. 1108)**

6.5   What is the *most* common cause of substance-induced violent behavior?

   A. Hallucinogens.
   B. Cocaine and amphetamines.
   C. Anticholinergic substances.
   D. Alcohol.

The correct response is option D: Alcohol.

Alcohol is the psychoactive substance most often associated with violence (option D is correct). Alcohol-related violence may result from a severely intoxicated state that produces gross impairment of judgment. Pathological intoxication, seen in vulnerable individuals who have had modest amounts of alcohol, may be associated with disorganized behavior, emotional lability, and violent outbursts. In severe cases, it may be accompanied by delirium with hyperarousal, hallucinations, and delusions, followed by amnesia after recovery. Alcohol withdrawal can be accompanied by irritability and low frustration tolerance, which predispose individuals to directed aggression. Alcohol withdrawal can also result in seizures that are followed by aggression during the postictal state.

   Cocaine and amphetamine use can produce impulsive, disinhibited intoxicated states during which violence may occur (option B is incorrect). Violence is far less common in intoxication from hallucinogens (option A is incorrect); in these cases, the aggressive behavior appears to relate to the severe perceptual disturbances. Violence as a consequence of anticholinergic intoxication is rare and is most often associated with acute delirium (option C is incorrect). **Chapter 6 (p. 175)**

6.6   What is the most common association between violence and ictal/postictal states in patients with epilepsy?

   A. Most violent behavior in patients with epilepsy occurs during the ictal state.
   B. Most violent behavior in patients with epilepsy occurs during the postictal state because of postictal psychosis.
   C. Most violent behavior in patients with epilepsy is not associated with preictal, ictal, or postictal states.
   D. Most violent behavior in patients with epilepsy occurs during preictal affective instability.

The correct response is option C: Most violent behavior in patients with epilepsy is not associated with preictal, ictal, or postictal states.

Ictal violence is rare, and most cases are characterized by spontaneous, undirected, stereotyped aggressive behaviors. Typically, the patient's consciousness is impaired, and the aggressive behavior is poorly directed and not purposeful (Marsh and Krauss 2000) (option A is incorrect). Although uncommon, a prodromal state of affective instability preceding a seizure episode by several hours or days may be associated with directed aggression (Marsh and Krauss 2000) (option D is incorrect). Violent behavior in epilepsy usually occurs in postictal confusional states, which are typically brief but vary in duration, shaped by the type and severity of the preceding seizures (option B is incorrect). Most violent behaviors in patients with epilepsy have no particular association with ictal or postictal states. They typically occur around other people and are purposeful, nonstereotyped, and highly coordinated. The aggression usually can be "explained" by the situation at hand, is associated with the buildup of negative emotions concerning some circumstance, and may be of relatively prolonged duration (option C is correct). **Chapter 6 (pp. 176–177)**

6.7   What is *most* characteristic of aggression among people with dementia?

A. Simple behaviors like throwing objects, pushing, kicking, pinching, biting, and scratching.
B. Destruction of property.
C. Aggressive sexual behaviors.
D. Complex, coordinated violent activity driven by a consistent goal.

The correct response is option A: Simple behaviors like throwing objects, pushing, kicking, pinching, biting, and scratching.

In dementia, aggression generally manifests as relatively simple behaviors such as throwing objects, pushing, kicking, pinching, biting, and scratching (Cohen-Mansfield and Billig 1986) (option A is correct). Destruction of property is uncommon (option B is incorrect). Intrusive, aggressive sexual behaviors have been reported, particularly in residential care settings, and intimacy-seeking behaviors can also be complicated by reactive aggression when the patient is thwarted (de Medeiros et al. 2008) (option C is incorrect). It is unusual for elderly persons with dementia to have well-coordinated and goal-directed physical aggression (option D is incorrect). **Chapter 6 (p. 178)**

6.8   Which of the following is true of routine screening for intimate partner violence?

A. The evidence suggests that all women should be routinely screened for intimate partner violence.
B. Victims prefer face-to-face questioning rather than self-completed questionnaires.
C. Computer screening in the emergency department (ED) setting is likely to be widely implemented.
D. Although the U.S. Preventive Services Task Force and many advocacy organizations advocate universal screening, there is a lack of evidence that such screening improves outcomes.

The correct response is option D: Although the U.S. Preventive Services Task Force and many advocacy organizations advocate universal screening, there is a lack of evidence that such screening improves outcomes.

Routine screening of all women, recommended by many advocacy organizations and professional associations, is controversial. Although the U.S. Preventive Services Task Force recommends that all women of childbearing age be screened for intimate partner violence, evidence is lacking that such screening leads to increased referrals to and women's engagement with support services, reduced violence, or improvements in women's health (O'Doherty et al. 2015; Rabin et al. 2009) (option A is incorrect; option D is correct). Victims may prefer self-completed questionnaires to face-to-face questioning (MacMillan et al. 2006) (option B is incorrect). Computer-based screening approaches can improve rates of detection in the ED (Trautman et al. 2007), but they are not likely to be widely implemented (option C is incorrect). **Chapter 6 (p. 180)**

6.9   What *best* describes the role of medication in the treatment of aggression?

A. There is no evidence for any particular pharmacological intervention in either acute or chronic aggressive behavior.
B. Although antipsychotics and benzodiazepines are most frequently used for acute agitation, a broad range of medications are used for chronic aggressive behavior depending on context.
C. Only valproate has demonstrated efficacy as a treatment for acute aggression.
D. Antipsychotics are never first-line medication choices for chronic aggressive behavior.

The correct response is option B: Although antipsychotics and benzodiazepines are most frequently used for acute agitation, a broad range of medications are used for chronic aggressive behavior depending on context.

Pharmacological agents are prescribed for both acute and chronic aggression. For acute aggression, the treatment goal is typically rapid tranquilization. A survey of U.S. psychiatrists who specialize in emergency psychiatry found that benzodiazepines (particularly lorazepam) were the preferred agents for treating acute aggression (Allen et al. 2005) because they are relatively free of the adverse effects typically associated with antipsychotics, such as acute dystonia, akathisia, and parkinsonism. Antipsychotics, especially haloperidol, were considered first-line agents as well, particularly for acute aggression associated with psychosis (option B is correct).

A broad range of medicines are used for the treatment of chronic aggression. Antipsychotics are the most widely used medication class. The relative dearth of evidence from placebo-controlled trials and the heterogeneity of aggression may explain the diversity of agents used (option B is correct; option D is incorrect). Considerable empirical support exists for the use of specific psychotropic classes in treating aggression (option A is incorrect). Anticonvulsants may be effective in reducing impulsive aggression. A Cochrane review (Huband et al. 2010) concluded that valproate/divalproex, carbamazepine, oxcarbazepine, and phenytoin can reduce recurrent impulsive aggression in a broad spectrum of patients, including male psychiatric outpatients, prison inmates, and adults with personality disorders (option C is incorrect). **Chapter 6 (pp. 184–185)**

6.10   Which of the following is characteristic of communication-based de-escalation techniques for aggressive behavior?

A. They are exclusively used in lieu of pharmacological management.
B. They should be deployed as an unstructured, instinctive intervention.
C. They are most useful in situations that involve patient-staff conflict.
D. The basic goal is to assume an authoritative stance that compels patients to acquiesce.

The correct response is option C: They are most useful in situations that involve patient-staff conflict.

Although verbal de-escalation should be conceptualized as a semistructured intervention, in practice it is often deployed as an instinctive, commonsense reaction to the patient's behavior rather than as a systematic intervention (option B is incorrect). The basic goal of de-escalation is to bring a supportive and problem-solving stance and to balance acknowledgment of the patient's autonomy with boundary and limit setting (Price and Baker 2012) (option D is incorrect). Verbal de-escalation techniques are most useful in situations that involve patient-staff conflict (option C is correct), but they also can be used to manage pathological aggression and to set the stage for pharmacological interventions (option A is incorrect). **Chapter 6 (p. 182)**

References

Allen MH, Currier GW, Carpenter D, et al; Expert Consensus Panel for Behavioral Emergencies 2005: The expert consensus guideline series. Treatment of behavioral emergencies 2005. J Psychiatr Pract 11(Suppl 1):5–108, quiz 110–112, 2005 16319571

Brower MC, Price BH: Neuropsychiatry of frontal lobe dysfunction in violent and criminal behaviour: a critical review. J Neurol Neurosurg Psychiatry 71(6):720–726, 2001 11723190

Coccaro EF, Siever LJ: Pathophysiology and treatment of aggression, in Neuropsychopharmacology: The Fifth Generation of Progress. Edited by Davis KL, Charney D, Coyle JT, et al. Philadelphia, PA, Lippincott, Williams & Wilkins, 2002, pp 1709–1723

Cohen-Mansfield J, Billig N: Agitated behaviors in the elderly. I. A conceptual review. J Am Geriatr Soc 34(10):711–721, 1986 3531296

Corrigan PW, Watson AC: Findings from the National Comorbidity Survey on the frequency of violent behavior in individuals with psychiatric disorders. Psychiatry Res 136(2-3):153–162, 2005 16125786

Davidson RJ, Putnam KM, Larson CL: Dysfunction in the neural circuitry of emotion regulation--a possible prelude to violence. Science 289(5479):591–594, 2000 10915615

Demaree HA, Harrison DW: Case study: topographical brain mapping in hostility following mild closed head injury. Int J Neurosci 87(1-2):97–101, 1996 8913823

de Medeiros K, Rosenberg PB, Baker AS, Onyike CU: Improper sexual behaviors in elders with dementia living in residential care. Dement Geriatr Cogn Disord 26(4):370–377, 2008 18931496

Elbogen EB, Johnson SC: The intricate link between violence and mental disorder: results from the National Epidemiologic Survey on Alcohol and Related Conditions. Arch Gen Psychiatry 66(2):152–161, 2009 19188537

Huband N, Ferriter M, Nathan R, et al: Antiepileptics for aggression and associated impulsivity. Cochrane Database Syst Rev (2):CD003499, 2010 20166067

MacMillan HL, Wathen CN, Jamieson E, et al; McMaster Violence Against Women Research Group: Approaches to screening for intimate partner violence in health care settings: a randomized trial. JAMA 296(5):530–536, 2006 16882959

Marsh L, Krauss GL: Aggression and violence in patients with epilepsy. Epilepsy Behav 1(3):160–168, 2000 12609149

Nelson RJ, Trainor BC: Neural mechanisms of aggression. Nat Rev Neurosci 8(7):536–546, 2007 17585306

O'Doherty L, Hegarty K, Ramsay J, et al: Screening women for intimate partner violence in healthcare settings. Cochrane Database Syst Rev (7):CD007007, 2015 26200817

Price O, Baker J: Key components of de-escalation techniques: a thematic synthesis. Int J Ment Health Nurs 21(4):310–319, 2012 22340073

Rabin RF, Jennings JM, Campbell JC, Bair-Merritt MH: Intimate partner violence screening tools: a systematic review. Am J Prev Med 36(5):439–445.e4, 2009 19362697

Siever LJ: Neurobiology of aggression and violence. Am J Psychiatry 165(4):429–442, 2008 18346997

Tonkonogy JM, Geller JL: Hypothalamic lesions and intermittent explosive disorder. J Neuropsychiatry Clin Neurosci 4(1):45–50, 1992 1627961

Trautman DE, McCarthy ML, Miller N, et al: Intimate partner violence and emergency department screening: computerized screening versus usual care. Ann Emerg Med 49(4):526–534, 2007 17276547

Valet M, Gündel H, Sprenger T, et al: Patients with pain disorder show gray-matter loss in pain-processing structures: a voxel-based morphometric study. Psychosom Med 71(1):49–56, 2009 19073757

CHAPTER 7

Depression

7.1   Which of the following depressive diagnoses was reclassified as a trauma- and stressor-related disorder in DSM-5?

A. Persistent depressive disorder.
B. Bereavement.
C. Adjustment disorder with depressed features.
D. Depressive disorder due to another medical condition.

The correct response is option C: Adjustment disorder with depressed features.

The eight major categories of depressive disorders specified in DSM-5 (American Psychiatric Association 2013) are major depressive disorder (MDD), persistent depressive disorder (formerly dysthymia), substance/medication–induced depressive disorder, depressive disorder due to another medical condition, disruptive mood dysregulation disorder (applicable only in children), premenstrual dysphoric disorder, other specified depressive disorder (formerly minor or subsyndromal depression), and unspecified depressive disorder (when insufficient information is available to make a specific diagnosis) (options A and D are incorrect).

DSM-5 no longer excludes recent bereavement from a diagnosis of MDD (option B is incorrect), although it should be noted that normative and nonpathological grief following a loss may meet all diagnostic criteria for a depressive episode (Horwitz and Wakefield 2007). Indeed, it may be argued that the onset, exacerbation, or progression of a serious medical illness may be experienced as a loss that can be at least as distressing as the loss of a loved one.

Notably, a diagnosis of adjustment disorder, which in DSM-5 is reconceptualized as one of the trauma- and stressor-related disorders, can be applied when a patient has symptoms of depression in reaction to a stressor, such as medical illness, that do not meet criteria for MDD or persistent depressive disorder (option C is correct). **Chapter 7 (pp. 194–195)**

7.2   Which of the following illnesses has the highest prevalence of major depressive disorder (MDD)?

A. Stroke.
B. HIV/AIDS.
C. Cancer.
D. Alzheimer's disease.

The correct response is option B: HIV/AIDS.

Stroke has a 15%–31% prevalence of MDD (Morris et al. 1990; Robinson and Jorge 2016) (option A is incorrect). HIV/AIDS has an 18%–50% prevalence of MDD (Arseniou et al. 2014) (option B is correct). Cancer has an 8%–24% prevalence of MDD (Mitchell et al. 2011) (option C is incorrect). Alzheimer's disease has a 13%–22% prevalence of MDD (Chi et al. 2015; Lyketsos et al. 1997) (option D is incorrect). **Chapter 7 (Table 7–1, p. 196)**

7.3   Inflammatory cytokine-associated depression is most likely to present with which of the following symptoms of depression?

A. Anhedonia.
B. Suicidality.
C. Guilty ruminations.
D. Fatigue.

The correct response is option D: Fatigue.

Immune-activated systemic inflammation (Miller et al. 2009), manifesting as cytokine-induced "sickness behavior," is another proposed common pathophysiological mechanism that may underlie depression in a wide range of medical disorders, including cancer (Raison and Miller 2003), cardiovascular disease (Parissis et al. 2007), diabetes (Musselman et al. 2003), Alzheimer's disease (Leonard 2007), stroke (Arbelaez et al. 2007), multiple sclerosis (Wallin et al. 2006), asthma (Van Lieshout et al. 2009), and infectious diseases such as HIV/AIDS (Leserman 2003). This association has led some to posit the existence of a specific subtype of depression—inflammatory cytokine-associated depression (Lotrich 2015), characterized by more neurovegetative, such as fatigue, and fewer core psychological symptoms (Capuron et al. 2009; Pasquini et al. 2008)—that is more common in individuals with medical conditions associated with inflammation (Dantzer et al. 2008) (option D is correct; options A, B, and C are incorrect). **Chapter 7 (pp. 197)**

7.4   Which of the following is more consistent with subthreshold depression than with normal sadness?

A. Potentially transient and self-limited, including mood episodes lasting less than 2 weeks.
B. Belief that things will get better.

C. Maintenance of will to live.

D. Sense of self-worth fluctuating with thoughts of illness.

The correct response is option A: Potentially transient and self-limited, including mood episodes lasting less than 2 weeks.

The psychological features of subthreshold depression include low mood similar to major depressive disorder but not meeting full criteria for symptom number or duration; these symptoms are potentially transient and self-limited, including mood episodes lasting <2 weeks (option A is correct). Belief that things will get better, maintenance of a will to live, and a sense of self-worth that fluctuates with thoughts of illness (such as cancer) are all characteristics of normal sadness (options B, C, and D are incorrect). **Chapter 7 (Table 7–2, p. 200)**

7.5   To what are the increased mortality rates among depressed patients with cardiovascular disease most attributable?

A. Cigarette smoking.

B. Alcohol use.

C. Severity of medical illness.

D. Effects on the autonomic nervous system.

The correct response is option D: Effects on the autonomic nervous system.

Depression has been associated with more rapid progression of HIV disease (Leserman 2003) and with increased all-cause mortality in cardiovascular disease (Carney and Freedland 2017), cancer (Batty et al. 2017; Pinquart and Duberstein 2010), organ transplant (Dew et al. 2015), and diabetes (Park et al. 2013). This increased mortality rate, which persists even after factors such as smoking, alcohol consumption, and disease severity (Schulz et al. 2000) are controlled for, may be attributable to several different factors (options A, B, and C are incorrect). Biological mechanisms in depression may increase mortality rates in the medically ill via effects on the autonomic nervous system and on related cardiac outcomes (option D is correct). **Chapter 7 (p. 201)**

7.6   Which of the following depression self-report measures includes the fewest somatic items?

A. Center for Epidemiologic Studies–Depression Scale (CES-D).

B. Hospital Anxiety and Depression Scale (HADS).

C. Beck Depression Inventory–II (BDI-II).

D. Patient Health Questionnaire–9 (PHQ-9).

The correct response is option B: Hospital Anxiety and Depression Scale (HADS).

The CES-D is a 20-item self-report measure of depressive symptoms, in which only 4 of the 20 items are somatic (option A is incorrect). Originally designed as a measure of depressive distress in community samples, the CES-D has also been extensively used in medically ill samples, with evidence of good psychometric properties. A cutoff score of 17 was originally recommended to identify clinically significant depression (Radloff 1977), but the low positive predictive value of the CES-D suggests that it might be a better measure of general distress than of depression. Reported cutoff scores in a variety of medical populations have varied between 14 and 23. Depending on cutoffs and medical illness, sensitivity ranges from 73% to 100% and specificity from 61% to 89%.

The HADS is a 14-item self-report scale specifically designed for use in the medically ill, with separate 7-item subscales for anxiety and depression. The depression subscale emphasizes anhedonia and does not include somatic items (option B is correct). The HADS is highly acceptable to patients and has been extensively used in the medically ill, with reported cutoff scores ranging from 8 to 16. Depending on cutoffs and medical illness, sensitivity ranges from 39% to 87% and specificity from 64% to 95%. The HADS does not discriminate well between depression and anxiety, and like the CES-D, it may be better used as a measure of emotional distress (Cosco et al. 2012; Norton et al. 2013).

The BDI-II was originally developed as a 21-item self-report measure of symptom severity in psychiatric patients, but this instrument has been used in numerous studies in the medically ill. Concerns have been raised about its validity in patients with medical illness because of its preponderance of somatic items and about the acceptability to patients of its forced-choice format and complex response alternatives (Koenig et al. 1992) (option C is incorrect).

The PHQ-9 measures each of the nine DSM-5 criteria for a major depressive episode (Kroenke et al. 2001) (option D is incorrect). It has three somatic symptom questions. **Chapter 7 (pp. 203–204)**

7.7   What is considered the most important clinical psychotherapeutic tool in treating depression in many medically ill patients?

A. Psychoeducation techniques.
B. Behavioral activation techniques.
C. Supportive-expressive psychotherapy.
D. Relationship with the primary medical provider.

The correct response is option D: Relationship with the primary medical provider.

Although the preponderance of research evidence supports cognitive-behavioral approaches to treatment of depression in medical illness (Baumeister et al. 2014; Hummel et al. 2017; Jassim et al. 2015; Orgeta et al. 2015; Ski et al. 2016), such approaches are rarely adopted in routine clinical practice. More commonly, an individualized eclectic approach is used, combining elements of psychoeducation, behavioral activation, problem solving, interpersonal therapy, mindfulness-based therapy, and supportive-expressive psychotherapy delivered on an individual or a group basis. The relationship with the primary medical caregiver may be the most important psychotherapeutic tool to prevent or treat depression for many patients with a serious medical illness (option D is correct; options A, B, and C are incorrect). **Chapter 7 (p. 208)**

7.8   Which of the following can lead to the overdiagnosis and treatment of depression in the medical setting?

A. Time-pressured medical visits.
B. Patients' comfort with spontaneous disclosure of psychological issues.
C. Practitioners' comfort with managing psychological issues.
D. Identification of depression as an understandable reaction to medical illness.

The correct response is option A: Time-pressured medical visits.

The structure of medical care—with medical visits often lasting less than 15 minutes, with multiple clinical concerns that may need to be addressed during each visit, and the frequent lack of privacy in clinic and hospital settings—may inhibit disclosure or elaboration of symptoms. Furthermore, some clinicians avoid emotional inquiry because they fear that they lack sufficient time or skill to manage emotional reactions (option C is incorrect). Some patients are reluctant to disclose depressive symptoms because of perceived stigma or anticipated lack of interest of their medical caregivers (option B is incorrect). However, most patients welcome the opportunity to discuss psychosocial issues that are raised by their health care providers (Rodin et al. 2009). In some cases, both patients and clinicians have difficulty differentiating the somatic symptoms of depression from those of medical disease. Even when clinically significant depression is recognized as being present, it may be perceived as an "understandable" reaction to medical illness and therefore not worth treating (option D is incorrect).

Paradoxically, time-pressured medical clinic visits that preclude adequate assessment of mood can lead to the overdiagnosis of depression and unnecessary pharmacotherapy (option A is correct). **Chapter 7 (p. 202)**

7.9   Which of the following statements about repetitive transcranial magnetic stimulation (rTMS) is correct?

A. rTMS treatment is associated with short-term memory impairment.
B. rTMS has a similar antidepressant effect to selective serotonin reuptake inhibitors (SSRIs) in patients with Parkinson's disease.
C. rTMS has a robust antidepressant effect for depression, but not in specific medical populations.
D. rTMS use is discouraged in patients with neurological disorders.

The correct response is option B: rTMS has a similar antidepressant effect to selective serotonin reuptake inhibitors (SSRIs) in patients with Parkinson's disease.

Repetitive transcranial magnetic stimulation (rTMS), which does not produce the short-term memory impairment associated with ECT, is sometimes used as an alternative to pharmacotherapy, with growing evidence supporting its use in the medically ill (option A is incorrect). Replicated evidence (i.e., more than 80 randomized controlled trials) supports a robust antidepressant effect of rTMS for depression alone and in specific medical populations (Brunoni et al. 2017) (option C is incorrect). Likewise, in a meta-analysis of eight randomized controlled trials (N=312) evaluating the effects of rTMS for depression in Parkinson's disease, Xie et al. (2015) found a positive pooled antidepressant effect for rTMS versus sham rTMS and a similar antidepressant effect for rTMS versus SSRIs (option B is correct). There is growing evidence to support the use of rTMS for depression in medically ill patients, particularly those with neurological disorders (McIntyre et al. 2016) (option D is incorrect). **Chapter 7 (p. 210)**

7.10 Which of the following antidepressants is most effective in treating hot flashes in breast cancer?

A. Milnacipran.
B. Bupropion.
C. Venlafaxine.
D. Mirtazapine.

The correct response is option C: Venlafaxine.

Venlafaxine is effective for treatment of hot flashes in breast cancer (Loprinzi et al. 2000) (option C is correct); venlafaxine, duloxetine, and milnacipran are effective for the treatment of pain syndromes (Jann and Slade 2007) (option A is incorrect); mirtazapine may be useful in treating nausea, insomnia, and anorexia (de Boer 1996) (option D is incorrect); and bupropion may be particularly useful in treating patients with prominent neurovegetative symptoms, such as fatigue (Raison et al. 2005) (option B is incorrect). **Chapter 7 (p. 209)**

References

American Psychiatric Association: Diagnostic and Statistical Manual of Mental Disorders, 5th Edition. Arlington, VA, American Psychiatric Association, 2013
Arbelaez JJ, Ariyo AA, Crum RM, et al: Depressive symptoms, inflammation, and ischemic stroke in older adults: a prospective analysis in the cardiovascular health study. J Am Geriatr Soc 55(11):1825–1830, 2007 17916124
Arseniou S, Arvaniti A, Samakouri M: HIV infection and depression. Psychiatry Clin Neurosci 68(2):96–109, 2014 24552630
Batty GD, Russ TC, Stamatakis E, et al: Psychological distress in relation to site specific cancer mortality: pooling of unpublished data from 16 prospective cohort studies. BMJ 356:j108, 2017
Baumeister H, Hutter N, Bengel J: Psychological and pharmacological interventions for depression in patients with diabetes mellitus: an abridged Cochrane review. Diabet Med 31(7):773–786, 2014 24673571
Brunoni AR, Chaimani A, Moffa AH, et al: Repetitive transcranial magnetic stimulation for the acute treatment of major depressive episodes: a systematic review with network meta-analysis. JAMA Psychiatry 74(2):143–152, 2017 28030740

Capuron L, Fornwalt FB, Knight BT, et al: Does cytokine-induced depression differ from idiopathic major depression in medically healthy individuals? J Affect Disord 119(1-3):181–185, 2009 19269036

Carney RM, Freedland KE: Depression and coronary heart disease. Nat Rev Cardiol 14(3):145–155, 2017 27853162

Chi S, Wang C, Jiang T, et al: The prevalence of depression in Alzheimer's disease: a systematic review and meta-analysis. Curr Alzheimer Res 12(2):189–198, 2015 25654505

Cosco TD, Doyle F, Ward M, McGee H: Latent structure of the Hospital Anxiety and Depression Scale: a 10-year systematic review. J Psychosom Res 72(3):180–184, 2012 22325696

Dantzer R, Capuron L, Irwin MR, et al: Identification and treatment of symptoms associated with inflammation in medically ill patients. Psychoneuroendocrinology 33(1):18–29, 2008 18061362

de Boer T: The pharmacologic profile of mirtazapine. J Clin Psychiatry 57(Suppl 4):19–25, 1996 8636062

Dew MA, Rosenberger EM, Myaskovsky L, et al: Depression and mortality as risk factors for morbidity and mortality after organ transplantation: a systematic review and meta-analysis. Transplantation 100(5):988–1003, 2015 26492128

Horwitz AV, Wakefield JC: The Loss of Sadness: How Psychiatry Transformed Normal Sorrow Into Depressive Disorder. New York, Oxford University Press, 2007

Hummel J, Weisbrod C, Boesch L, et al: AIDE–Acute Illness and Depression in Elderly patients. Cognitive behavioral group psychotherapy in geriatric patients with comorbid depression: a randomized controlled trial. J Am Med Dir Assoc 18(4):341–349, 2017 27956074

Jann MW, Slade JH: Antidepressant agents for the treatment of chronic pain and depression. Pharmacotherapy 27(11):1571–1587, 2007 17963465

Jassim GA, Whitford DL, Hickey A, Carter B: Psychological interventions for women with non-metastatic breast cancer. Cochrane Database Syst Rev (5):CD008729, 2015 26017383

Koenig HG, Cohen HJ, Blazer DG, et al: A brief depression scale for use in the medically ill. Int J Psychiatry Med 22(2):183–195, 1992 221517023

Kroenke K, Spitzer RL, Williams JB: The PHQ-9: validity of a brief depression severity measure. J Gen Intern Med 16(9):606–613, 2001 11556941

Leonard BE: Inflammation, depression and dementia: are they connected? Neurochem Res 32(10):1749–1756, 2007 17705097

Leserman J: HIV disease progression: depression, stress, and possible mechanisms. Biol Psychiatry 54(3):295–306, 2003 12893105

Loprinzi CL, Kugler JW, Sloan JA, et al: Venlafaxine in management of hot flashes in survivors of breast cancer: a randomised controlled trial. Lancet 356(9247):2059–2063, 2000 11145492

Lotrich FE: Inflammatory cytokine-associated depression. Brain Res 1617:113–125, 2015 25003554

Lyketsos CG, Steele C, Baker L, et al: Major and minor depression in Alzheimer's disease: prevalence and impact. J Neuropsychiatry Clin Neurosci 9(4):556–561, 1997 9447496

McIntyre A, Thompson S, Burhan A, et al: Repetitive Transcranial Magnetic Stimulation for depression due to cerebrovascular disease: a systematic review. J Stroke Cerebrovasc Dis 25(12):2792–2800, 2016 27743927

Miller AH, Maletic V, Raison CL: Inflammation and its discontents: the role of cytokines in the pathophysiology of major depression. Biol Psychiatry 65(9):732–741, 2009 19150053

Mitchell AJ, Chan M, Bhatti H, et al: Prevalence of depression, anxiety, and adjustment disorder in oncological, haematological, and palliative-care settings: a meta-analysis of 94 interview-based studies. Lancet Oncol 12(2):160–174, 2011 21251875

Morris PLP, Robinson RG, Raphael B: Prevalence and course of depressive disorders in hospitalized stroke patients. Int J Psychiatry Med 20(4):349–364, 1990 2086522

Musselman DL, Betan E, Larsen H, Phillips LS: Relationship of depression to diabetes types 1 and 2: epidemiology, biology, and treatment. Biol Psychiatry 54(3):317–329, 2003 12893107

Norton S, Cosco T, Doyle F, et al: The Hospital Anxiety and Depression Scale: a meta confirmatory factor analysis. J Psychosom Res 74(1):74–81, 2013 23272992

Orgeta V, Qazi A, Spector A, Orrell M: Psychological treatments for depression and anxiety in dementia and mild cognitive impairment: systematic review and meta-analysis. Br J Psychiatry 207(4):293–298, 2015 26429684

Parissis JT, Fountoulaki K, Filippatos G, et al: Depression in coronary artery disease: novel pathophysiologic mechanisms and therapeutic implications. Int J Cardiol 116(2):153–160, 2007 16822560

Park M, Katon WJ, Wolf FM: Depression and risk of mortality in individuals with diabetes: a meta-analysis and systematic review. Gen Hosp Psychiatry 35(3):217–225, 2013 23415577

Pasquini M, Speca A, Mastroeni S, et al: Differences in depressive thoughts between major depressive disorder, IFN-alpha-induced depression, and depressive disorders among cancer patients. J Psychosom Res 65(2):153–156, 2008 18655860

Pinquart M, Duberstein PR: Depression and cancer mortality: a meta-analysis. Psychol Med 40(11):1797–1810, 2010 20085667

Radloff L: The CES-D Scale: a self-report depression scale for research in the general population. Appl Psychol Meas 1(3):385–401, 1977

Raison CL, Miller AH: Depression in cancer: new developments regarding diagnosis and treatment. Biol Psychiatry 54(3):283–294, 2003 12893104

Raison CL, Demetrashvili M, Capuron L, Miller AH: Neuropsychiatric adverse effects of interferon-α: recognition and management. CNS Drugs 19(2):105–123, 2005 15697325

Robinson RG, Jorge RE: Post-stroke depression: a review. Am J Psychiatry 173(3):221–231, 2016 26684921

Rodin G, Mackay JA, Zimmermann C, et al: Clinician-patient communication: a systematic review. Support Care Cancer 17(6):627–644, 2009 19259706

Schulz R, Beach SR, Ives DG, et al: Association between depression and mortality in older adults: the Cardiovascular Health Study. Arch Intern Med 160(12):1761–1768, 2000 10871968

Ski CF, Jelinek M, Jackson AC, et al: Psychosocial interventions for patients with coronary heart disease and depression: a systematic review and meta-analysis. Eur J Cardiovasc Nurs 15(5):305–316, 2016 26475227

Van Lieshout RJ, Bienenstock J, MacQueen GM: A review of candidate pathways underlying the association between asthma and major depressive disorder. Psychosom Med 71(2):187–195, 2009 19073754

Wallin MT, Wilken JA, Turner AP, et al: Depression and multiple sclerosis: review of a lethal combination. J Rehabil Res Dev 43(1):45–62, 2006 16847771

Xie CL, Chen J, Wang XD, et al: Repetitive transcranial magnetic stimulation (rTMS) for the treatment of depression in Parkinson disease: a meta-analysis of randomized controlled clinical trials. Neurol Sci 36(10):1751–1761, 2015 26209930

CHAPTER 8

Suicidality

8.1   Which of the following statements is true regarding gender differences in suicide rates?

A. Men age 75 years and older have the highest suicide rate.
B. Suicide rates in women are high in younger ages, decline in midlife, and peak as they get older.
C. Suicide rates in men decrease with age.
D. Men consistently have a lower suicide rate than women.

The correct response is option A: Men age 75 years and older have the highest suicide rate.

The suicide rate in 2015 was 3.4 times higher for men than for women (option D is incorrect), and the rate for nonwhite Americans was less than half the rate for white Americans (Drapeau and McIntosh 2016). Over the course of the life cycle, men and women show different suicide patterns. For men, suicide rates rise gradually from adolescence onward (option C is incorrect). In 2014, the rate was 18.2 suicides per 100,000 population for men ages 15–24 years, jumping to 24.3 per 100,000 for men ages 25–44 years and 29.7 per 100,000 for men ages 45–64 years, dipping slightly to 26.6 per 100,000 for men ages 65–74 years, and culminating in a dramatic leap to 38.8 per 100,000 for men ages 75 years and older (option A is correct). For women, suicide rates start low, peak in midlife, and then decline (option B is incorrect). In 2014, the rate was 4.6 suicides per 100,000 population for women ages 15–24 years, jumping to 9.8 per 100,000 for women in midlife (ages 45–64 years), and then gradually declining to 4.0 per 100,000 for women 75 years and older (Curtin et al. 2016). **Chapter 8 (pp. 224–225)**

8.2   Which of the following is *true* regarding predicting suicide risk?

A. Chronically suicidal individuals rarely end up committing suicide.
B. History of suicide attempts is an important predictor of future suicide risk.
C. Active alcohol use and other substances play an insignificant role in predicting suicide risk.
D. Opiate use disorder does not increase suicide risk.

The correct response is option B: History of suicide attempts is an important predictor of future suicide risk.

A history of suicide attempt is an important predictor of future suicide risk (Pokorny 1983). One in 100 survivors of a suicide attempt will die by suicide within the year of index attempt, a mortality risk 100 times that in the general population (Hawton 1992) (option B is correct). Twenty-five percent of chronically suicidal or self-destructive individuals will end up committing suicide (Litman 1989). Among those who complete suicide, 25%–50% had made a previous attempt (Patterson et al. 1983) (option A is incorrect). Active alcohol use and substance use disorder figure prominently in many suicides. An Australian study of completed suicide found evidence of alcohol use in 41% of cases and illicit drug use in 20% (Darke et al. 2009) (option C is incorrect). Over the past 18 years, the annual death rate from suicide by opiate poisoning has doubled from 0.3 per 100,000 in 1999 to 0.6 per 100,000 in 2014 (Braden et al. 2017) (option D is incorrect). **Chapter 8 (pp. 225–226)**

8.3   Which of the following statements is *true* regarding the demographics of suicide attempts?

A. Medical illness in those who attempt suicide is uncommon.
B. Those who attempt suicide have very different predictors compared with those who complete suicide.
C. Life-threatening illness and chronic deteriorating illness are rare in those who attempt suicide.
D. The ratio of attempts to completed suicides narrows precipitously in old age.

The correct response is option D: The ratio of attempts to completed suicides narrows precipitously in old age.

The ratio of attempts to completed suicide in the young is 25:1 and narrows precipitously in the elderly to 4:1 (American Foundation for Suicide Prevention 2015) (option D is correct). Medical illness is common among those who attempt suicide who are admitted to general psychiatric units. In a yearlong study of patients sequentially admitted to a Danish psychiatric unit after a suicide attempt, 52% carried a somatic diagnosis and 21% took daily analgesic medication for pain (option A is incorrect). In a New Zealand study comparing those who completed suicide with survivors of serious attempts, Beautrais (2001) found that the two groups shared the same predictors, including current psychiatric disorder, previous suicide attempts, previous psychiatric contact, social disadvantage, and exposure to recent stressful life events (option B is incorrect). Hall et al. (1999) found that among 100 cases of serious suicide attempts, 41% had chronic deteriorating medical illness and 9% had recently been diagnosed with a life-threatening illness (option C is incorrect). **Chapter 8 (p. 226)**

8.4   What is the focus when assessing suicide risk in medically ill patients?

A. The medical diagnosis.
B. Understanding that comorbid psychiatric illnesses play only a limited role in suicide risk.
C. Assessment of psychiatric conditions associated with suicide.
D. Understanding that there is a high risk of completed suicides in inpatient units.

The correct response is option C: Assessment of psychiatric conditions associated with suicide.

Rather than focusing on particular medical diagnoses, the medical psychiatrist will find it more fruitful to determine whether psychiatric conditions associated with suicide are present, whether patients are at emotionally difficult times in their illness courses, and whether secondary effects of medical illnesses—pain, physical disfigurement, cognitive dysfunction, and disinhibition—are augmenting risk (option C is correct). The U.S. National Comorbidity Survey identified 12 medical diagnostic categories with odds ratio of 1.1–3.2 for suicide attempts (Goodwin et al. 2003), but ultimately, this offers little help when assessing suicide risk in medically ill patients (option A is incorrect). What is useful is evidence that suicides in the medically ill—as in the general population—appear to be related to frequently unrecognized comorbid psychiatric illnesses (option B is incorrect). Completed suicides are very rare on inpatient units. One Finish study (Suominen et al. 2002) found that about 2% of suicides in that country occurred in medical or surgical inpatient settings (option D is incorrect). **Chapter 8 (pp. 228–229)**

8.5   Suicide risk is the highest in which of the following groups of cancer patients?

A. Good prognosis group.
B. Patients with lung and bronchial cancer.
C. Patients with laryngeal cancer.
D. Patients in the later stages of cancer illness.

The correct response is option B: Patients with lung and bronchial cancer.

In a cohort of 3.6 million individuals diagnosed with cancer between 1973 and 2002, the standardized mortality ratio (SMR) for suicide was 1.9 (Misono et al. 2008). The highest rate was found in lung and bronchial cancer (SMR=5.7) (option B is correct), stomach (SMR=4.68), oral pharyngeal (SMR=3.66), and laryngeal (SMR=2.83) (option C is incorrect) cancer. In an Australian study examining incidence and risk of suicide among cancer patients (Dormer et al. 2008), suicide risk in the poor-prognosis group (SMR=3.39) was nearly four times the risk in the good prognosis group (SMR=0.86) (option A is incorrect). The lower the survival rate of cancer, the higher the suicide rate, with the highest rate found in pancreatic, esophageal, hepatocellular, and pulmonary cancer, conditions known for being particularly painful and destructive of quality of life. In a U.S. Study of 871,320 cases of lung cancer diagnosed between 1973 and 2008, Urban et al. (2013) found an overall SMR of 4.95 with suicide risk dramatically heightened, at 13.4, within the first 3 months after diagnosis but dropping to 3.8 thereafter (option D is incorrect). **Chapter 8 (pp. 230–231)**

8.6 The suicide rates in people with HIV/AIDS have decreased but remain elevated. Which factors contribute to this elevated risk?

A. Treatment with highly active antiretroviral therapy (HAART).
B. Living with long-term AIDS.
C. Substance abuse, psychiatric illness, and intimate partner violence contribute independently to elevated suicide risk.
D. Lack of intimate partner violence does not protect against the risk of a suicide attempt.

The correct response is option C: Substance abuse, psychiatric illness, and intimate partner violence contribute independently to elevated suicide risk.

Tracking the association between the debut of HAART in 1996 and suicide rates in patients with HIV/AIDS, Gurm et al. (2015) found that suicide rates in British Columbia declined more than 300-fold after the introduction of effective treatment, from a peak of 961 per 100,000 person-years in 1998 to 2.81 in 100,000 person-years in 2010 (option A is incorrect). As with cancer, earlier studies showed increases in suicide attempts around the time that physical symptoms first appeared and around the time full-blown AIDS emerged, with the rate dropping for those living with long-term AIDS (McKegney and O'Dowd 1992) (option B is incorrect). Men having sex with men, injection drug use, poor minority heterosexual woman, intimate partner violence, and psychiatric illness contribute to higher suicide risk in HIV/AIDS patients (option C is correct). A 2005 study (Gielen et al. 2005) looked at suicidal thoughts and attempts, anxiety, and depression among four subgroups of women based on HIV status and intimate partner violence. Women who were HIV positive and experienced intimate partner violence had three times the rate of suicidal ideations, eight times the rate of suicide attempts, and four times the rate of anxiety and depression compared with HIV-negative women who had not experienced intimate partner violence (option D is incorrect). **Chapter 8 (pp. 232–233)**

8.7 Along with early detection and treatment of comorbid psychiatric disorders, which of the following is helpful in preventing suicide in the medically ill?

A. Always prescribing antidepressant medications for medically ill patients expressing suicidal ideation.
B. Diagnosing depression when patients are fatigued, have trouble concentrating, and are expressing disappointment.

C. Avoiding any direct questions about suicidal ideations.

D. Advocating psychotherapy.

The correct response is option D: Advocating psychotherapy.

Direct questions and frank discussions about suicidal thoughts can reduce suicidal pressure. Patient and family education about illness and treatment can help prevent excessive fear and pessimism (option C is incorrect). One important role for psychiatrists is to discourage other physicians from automatically prescribing antidepressant medication for every medically ill patient who expresses a wish to die, particularly without also recommending psychotherapy to address cognitive misconceptions that may be encouraging hopelessness or impulsivity (Mann et al. 2005) (option A is incorrect). Overdiagnosis of depression leads to inappropriate pharmacotherapy and pathologizes normal feelings or neglect of relevant personality traits potentially amenable to psychotherapeutic interventions (option B is incorrect). In addition to treating psychiatric symptoms, psychiatrists can monitor for illicit drug use, medication side effects, and emergent neuropsychiatric complications of the underlying medical illness. Psychotherapy can facilitate the exploration and expression of grief and help restore a sense of meaning in life (Chochinov 2002; Frierson and Lippmann 1988) (option D is correct). **Chapter 8 (pp. 233–234)**

8.8 What is the most important factor to consider for managing a patient admitted to a medical unit after a suicide attempt?

A. Psychiatrists should trust the judgment of the primary team about whether patients are medically cleared for transfer.

B. Hospital environments are generally safe.

C. Attention should be paid to items that could be used for self-strangulation.

D. One-to-one observation by sitters is not cost-effective and should be avoided.

The correct response is option C: Attention should be paid to items that could be used for self-strangulation.

Whatever the setting, psychiatrists must form their own judgment about whether a patient is medically stable for transfer. Countertransference reactions may lead to prematurely "clearing" patients. Once a patient is labeled "psychiatric," an appropriate medical workup might be precluded (option A is incorrect). Staff must secure patients' immediate surroundings. In doing so, they must "think like suicide" (Bostwick and Lineberry 2009)—that is, anything potentially usable for self-injury must be removed. Rooms in general medical hospitals often lack safeguards that are now routine on inpatient psychiatric units (option B is incorrect). Despite the absence of published data on constant observations (Jaworowski et al. 2008), prudent risk management supports its use (Cardell and Pitula 1999), while avoiding overuse and underuse (option D is incorrect). Special attention should be paid to items that could be used for self-strangulation, such as drapery cords, belt, shoelaces, ties, and other clothing items (Tishler and Reiss 2009) (option C is correct). Imported objects (e.g., phlebotomists' needles, pop-tops from soft drink cans, custodian disinfectants, meal utensils) should be regarded as potential hazards. **Chapter 8 (pp. 234–235)**

8.9   A competent, terminally ill patient whose decision-making ability is not compromised by psychiatric illness can request hastened death or physician-assisted suicide (PAS) in which of the following states?

A. Massachusetts, New York, New Hampshire, Maryland, and Maine.
B. The majority of states because voters have passed PAS ballot measures even though the states have not put the legislation into effect.
C. Oregon, Washington, Vermont, Colorado, California, and the District of Columbia.
D. Arizona, New Mexico, Texas, Montana, and Idaho.

The correct response is option C: Oregon, Washington, Vermont, Colorado, California, and the District of Columbia.

Although the U.S. Supreme Court ruled in 1997 that there is no constitutional right for PAS (Burt 1997), it endorsed making palliative care more available and permitted the states wide latitude in legislating their own statutes regarding PAS (Quill et al. 1997). Five states, Oregon (1997), Washington (2008), Vermont (2013), California (2016), Colorado (2016), and the District of Columbia (2017) have legalized PAS (option C is correct; options A and D are incorrect). Voters and legislators in majority of states have rejected PAS ballot measures (option B is incorrect). Canada's Supreme Court legalized PAS in 2015, and in 2016, the Canadian Parliament legalized both passive and active euthanasia. The Netherlands, Belgium, Luxemburg, Switzerland, and Colombia permit variations of PAS. **Chapter 8 (p. 237)**

8.10   Within the ethos and practice of palliative care, which of the following is correct in the assessment of patients requesting PAS?

A. Depression and cognitive impairment play no role when assessing patients requesting PAS.
B. The Oregon experience has shown that offering palliative interventions results in higher PAS requests.
C. Pain, mental anguish, strained interpersonal relationships, spiritual despair, and iatrogenic anxiety about the dying process should be addressed.
D. Physical distress motivates desire for hastened death.

The correct response is option C: Pain, mental anguish, strained interpersonal relationships, spiritual despair, and iatrogenic anxiety about the dying process should be addressed.

It is universally agreed that if the patient is seeking PAS to avoid physical pain, mental anguish, strained interpersonal relationships, spiritual uncertainty, or the dying process itself, these should be considered prior to considering PAS (option C is correct). The psychiatrist's role in PAS is to be available for consultation, specifically if depression, cognitive impairment, or other psychiatric factors may be interfering with patient capacity (option A is incorrect). Concerns that patients would not avail themselves of hospice care have not been borne out, with 92.2% in care at the time of their deaths (Blanke et al. 2017) (option B is incorrect). Thought leaders opining on the appropriate deployment of PAS since its inception now concur that "patients with serious illness wish to have control over their own bodies, their own lives, and concern about future physical and psychosocial distress" (Quill et al. 2016, p. 246). In other words, existential concerns rather than physical distress motivate requests for hastened death (Herx 2015) (option D is incorrect). **Chapter 8 (pp. 239–240)**

References

American Foundation for Suicide Prevention: Suicide statistics. 2015. Available at: https://afsp.org/about-suicide/suicide-statistics. Accessed June 4, 2017.

Beautrais AL: Suicides and serious suicide attempts: two populations or one? Psychol Med 31(5):837–845, 2001 11459381

Blanke C, LeBlanc M, Hershman D, et al: Characterizing 18 Years of the Death With Dignity Act in Oregon. JAMA Oncol 3(10):1403–1406, 2017 28384683

Bostwick JM, Lineberry TW: Editorial on "Inpatient suicide: preventing a common sentinel event." Gen Hosp Psychiatry 31(2):101–102, 2009 19269528

Braden JB, Edlund MJ, Sullivan MD: Suicide deaths with opioid poisoning in the United States: 1999–2014. Am J Public Health 107(3):421–426, 2017 28103068

Burt RA: The Supreme Court speaks--not assisted suicide but a constitutional right to palliative care. N Engl J Med 337(17):1234–1236, 1997 9337388

Cardell R, Pitula CR: Suicidal inpatients' perceptions of therapeutic and nontherapeutic aspects of constant observation. Psychiatr Serv 50(8):1066–1070, 1999 10445656

Chochinov HM: Dignity-conserving care--a new model for palliative care: helping the patient feel valued. JAMA 287(17):2253–2260, 2002 11980525

Curtin S, Warner M, Hedegaard H: Increase in suicide in the United States, 1999–2014. NCHS Data Brief No 241. DHHS Publ No 2016–1209. Hyattsville, MD, National Center for Health Statistics, Centers for Disease Control and Prevention, April 2016. Available at: https://www.cdc.gov/nchs/data/databriefs/db241.pdf. Accessed July 26, 2017.

Darke S, Duflou J, Torok M: Drugs and violent death: comparative toxicology of homicide and non-substance toxicity suicide victims. Addiction 104(6):1000–1005, 2009 19466923

Dormer NR, McCaul KA, Kristjanson LJ: Risk of suicide in cancer patients in Western Australia, 1981-2002. Med J Aust 188(3):140–143, 2008 18241168

Drapeau CW, McIntosh JL: U.S.A. Suicide: 2015 Official Final Data. Washington, DC, American Association of Suicidology, 2016. Available at: http://www.suicidology.org/Portals/14/docs/Resources/FactSheets/2015/2015datapgsv1.pdf?ver=2017-01-02-220151-870. Accessed July 26, 2017.

Frierson RL, Lippmann SB: Suicide and AIDS. Psychosomatics 29(2):226–231, 1988 3368568

Gielen AC, McDonnell KA, O'Campo PJ, Burke JG: Suicide risk and mental health indicators: do they differ by abuse and HIV status? Womens Health Issues 15(2):89–95, 2005 15767199

Goodwin RD, Marusic A, Hoven CW: Suicide attempts in the United States: the role of physical illness. Soc Sci Med 56(8):1783–1788, 2003 12639594

Gurm J, Samji H, Nophal A, et al: Suicide mortality among people accessing highly active antiretroviral therapy for HIV/AIDS in British Columbia: a retrospective analysis. CMAJ Open 3(2):E140–E148, 2015 26389091

Hall RC, Platt DE, Hall RC: Suicide risk assessment: a review of risk factors for suicide in 100 patients who made severe suicide attempts. Evaluation of suicide risk in a time of managed care. Psychosomatics 40(1):18–27, 1999 9989117

Hawton K: Suicide and attempted suicide, in Handbook of Affective Disorders. Edited by Paykel E. New York, Guilford, 1992, pp 635–650

Herx L: Physician-assisted death is not palliative care. Curr Oncol 22(2):82–83, 2015 25908906

Jaworowski S, Raveh D, Lobel E, et al: Constant Observation in the general hospital: a review. Isr J Psychiatry Relat Sci 45(4):278–284, 2008 19439833

Litman R: Suicides: what do they have in mind? in Suicide: Understanding and Responding. Edited by Jacobs D, Brown H. Madison, CT, International Universities Press, 1989, pp 143–154

Mann JJ, Apter A, Bertolote J, et al: Suicide prevention strategies: a systematic review. JAMA 294(16):2064–2074, 2005 16249421

McKegney FP, O'Dowd MA: Suicidality and HIV status. Am J Psychiatry 149(3):396–398, 1992 1536281

Misono S, Weiss NS, Fann JR, et al: Incidence of suicide in persons with cancer. J Clin Oncol 26(29):4731–4738, 2008 18695257

Patterson WM, Dohn HH, Bird J, Patterson GA: Evaluation of suicidal patients: the SAD PERSONS scale. Psychosomatics 24(4):343–345, 348–349, 1983

Pokorny AD: Prediction of suicide in psychiatric patients. Report of a prospective study. Arch Gen Psychiatry 40(3):249–257, 1983 6830404

Quill TE, Lo B, Brock DW: Palliative options of last resort: a comparison of voluntarily stopping eating and drinking, terminal sedation, physician-assisted suicide, and voluntary active euthanasia. JAMA 278(23):2099–2104, 1997 9403426

Quill TE, Back AL, Block SD: Responding to patients requesting physician-assisted death: physician involvement at the very end of life. JAMA 315(3):245–246, 2016 26784762

Suominen K, Isometsä E, Heilä H, et al: General hospital suicides--a psychological autopsy study in Finland. Gen Hosp Psychiatry 24(6):412–416, 2002 12490343

Tishler CL, Reiss NS: Inpatient suicide: preventing a common sentinel event. Gen Hosp Psychiatry 31(2):103–109, 2009 19269529

Urban D, Rao A, Bressel M, et al: Suicide in lung cancer: who is at risk? Chest 144(4):1245–1252, 2013 23681288

CHAPTER 9

Psychosis, Mania, and Catatonia

9.1   Which of the following would be considered a secondary psychosis in a medically hospitalized patient?

A. Acute exacerbation of schizophrenia.
B. A patient with schizophrenia and Grave's disease with psychosis due to thyroid abnormalities.
C. Psychosis due to epilepsy.
D. Psychosis with no Schneiderian first-rank symptoms.

The correct response is option C: Psychosis due to epilepsy.

Psychotic symptoms in a medically hospitalized patient fall into one of three possibilities: 1) primary psychiatric illness—new-onset or an acute exacerbation of psychiatric illness associated with psychosis (option A is incorrect); 2) secondary psychosis—psychosis due to general medical condition (systemic or brain based; option C is correct), substance-induced psychosis, or medication-induced psychosis; or 3) "secondary on primary"—a patient with a primary psychotic disorder has psychosis unrelated to his or her primary psychotic disorder (option B is incorrect).

Unfortunately, no pathognomonic signs or symptoms differentiate primary from secondary psychosis or allow clinicians to determine the presence of a secondary psychosis on clinical grounds alone. For example, the presence of Schneiderian first-rank symptoms has been reported in a wide variety of "organic" conditions, particularly epilepsy and endocrine disturbances (Marneros 1988) (option D is incorrect). **Chapter 9 (pp. 251–252)**

9.2   How can psychosis affect care in the medical setting?

A. Need for legal intervention can result in treatment delays.
B. Staff may increase interaction and become more responsive to the patient.
C. Patients with dementia may be less likely to be admitted to a nursing home.
D. Life span of patients with schizophrenia may improve.

The correct response is option A: Need for legal intervention can result in treatment delays.

The presence of psychosis can greatly jeopardize the cooperation necessary for a successful hospital stay. Lack of insight into the need for psychiatric treatment can require legal intervention, resulting in treatment delays (option A is correct). Because patients who are overtly psychotic and agitated may pose a risk to themselves and others on the ward, staff might be rightly afraid and limit interactions (option B is incorrect). However, patients also can be quietly psychotic and appear withdrawn (i.e., secondary negative symptoms). Patients who are suspicious, mildly disorganized, or apathetic can get "blamed" for their inability to conform to ward routines or to participate in their own treatment (Freudenreich and Stern 2003). The emergence of psychosis is a major cause of nursing home admissions in patients with dementia who were being cared for at home (Ballard et al. 2008) (option C is incorrect). Poorly controlled psychosis is a major impediment to medical care and contributes to premature death in patients with schizophrenia (Colton and Manderscheid 2006) (option D is incorrect). **Chapter 9 (p. 257)**

9.3   Which of the following considerations are *true* when making recommendations for managing psychosis in a patient with dementia who has Parkinson's disease?

A. Benzodiazepines are the treatment of choice for secondary psychosis.
B. Clozapine has few potential side effects in patients with Parkinson's disease.
C. There may be an increased risk of death in patients with dementia treated with antipsychotics.
D. No selective serotonin reuptake inhibitors (SSRIs) have shown efficacy in treating psychotic agitation.

The correct response is option C: There may be an increased risk of death in patients with dementia treated with antipsychotics.

Often, antipsychotics are needed to treat secondary psychosis. Some, but not all, studies (Rafaniello et al. 2014) show an increased risk of death in patients with dementia who are prescribed antipsychotics (Maust et al. 2015) (option C is correct). Antipsychotics may be withheld if psychosis is mild and expected to resolve within hours (e.g., substance-induced psychosis). Instead, benzodiazepines such as diazepam (10 mg orally) can be given to alleviate distress. However, in instances when distress from psychosis is severe; when psychosis can be expected to last longer than a few hours; or when psychosis jeopardizes the medical treatment and safety of patients, staff, or visitors, antipsychotics are the treatment of choice (option A is incorrect). Clozapine and quetiapine have traditionally been used for psychosis in Parkinson's patients, but side-effect management in the former and questionable antipsychotic efficacy in the latter have created treatment challenges (option B is incorrect). The combination drug dextromethorphan/quinidine, although not an antipsychotic, has recently shown some promise in the management of agitation in patients with dementia, as has the SSRI citalopram (Cummings and

Zhong 2015). Use of these medications in agitated psychotic patients with dementia may at least reduce the antipsychotic dosage requirement (option D is incorrect). **Chapter 9 (pp. 258–259)**

9.4   What is the best way to distinguish delirium from secondary mania?

A. The gradual onset of delirium.
B. The waxing and waning course of delirium.
C. The sleep disturbance found in mania.
D. The presence of psychosis in mania.

The correct response is option B: The waxing and waning course of delirium.

Because delirium and mania have similar clinical presentations, their differentiation can be difficult. Both syndromes are abrupt in onset (option A is incorrect) and have accompanying symptoms of inattention, agitation, erratic sleep (option C is incorrect), and the presence of paranoia and psychosis (option D is incorrect). The waxing and waning course of delirium, along with decreased arousal and clouding of consciousness, should help differentiate it from secondary mania (option B is correct). **Chapter 9 (pp. 260–261)**

9.5   Which of the following is a *rare* cause of secondary mania?

A. Frontotemporal dementia.
B. Epilepsy.
C. Alzheimer's disease.
D. Central nervous system infection.

The correct response is option C: Alzheimer's disease.

Secondary mania has been ascribed to numerous conditions. Mania tends to be rare in Alzheimer's disease; it has been reported to occur in greater frequency in patients with frontotemporal dementia (option C is correct; option A is incorrect). In those with epilepsy, investigators have reported a frequency of bipolar illness of 3%–22% (Robertson 1992) (option B is incorrect). Several infections involving the central nervous system may produce manic syndromes (option D is incorrect). **Chapter 9 (pp. 261–263; Table 9–4, p. 262)**

9.6   Which of the following conditions is *most* likely to cause secondary mania?

A. Hypothyroidism.
B. Alzheimer's disease.
C. Cushing's disease.
D. Epilepsy.

The correct response is option C: Cushing's disease.

Although mania tends to be rare in Alzheimer's disease, it has been reported to occur in greater frequency in patients with frontotemporal dementia (Arciniegas 2006; Gálvez-Andres et al. 2007; Woolley et al. 2007) (option B is incorrect). Several endocrine diseases have been associated with the development of manic states, including Cushing's disease and hyperthyroidism (Clower 1984; Lee and Hutto 2008; Villani and Weitzel 1979) (option C is correct) and in rare cases hypothyroidism (Stowell and Barnhill 2005) (option A is incorrect). Although depression is more common in those with epilepsy, mania also may arise. Investigators have reported a frequency of bipolar illness of 3%–22% (Robertson 1992) in depressed patients with epilepsy (option D is incorrect). **Chapter 9 (pp. 263–264)**

9.7   In which of the following patient populations does catatonia have the *highest* incidence?

A. Patients hospitalized with acute psychotic episodes.
B. Patients with mood disorders.
C. Patients with medical illness.
D. Patients with mental retardation and autistic spectrum disorders.

The correct response is option C: Patients with medical illness.

Catatonia secondary to medical illness with a variety of "organic" etiologies accounts for 4%–46% of cases in various series, underscoring the need for a thorough medical evaluation when catatonic signs are present (option C is correct). In a series of prospective studies of patients hospitalized with acute psychotic episodes, the incidence of catatonia was within the 7%–17% range (Caroff et al. 2004) (option A is incorrect). When mood disorders were the focus, rates ranged from 13% to 31% (option B is incorrect). In pediatric settings, catatonia is sometimes reported in patients with mental retardation and autistic spectrum disorders (Wing and Shah 2006) (option D is incorrect). **Chapter 9 (p. 265)**

9.8   What is the *most* effective treatment for catatonia?

A. Benzodiazepines.
B. First-generation high-potency antipsychotics.
C. Electroconvulsive therapy (ECT).
D. Second-generation antipsychotics.

The correct response is option C: Electroconvulsive therapy (ECT).

ECT is the most effective treatment for catatonia (option C is correct). Clinical experience and case series have determined that ECT produces remission of catatonia even when other treatments such as lorazepam have failed (Girish and Gill 2003) (option A is incorrect). An added benefit of ECT is its effectiveness for the mood or psychotic disorders frequently associated with the catatonic syndrome. When properly treated, catatonia typically resolves completely. Benzodiazepines and ECT are the most frequently recommended treatments.

One damaging consequence of the nosological error of linking catatonia prominently to schizophrenia was the reflexive use of neuroleptic medication in catatonic patients. Many patients have been pushed into neuroleptic malignant syndrome (NMS) as a result. The use of antipsychotics for catatonia requires caution because of the risk of transforming a simple catatonia into a malignant one. Several reports indicated that both the older high-potency agents, such as haloperidol, and the second-generation antipsychotics failed to improve catatonia, induced or worsened catatonia, or led to progression from catatonia to NMS (Lopez-Canino and Francis 2004; Rosebush and Mazurek 2004; White and Robins 1991) (options B and D are incorrect). Nevertheless, second-generation antipsychotics may have a role in the treatment of catatonia (Van Den Eede et al. 2005). If antipsychotic medications are prescribed for psychotic patients with current or recent catatonia, consideration should be given to coadministration of lorazepam to prevent progression to malignant catatonia or recurrence of catatonia. **Chapter 9 (pp. 272–273)**

9.9   Which of the following is a secondary catatonia?

A. Neuroleptic malignant syndrome (NMS).
B. Stiff person syndrome.
C. Malignant hyperthermia.
D. Locked-in syndrome.

The correct response is option A: Neuroleptic malignant syndrome (NMS).

Certain conditions may increase the risk of developing NMS—an important iatrogenic form of catatonia (Mann et al.1994) (option A is correct). A history of simple catatonia is a major risk factor for progression to NMS (White and Robins 1991). Other entities to consider in the differential diagnosis that are not secondary catatonia but may be mistaken for it include stiff-person syndrome (option B is incorrect), malignant hyperthermia (option C is incorrect), locked-in syndrome (option D is incorrect), and other hyperkinetic and hypokinetic states. **Chapter 9 (pp. 266, 268)**

9.10   Which of the following is an example of malignant catatonia?

A. Bell's mania.
B. Kahlbaum's syndrome.
C. A score of at least 9/14 on the Bush-Francis Catatonia Rating Scale (BFCRS).
D. Catatonia causing critical illness with hyperthermia or autonomic instability.

The correct response is option D: Catatonia causing critical illness with hyperthermia or autonomic instability.

In 1934, Stauder (1934) described a syndrome of "lethal catatonia." It was marked by the acute onset of a manic delirium, high fever, and catatonic stupor and a mortality rate of greater than 50%. Because not all cases are lethal, Philbrick and Rummans (1994) suggested the term *malignant catatonia* to describe critically ill cases marked by autonomic instability or hyperthermia, in contrast to cases of "simple, nonmalignant catatonia" (option D is correct). Catatonic excitement has at times been called "delirious mania" or "Bell's mania" (Bell 1849) (option A is incorrect). Catatonic withdrawal, with posturing, rigidity, mutism, and repetitive actions, is the most commonly recognized form, and the term *catatonia* is sometimes used as shorthand for this retarded motor state, occasionally referred to as "Kahlbaum's syndrome" (Fink and Taylor 2009) (option B is incorrect). With the BFCRS, a case is defined by the presence of at least 2 of the first 14 items from this scale. However, the number of signs and symptoms required to make a diagnosis is controversial, and the structure of catatonia remains to be defined (Wilson et al. 2015) (option C is incorrect). **Chapter 9 (p. 266)**

References

Arciniegas DB: New-onset bipolar disorder in late life: a case of mistaken identity. Am J Psychiatry 163(2):198–203, 2006 16449470

Ballard C, Day S, Sharp S, et al: Neuropsychiatric symptoms in dementia: importance and treatment considerations. Int Rev Psychiatry 20(4):396–404, 2008 18925489

Bell L: On a form of disease resembling some advanced stages of mania and fever. Am J Insanity 6(2):97–127, 1849

Caroff SN, Mann SC, Campbell EC, et al: Epidemiology in catatonia: from psychopathology to neurobiology, in Catatonia: From Psychopathology to Neurobiology. Edited by Caroff SN, Mann SC, Francis A, et al. Washington, DC, American Psychiatric Publishing, 2004, pp 15–31

Clower CG: Organic affective syndromes associated with thyroid dysfunction. Psychiatr Med 2(2):177–181, 1984 6571621

Colton CW, Manderscheid RW: Congruencies in increased mortality rates, years of potential life lost, and causes of death among public mental health clients in eight states. Prev Chronic Dis 3(2):A42, 2006 16539783

Cummings J, Zhong K: Trial design innovations: Clinical trials for treatment of neuropsychiatric symptoms in Alzheimer's Disease. Clin Pharmacol Ther 98(5):483–485, 2015 26206713

Fink M, Taylor MA: The catatonia syndrome: forgotten but not gone. Arch Gen Psychiatry 66(11):1173–1177, 2009 19884605

Freudenreich O, Stern TA: Clinical experience with the management of schizophrenia in the general hospital. Psychosomatics 44(1):12–23, 2003 12515833

Gálvez-Andres A, Blasco-Fontecilla H, González-Parra S, et al: Secondary bipolar disorder and Diogenes syndrome in frontotemporal dementia: behavioral improvement with quetiapine and sodium valproate. J Clin Psychopharmacol 27(6):722–723, 2007 18004150

Girish K, Gill NS: Electroconvulsive therapy in Lorazepam non-responsive catatonia. Indian J Psychiatry 45(1):21–25, 2003 21206808

Lee CS, Hutto B: Recognizing thyrotoxicosis in a patient with bipolar mania: a case report. Ann Gen Psychiatry 7:3, 2008 18284661

Lopez-Canino A, Francis A: Drug induced catatonia, in Catatonia: From Psychopathology to Neurobiology. Edited by Caroff SN, Mann SC, Francis A, et al. Washington, DC, American Psychiatric Publishing, 2004, pp 129–140

Mann SC, Caroff SN, Keck PE, et al: Neuroleptic Malignant Syndrome and Related Conditions, 2nd Edition. Washington, DC, American Psychiatric Press, 1994

Marneros A: Schizophrenic first-rank symptoms in organic mental disorders. Br J Psychiatry 152:625–628, 1988 3167434

Maust DT, Kim HM, Seyfried LS, et al: Antipsychotics, other psychotropics, and the risk of death in patients with dementia: number needed to harm. JAMA Psychiatry 72(5):438–445, 2015 25786075

Philbrick KL, Rummans TA: Malignant catatonia. J Neuropsychiatry Clin Neurosci 6(1):1–13, 1994 7908547

Rafaniello C, Lombardo F, Ferrajolo C, et al: Predictors of mortality in atypical antipsychotic-treated community-dwelling elderly patients with behavioural and psychological symptoms of dementia: a prospective population-based cohort study from Italy. Eur J Clin Pharmacol 70(2):187–195, 2014 24145814

Robertson MM: Affect and mood in epilepsy: an overview with a focus on depression. Acta Neurol Scand Suppl 140:127–132, 1992 1441907

Rosebush P, Mazurek M: Pharmacotherapy, in Catatonia: From Psychopathology to Neurobiology. Edited by Caroff SN, Mann SC, Francis A, et al. Washington, DC, American Psychiatric Publishing, 2004, pp 141–150

Stauder K: Die tödliche Katatonie. Arch Psychiatr Nervenkr 102:614–634, 1934

Stowell CP, Barnhill JW: Acute mania in the setting of severe hypothyroidism. Psychosomatics 46(3):259–261, 2005 15883148

Van Den Eede F, Van Hecke J, Van Dalfsen A, et al: The use of atypical antipsychotics in the treatment of catatonia. Eur Psychiatry 20(5-6):422–429, 2005 15964746

Villani S, Weitzel WD: Secondary mania. Arch Gen Psychiatry 36(9):1031, 1979 582361

White DA, Robins AH: Catatonia: harbinger of the neuroleptic malignant syndrome. Br J Psychiatry 158:419–421, 1991 1674666

Wilson JE, Niu K, Nicolson SE, et al: The diagnostic criteria and structure of catatonia. Schizophr Res 164(1-3):256–262, 2015 25595653

Wing L, Shah A: A systematic examination of catatonia-like clinical pictures in autism spectrum disorders. Int Rev Neurobiol 72:21–39, 2006 16697289

Woolley JD, Wilson MR, Hung E, et al: Frontotemporal dementia and mania. Am J Psychiatry 164(12):1811–1816, 2007 18056235

CHAPTER 10

Anxiety Disorders

10.1 What percentage of primary care patients with generalized anxiety disorder (GAD) are correctly diagnosed?

A. 14%.
B. 24%.
C. 34%.
D. 44%.

The correct response is option C: 34%.

A 2002 study of more than 20,000 primary care patients found that only 34% of patients with GAD were correctly diagnosed (Wittchen et al. 2002) (option C is correct; options A, B, and D are incorrect). **Chapter 10 (p. 282)**

10.2 Which measure is considered the *gold standard* for diagnosis of an anxiety disorder?

A. A clinical interview using DSM-5 criteria.
B. The Generalized Anxiety Disorder–7 (GAD-7) scale.
C. The Hospital Anxiety and Depression Scale (HADS).
D. The Patient Health Questionnaire–4 (PHQ-4).

The correct response is option A: A clinical interview using DSM-5 criteria.

An interview in which DSM-5 (American Psychiatric Association 2013) criteria are used is the gold standard for diagnosis of anxiety disorder (option A is correct). In primary care settings, it is often useful to ask brief screening questions to determine whether a full diagnostic assessment is necessary. A seven-item anxiety inventory, the GAD-7 scale, has been reported to be an effective screen for GAD, panic, posttraumatic stress disorder (PTSD), and social phobia (Herr et al. 2014) (option B is incorrect). The HADS (Bjelland et al. 2002), a 14-item scale, and the PHQ-4 (Kroenke et al. 2009), a 4-item scale, have also been shown to be valid screening instruments for both anxiety and depression (options C and D are incorrect). **Chapter 10 (p. 282)**

10.3   Which type of anxiety disorder is quite common but rarely comes to the attention of primary care physicians?

A. GAD.
B. Panic disorder.
C. Specific phobia.
D. Posttraumatic stress disorder.

The correct response is option C: Specific phobia.

Although specific phobias are quite common, they rarely come to the attention of physicians (option C is correct). Although the 12-month prevalence rate of GAD in community samples is approximately 2.0% (Kessler et al. 2012), an international study found the 1-month prevalence rate in primary care to be 7.9% (Maier et al. 2000). GAD may lead to excessive health care use (Jones et al. 2001). GAD somatic symptoms such as fatigue, muscle tension, and insomnia, often lead patients to present initially to a primary care physician (option A is incorrect). Primary care patients with panic attacks are high utilizers of medical care (Roy-Byrne et al. 1999) (option B is incorrect). Trauma victims and individuals with PTSD are frequent users of health care (Seng et al. 2006). The National Comorbidity Survey Replication estimated the 12-month prevalence of PTSD in the general population to be 3.7% (Kessler et al. 2012). Prevalence in medical settings may be higher (option D is incorrect). **Chapter 10 (pp. 283–284)**

10.4   Which of the following scenarios should prompt consideration of a medical cause for anxiety?

A. When there is a personal or family history of primary anxiety disorder.
B. When the onset of anxiety is at a younger age.
C. When psychosocial stressors are present.
D. When anxiety is accompanied by disproportionate or atypical physical symptoms.

The correct response is option D: When anxiety is accompanied by disproportionate or atypical physical symptoms.

It is important to evaluate medical causes when anxiety is accompanied by disproportionate physical symptoms (e.g., marked dyspnea, tachycardia, tremor) or atypical ones (e.g., syncope, confusion, focal neurological symptoms) (option D is correct). It is particularly important to consider medical causes of anxiety when the history is atypical for a primary anxiety disorder (e.g., lack of personal or family history [option A is incorrect], lack of psychosocial stressors [option C is incorrect], and when onset of anxiety is at a later age [option B is incorrect]). **Chapter 10 (pp. 284–285)**

10.5 How can one distinguish between anxiety secondary to hyperthyroidism and a primary anxiety disorder?

A. Hyperthyroidism is associated with persistent tachycardia.
B. Hyperthyroidism is associated with cold intolerance.
C. Anxiety associated with hyperthyroidism is alleviated by treatment with beta-blockers.
D. Hyperthyroidism is accompanied by adrenergic overreactivity.

The correct response is option A: Hyperthyroidism is associated with persistent tachycardia.

Hyperthyroidism causing anxiety can be difficult to distinguish from a primary anxiety disorder; signs of hyperthyroidism, such as persistent tachycardia (option A is correct) and heat intolerance (option B is incorrect), help identify the former. However, differentiating the two can be challenging (see Iacovides et al. 2000). Beta-blockers alleviate symptoms of both hyperthyroidism and anxiety (option C is incorrect). The adrenergic overactivity that accompanies hyperthyroidism provides a ready explanation for its association with anxiety (option D is incorrect). **Chapter 10 (p. 285)**

10.6 How does PTSD based on the trauma of a medical experience, such as cancer or myocardial infarction, differ from more usual PTSD stressors such as rape?

A. In PTSD associated with a medical experience, the stressor is related to memory of a past event rather than fear of recurrence.
B. In PTSD associated with a medical experience, the threat arises from one's own body.
C. PTSD associated with a medical experience does not arise out of a perceived trauma.
D. Development of PTSD in medical illness is predicted by disease severity.

The correct response is option B: In PTSD associated with a medical experience, the threat arises from one's own body.

Myocardial infarction, cancer, and other life-threatening illnesses can precipitate PTSD. A recent meta-analysis underscored that cancer survivors frequently develop PTSD based on the trauma of their experience with cancer (Abbey et al. 2015). Other medical interventions can be experienced by patients as traumatic. For example, receiving treatment in intensive care units has been associated with development of PTSD (Davydow et al. 2008; Hatch et al. 2011), and there have been numerous studies of PTSD following organ transplantation (option C is incorrect). However, this trauma is different from the more usual PTSD stressors such as rape in two principal ways: the threat arises from one's own body (option B is correct) and once the patient has been treated, the ongoing stressor is often not the memory of past events but rather the fear of recurrence (Green et al. 1997) (option A is incorrect). As is the case with other medical illnesses, severity of cancer is not a strong predictor of the development of PTSD (option D is incorrect). **Chapter 10 (pp. 285–287)**

10.7 Which class of medication might contribute to anxiety both with therapeutic use as well as during withdrawal?

A. Antidepressants.
B. Antineoplastic agents.
C. Phenethylamines.
D. Interferons.

The correct response is option A: Antidepressants.

In evaluating the anxious medical patient, it is important to consider whether medications or their withdrawal might be contributory. The most important drug classes that are associated with anxiety are summarized in Table 10–1, which includes examples of specific substances in each class. Antidepressants (option A is correct), including bupropion, serotonin-norepinephrine reuptake inhibitors, selective serotonin reuptake inhibitors, and tricyclics, may cause anxiety, and anxiety may also result from withdrawal of these medications. Antineoplastic agents such as vinblastine, phenethylamines such as ephedrine, pseudoephedrine, and epinephrine, and interferons may all cause anxiety in patients as well (options B, C, and D are incorrect). **Chapter 10 (pp. 287–289; Table 10–1, pp. 288–289)**

10.8 Which modality of psychotherapeutic treatment for anxiety involves promoting the patient's adaptive defenses and challenging only clearly maladaptive defenses?

A. Cognitive-behavioral therapy.
B. Psychodynamic therapy.
C. Supportive psychotherapy.
D. Mindfulness-based stress reduction.

The correct response is option C: Supportive psychotherapy.

In supportive work, the psychotherapist promotes the patient's adaptive defenses and challenges only those defenses that are clearly maladaptive (option C is correct).

In cognitive-behavioral therapy, cognitive techniques are used to uncover and correct misinterpretations and irrational thoughts that lead to increased anxiety and distress. Behavioral techniques can be used to help overcome fears that can interfere with effective treatment (Munn and Jordan 2012).

For patients who are not too ill and who have sufficient emotional resilience, brief dynamic psychotherapy can be useful in uncovering conscious and unconscious meaning of the illness to the patient. Understanding patients' developmental history, interpersonal dynamics, and defense mechanisms can help the psychiatrist to assist them in finding healthier ways to cope with medical illness (Viederman 2000) (option B is incorrect).

Mindfulness-based stress reduction is widely used for many medical and psychiatric problems to improve patient well-being. Often given in a group format, it may incorporate mindfulness meditation, body scanning, and yoga (option D is incorrect). **Chapter 10 (pp. 292–294)**

10.9 Which statement best reflects the recommended treatment approach for managing death anxiety in patients confronting life-threatening or terminal illnesses such as cancer?

A. Open discussions about death should be avoided, as they increase anxiety and distress.
B. Emphasizing the importance of patients to their families can potentially increase anxiety and distress.
C. The primary goal should remain full recovery.
D. Helping patients find meaning despite their suffering is an important therapy goal.

The correct response is option D: Helping patients find meaning despite their suffering is an important therapy goal.

Patients confronting life-threatening or terminal illnesses may experience death anxiety (Yalom 1980). Open discussions with patients about death help to reduce anxiety and distress (Spiegel et al. 1981) (option A is incorrect). Helping patients find meaning and value in their lives, despite their suffering, helps to relieve emotional distress (Frankl 1987) (option D is correct). For example, anxiety can be reduced when patients see that they are still important to their families or that they still have unfinished business to address (option B is incorrect). Maintaining hope is an important aspect of minimizing anxiety, although the primary goal can change from full recovery to having more time for specific short-term accomplishments (option C is incorrect). **Chapter 10 (p. 293)**

10.10 Which benzodiazepine has the advantages of oral, intravenous, or intramuscular administration?

A. Diazepam.
B. Oxazepam.
C. Lorazepam.
D. Midazolam.

The correct response is option C: Lorazepam.

Because lorazepam can be given orally, intravenously, or intramuscularly and does not have an active metabolite, it is often a preferred medication in hospitalized patients. Lorazepam can be given in an intravenous bolus or drop; however, as doses increase to provide sedation and treat delirium tremens, respiratory status must be watched closely. Lorazepam and oxazepam are metabolized through conjugation, and temazepam is metabolized almost exclusively through conjugation (Trevor and Way 2007). As a result, those benzodiazepines may be less problematic in patients with liver disease than are the other benzodiazepines, which are oxidatively metabolized (Crone et al. 2006) (option C is correct).

Diazepam is available via oral and intravenous routes and has a long elimination half-life of 30–100 hours, including metabolites (option A is incorrect).

Oxazepam is metabolized through conjugation but is only available via the oral route (option B is incorrect).

Midazolam is a benzodiazepine with a very short half-life that can only be given intravenously or intramuscularly; it is used for short-term procedures such as bone marrow biopsies, endoscopies, and magnetic resonance imaging scans in claustrophobic patients (option D is incorrect). **Chapter 10 (p. 295; Table 10–2, p. 296)**

References

Abbey G, Thompson SB, Hickish T, Heathcote D: A meta-analysis of prevalence rates and moderating factors for cancer-related post-traumatic stress disorder. Psychooncology 24(4):371–381, 2015 25146298

American Psychiatric Association: Diagnostic and Statistical Manual of Mental Disorders, 5th Edition. Arlington, VA, American Psychiatric Association, 2013

Bjelland I, Dahl AA, Haug TT, Neckelmann D: The validity of the Hospital Anxiety and Depression Scale. An updated literature review. J Psychosom Res 52(2):69–77, 2002 11832252

Crone CC, Gabriel GM, DiMartini A: An overview of psychiatric issues in liver disease for the consultation-liaison psychiatrist. Psychosomatics 47(3):188–205, 2006 16684936

Davydow DS, Gifford JM, Desai SV, et al: Posttraumatic stress disorder in general intensive care unit survivors: a systematic review. Gen Hosp Psychiatry 30(5):421–434, 2008 18774425

Frankl V: Man's Search for Meaning. London, Hoddard-Stoughton, 1987

Green BL, Epstein SA, Krupnick JL, et al: Trauma and medical illness: assessing trauma-related disorders in medical settings, in Assessing Psychological Trauma and PTSD. Edited by Wilson JP, Keane TM. New York, Guilford, 1997, pp 160–191

Hatch R, McKechnie S, Griffiths J: Psychological intervention to prevent ICU-related PTSD: who, when and for how long? Crit Care 15(2):141, 2011 21542870

Herr NR, Williams JW Jr, Benjamin S, McDuffie J: Does this patient have generalized anxiety or panic disorder?: The Rational Clinical Examination systematic review. JAMA 312(1):78–84, 2014 25058220

Iacovides A, Fountoulakis KN, Grammaticos P, Ierodiakonou C: Difference in symptom profile between generalized anxiety disorder and anxiety secondary to hyperthyroidism. Int J Psychiatry Med 30(1):71–81, 2000 10900562

Jones GN, Ames SC, Jeffries SK, et al: Utilization of medical services and quality of life among low-income patients with generalized anxiety disorder attending primary care clinics. Int J Psychiatry Med 31(2):183–198, 2001 11760862

Kessler RC, Petukhova M, Sampson NA, et al: Twelve-month and lifetime prevalence and lifetime morbid risk of anxiety and mood disorders in the United States. Int J Methods Psychiatr Res 21(3):169–184, 2012 22865617

Kroenke K, Spitzer RL, Williams JB, Löwe B: An ultra-brief screening scale for anxiety and depression: the PHQ-4. Psychosomatics 50(6):613–621, 2009 19996233

Maier W, Gänsicke M, Freyberger HJ, et al: Generalized anxiety disorder (ICD-10) in primary care from a cross-cultural perspective: a valid diagnostic entity? Acta Psychiatr Scand 101(1):29–36, 2000 10674948

Munn Z, Jordan Z: The effectiveness of interventions to reduce anxiety, claustrophobia, sedation and non-completion rates of patients undergoing high technology medical imaging. JBI Library Syst Rev 10(19):1122–1185, 2012 27820328

Roy-Byrne PP, Stein MB, Russo J, et al: Panic disorder in the primary care setting: comorbidity, disability, service utilization, and treatment. J Clin Psychiatry 60(7):492–499, quiz 500, 1999

Seng JS, Clark MK, McCarthy AM, Ronis DL: PTSD and physical comorbidity among women receiving Medicaid: results from service-use data. J Trauma Stress 19(1):45–56, 2006 16568470

Spiegel D, Bloom JR, Yalom I: Group support for patients with metastatic cancer. A randomized outcome study. Arch Gen Psychiatry 38(5):527–533, 1981 7235853

Trevor AJ, Way WL: Sedative-hypnotic drugs, in Basic and Clinical Pharmacology, 10th Edition. Edited by Katzung BG. New York, McGraw-Hill, 2007, pp 347–362

Viederman M: The supportive relationship, the psychodynamic narrative, and the dying patient, in Handbook of Psychiatry in Palliative Medicine. Edited by Chochinov HM, Breitbart W. New York, Oxford University Press, 2000, pp 215–222

Wittchen HU, Kessler RC, Beesdo K, et al: Generalized anxiety and depression in primary care: prevalence, recognition, and management. J Clin Psychiatry 63(Suppl 8):24–34, 2002 12044105

Yalom I: Death and Dying. New York, Basic Books, 1980

CHAPTER 11

Somatic Symptom Disorder and Illness Anxiety Disorder

11.1   Which of the following is a major change in the DSM-5 diagnostic criteria for somatic symptom disorders?

A. Positive psychobehavioral features in criterion B have been eliminated.
B. Multiple distressing bodily symptoms are a requirement for the diagnosis.
C. The diagnosis rests on the determination that the bodily symptoms be medi-
cally unexplained.
D. Illness anxiety disorder (IAD) replaces hypochondriasis in older *Diagnostic
and Statistical Manual of Mental Disorders* (DSM) editions.

**The correct response is option D: Illness anxiety disorder (IAD) replaces hypo-
chondriasis in older *Diagnostic and Statistical Manual of Mental Disorders*
(DSM) editions.**

Tables 11–1 and 11–2 list the DSM-5 (American Psychiatric Association 2013) diagnostic criteria for somatic symptom disorder (SSD) and IAD, respectively. The
psychopathological features of the two disorders (SSD criterion B; IAD criteria A,
C, and D) are essentially similar—that is, dysfunctional mental and behavioral aspects of health anxiety and health-related behavior. It is these features that turn
the diagnoses into legitimately mental ones. The main distinction between the two
diagnoses is that SSD requires the presence of distressing bodily symptoms and
IAD does not. The two new diagnoses mark major changes in the diagnostic tradi-
tion in this field (Figure 11–1): Somatic Symptom and Related Disorders replaces
the category of Somatoform Disorders, which had been part of the DSM classification since 1980, appearing in the third (DSM-III [American Psychiatric Association
1980]), revised third (DSM-III-R [American Psychiatric Association 1987]), and
fourth editions (DSM-IV [American Psychiatric Association 1994]) and including
the subcategories of somatization disorder, undifferentiated somatoform disorder,
and pain disorder. Whereas a DSM-5 SSD diagnosis requires the presence of only
one distressing bodily symptom (option B is incorrect), the prototypic somatization disorder diagnoses required the presence of multiple distressing bodily symptoms (DSM-III: 14 symptoms in men, 12 in women; DSM-III-R: 13 symptoms for

both sexes; DSM-IV: four pain, two gastrointestinal, one sexual, and one neurological symptom)—a major reason why this category remained rare in research. The diagnosis of somatoform disorder primarily rested on the determination that the bodily symptoms be medically unexplained, and this central requirement has been dropped in DSM-5 SSD criterion A (option C is incorrect). By contrast, the inclusion of positive psychobehavioral features in criterion B is new for SSD compared with the former somatoform disorder diagnoses (option A is incorrect). IAD is a follow-up category that replaces hypochondriasis in the older DSM editions (option D is correct). Whereas most patients previously diagnosed with hypochondriasis also reported distressing bodily symptoms and hence will in future qualify for SSD in DSM-5, a minority of these patients (about 25%) showed only the preoccupation with having a serious illness, without suffering from bodily distress; hence, this subgroup would now qualify for IAD in DSM-5 (Dimsdale et al. 2013; see also Figure 11–1). **Chapter 11 (p. 307; Table 11–1, p. 308; Table 11–2, p. 309; Figure 11–1)**

TABLE 11–1. DSM-5 diagnostic criteria for somatic symptom disorder

A. One or more somatic symptoms that are distressing or result in significant disruption of daily life.

B. Excessive thoughts, feelings, or behaviors related to the somatic symptoms or associated health concerns as manifested by at least one of the following:

1. Disproportionate and persistent thoughts about the seriousness of one's symptoms.

2. Persistently high level of anxiety about health or symptoms.

3. Excessive time and energy devoted to these symptoms or health concerns.

C. Although any one somatic symptom may not be continuously present, the state of being symptomatic is persistent (typically more than 6 months).

Specify if:

With predominant pain (previously pain disorder): This specifier is for individuals whose somatic symptoms predominantly involve pain.

Specify if:

Persistent: A persistent course is characterized by severe symptoms, marked impairment, and long duration (more than 6 months).

Specify current severity:

Mild: Only one of the symptoms specified in Criterion B is fulfilled.

Moderate: Two or more of the symptoms specified in Criterion B are fulfilled.

Severe: Two or more of the symptoms specified in Criterion B are fulfilled, plus there are multiple somatic complaints (or one very severe somatic symptom).

Source. Reprinted from American Psychiatric Association: *Diagnostic and Statistical Manual of Mental Disorders*, 5th Edition, Arlington, VA, American Psychiatric Association, 2013, p. 311. Copyright 2013, American Psychiatric Association. Used with permission.

TABLE 11–2. DSM-5 diagnostic criteria for illness anxiety disorder

A. Preoccupation with having or acquiring a serious illness.

B. Somatic symptoms are not present or, if present, are only mild in intensity. If another medical condition is present or there is a high risk for developing a medical condition (e.g., strong family history is present), the preoccupation is clearly excessive or disproportionate.

C. There is a high level of anxiety about health, and the individual is easily alarmed about personal health status.

D. The individual performs excessive health-related behaviors (e.g., repeatedly checks his or her body for signs of illness) or exhibits maladaptive avoidance (e.g., avoids doctor appointments and hospitals).

E. Illness preoccupation has been present for at least 6 months, but the specific illness that is feared may change over that period of time.

F. The illness-related preoccupation is not better explained by another mental disorder, such as somatic symptom disorder, panic disorder, generalized anxiety disorder, body dysmorphic disorder, obsessive-compulsive disorder, or delusional disorder, somatic type.

Specify whether:

  Care-seeking type: Medical care, including physician visits or undergoing tests and procedures, is frequently used.

  Care-avoidant type: Medical care is rarely used.

Source. Reprinted from American Psychiatric Association: *Diagnostic and Statistical Manual of Mental Disorders,* 5th Edition, Arlington, VA, American Psychiatric Association, 2013, p. 315. Copyright 2013, American Psychiatric Association. Used with permission.

11.2   Which of the following is a predisposing factor for bodily distress and somatization?

   A. Childhood adversity.
   B. Ability to read one's own emotional states.
   C. Attachment security.
   D. Single gene inheritance.

The correct response is option A: Childhood adversity.

Genetic factors contribute to a predisposition to bodily distress as well as to chronic pain in general, but only to a limited extent, explaining up to 30% of the variance (Denk et al. 2014; Kato et al. 2010). Thus far, genome-wide and other studies attempting to identify single genes responsible for this predisposition have yielded inconsistent results (option D is incorrect); epigenetic mechanisms are increasingly seen as also being highly relevant (Denk et al. 2014). Such mechanisms offer a potential link to the well-established role played by childhood adversity (option A is correct) as a predisposing factor for bodily distress, raising the odds of developing bodily distress up to fourfold (Afari et al. 2014). Attachment patterns form another link between childhood adversity and somatization, with maternal insensitivity at 18 months predicting somatization in 5-year-old children, and attachment insecurity in adults predicting somatization (option C is incorrect), with the strongest links found between attachment anxiety and health anxiety (Maunder et al. 2017). Another developmentally grounded deficiency—in emotion recognition and regulation—has also long been linked to various facets of bodily distress, with alexithymic cultural patterns as the most prominent concept—*alexithymia* refers to an inability to "read" (i.e., perceive and name) one's own emotional states (option B is incorrect). **Chapter 11 (pp. 311–312)**

11.3 What advice would be most appropriate for an internist regarding management of a patient with somatic symptom disorder?

A. Repetitive investigations should be undertaken to reassure and calm the patient.
B. Persistent physical symptoms should be equated with malingering.
C. Pay attention to patient clues indicating distress beyond the current main symptom.
D. Do not screen for anxiety and depression as it is outside your specialist field.

The correct response is option C: Pay attention to patient clues indicating distress beyond the current main symptom.

The following recommendations are aimed at primary care physicians and somatic specialists; they also form a basis for interventions by mental health care specialists (see also Academic Health Science Network for the North East and North Cumbria 2015; Schäfert et al. 2012):

- Consider the possibility of SSD in a patient with persistent physical symptoms as early as possible; do not equate such symptoms with malingering (option B is incorrect).
- Avoid repetitive, especially risky investigations undertaken solely to reassure and calm the patient or yourself; bear in mind that negative findings rarely provide lasting reassurance, and excessive evaluation introduces risk of additional complications and "incidentalomas" (Chidiac and Aron 1997) (option A is incorrect).
- Be attentive to patient clues indicating bodily or emotional distress beyond the current main symptom and outside your specialist field (option C is correct).
- Screen for other physical symptoms, anxiety, and depression (option D is incorrect).
- Do not miss potential medication or alcohol misuse or suicidal ideation.

Chapter 11 (p. 313)

11.4 Which of the following is a helpful theragnostic principle for management of patients with IAD?

A. Avoid taking bodily complaints seriously when no well-defined organic pathology is demonstrated.
B. Frame context factors as amplifiers rather than causes of symptoms.

C. Symptomatic measures from complementary medicine should be strictly prohibited.

D. Wait for the patient to initiate appointments.

The correct response is option B: Frame context factors as amplifiers rather than causes of symptoms.

Good management of patients with SSD or IAD should avoid the trap of en-
trenched dualistic "either mental or physical" thinking. The bodily complaints of
patients need to be taken seriously even if no well-defined organic pathology is
demonstrated and no clear-cut (other) mental disorder is present (option A is incorrect). In mild cases, these theragnostic principles and techniques may be helpful:

- Frame context factors as amplifiers rather than causes of the patient's symptoms (option B is correct).
- Build an effective, blame-free narrative that is linked to physical as well as
  psychosocial mechanisms and that makes sense to the patient.
- Provide symptomatic treatment measures such as nonsteroidal pain relief or
  laxatives; allow measures from complementary medicine according to the patient's wishes; explain that these measures are temporarily helpful but are less
  effective than self-management (option C is incorrect).
- If appropriate, set appointments at regular intervals rather than waiting for
  the patient to initiate, so that the patient does not "need" symptom exacerbations as an entry ticket for a visit (option D is incorrect).

Chapter 11 (pp. 314–315)

11.5 Which of the following is a rigorously evidence-based intervention for somatic
symptom disorder (SSD)?

A. Cognitive-behavioral interventions.

B. Tricyclic antidepressants.

C. St. John's wort.

D. Training in enhanced care for primary care physicians.

The correct response is option A: Cognitive-behavioral interventions.

Two Cochrane reviews on nonpharmacological and pharmacological interventions for somatoform disorders and medically unexplained physical symptoms
(Kleinstäuber et al. 2014; van Dessel et al. 2014) documented consistently low- to
moderate-quality evidence for the efficacy of different forms of short-term psychotherapy and self-help interventions, and follow-up—effect sizes usually were
in the low to medium range (0.3–0.5). Most evidence refers to cognitive-behavioral
interventions (option A is correct), but there is also evidence for psychodynamic
and other psychosocial interventions. In terms of pharmacotherapy, there is some
very low quality evidence for the efficacy of newer-generation and tricyclic anti-

depressants and of natural products such as St. John's wort in this group of patients (options B and C are incorrect). However, this evidence must be balanced against a relatively high rate of adverse effects, because these patients, as a result of their sensitivity to somatic sensations, are prone to unusual side effects of medications, including multiple types of "allergies" to drugs. It must also be borne in mind that none (!) of the pharmacological trials provided follow-up data. No evidence is yet available for the efficacy of training in enhanced care for primary care physicians (Rosendal et al. 2013) (option D is incorrect). **Chapter 11 (pp. 316–317)**

11.6   What is the prevalence of health anxiety across the life span?

A. 3.4%.
B. 5.7%.
C. 7%.
D. 20%.

The correct response is option B: 5.7%.

Health anxiety affects approximately 5.7% of the population across the life span (option B is correct); there is a 3.4% prevalence at the time of the interview (Sunderland et al. 2013) (option A is incorrect)). A U.K. study of 28,991 medical clinic patients found that almost 20% had high health anxiety (Tyrer et al. 2011) (option D is incorrect). For IAD, the prevalence will probably be around 25% of the prevalence formerly found for hypochondriasis according to DSM-IV, which had variable rates in the population of up to 7% (Bailer et al. 2016; Creed and Barsky 2004) (option C is incorrect). **Chapter 11 (p. 311)**

11.7   What is the most relevant disorder in the differential diagnosis of IAD?

A. Factitious disorder.
B. Depressive disorder.
C. Generalized anxiety disorder.
D. Personality disorder.

The correct response is option C. Generalized anxiety disorder.

For IAD, the most relevant disorders in the differential diagnoses are generalized anxiety disorder (DSM-5 300.02) (option C is correct), wherein excessive worry and anxiety are focused on several events and issues, not just on illness in particular, and delusional disorder, somatic type. Depressive and anxiety disorders are commonly present in patients with SSD (option B is incorrect). Rare conditions to consider in the differential diagnosis of SSD are factitious disorder (DSM-5 300.19) and malingering (option A is incorrect). In more severe cases of SSD, personality disorders are frequently present (Garcia-Campayo et al. 2007) (option D is incorrect). **Chapter 11 (p. 314)**

11.8   Which recommendation is most appropriate for the initial phase of psychotherapy in patients with SSD/IAD?

A. Establish "cure" as a treatment goal.
B. Listen attentively to bodily complaints.
C. Concentrate on psychosocial issues independently of lead complaints.
D. Avoid discussing the patient with others involved in his or her care.

The correct response is option B: Listen attentively to bodily complaints.

The following recommendations for these initial phases of psychotherapy aim at building a sustainable therapeutic relationship independent of later differentiations according to the pattern of patient problems and school of psychotherapy:

- Listen attentively to bodily complaints and relationship experiences connected to them (option B is correct). Give feedback on the emotional aspects of these experiences (e.g., anger, disappointment, fear).
- Negotiate realistic (i.e., modest) treatment goals. Advocate "better adaptation" and "coping"; avoid "cure" as a treatment goal (option A is incorrect).
- Resist the temptation to concentrate on psychosocial issues too early and too independently of lead complaints (option C is incorrect).
- Liaise with others involved in the care of the patient to obtain relevant information, especially regarding the necessity of further somatic diagnostic and therapeutic interventions, but also to send the message to the patient that constructive cooperation in caring for him or her is possible (option D is incorrect).

Chapter 11 (pp. 315–316)

References

Academic Health Science Network for the North East and North Cumbria: We need to talk about symptoms: an introduction. Information for health professionals on Persistent Physical Symptoms, Version 1. October 2015. Available at: http://www.ahsn-nenc.org.uk/wpcontent/uploads/sites/3/2014/12/We-need-to-talk-about-symptons-an-introduction.pdf. Accessed April 24, 2017.

Afari N, Ahumada SM, Wright LJ, et al: Psychological trauma and functional somatic syndromes: a systematic review and meta-analysis. Psychosom Med 76(1):2–11, 2014 24336429

American Psychiatric Association: Diagnostic and Statistical Manual of Mental Disorders, 3rd Edition. Washington, DC, American Psychiatric Association, 1980

American Psychiatric Association: Diagnostic and Statistical Manual of Mental Disorders, 3rd Edition, Revised. Washington, DC, American Psychiatric Association, 1987

American Psychiatric Association: Diagnostic and Statistical Manual of Mental Disorders, 4th Edition. Washington, DC, American Psychiatric Association, 1994

American Psychiatric Association: Diagnostic and Statistical Manual of Mental Disorders, 5th Edition, Arlington, VA, American Psychiatric Association, 2013

Bailer J, Kerstner T, Witthöft M, et al: Health anxiety and hypochondriasis in the light of DSM-5. Anxiety Stress Coping 29(2):219–239, 2016 25846805

Chidiac RM, Aron DC: Incidentalomas. A disease of modern technology. Endocrinol Metab Clin North Am 26(1):233–253, 1997 9074861

Creed F, Barsky A: A systematic review of the epidemiology of somatisation disorder and hypochondriasis. J Psychosom Res 56(4):391–408, 2004 15094023

Denk F, McMahon SB, Tracey I: Pain vulnerability: a neurobiological perspective. Nat Neurosci 17(2):192–200, 2014 24473267

Dimsdale JE, Creed F, Escobar J, et al: Somatic symptom disorder: an important change in DSM. J Psychosom Res 75(3):223–228, 2013 23972410

Garcia-Campayo J, Alda M, Sobradiel N, et al: Personality disorders in somatization disorder patients: a controlled study in Spain. J Psychosom Res 62(6):675–680, 2007 17540225

Kato K, Sullivan PF, Pedersen NL: Latent class analysis of functional somatic symptoms in a population-based sample of twins. J Psychosom Res 68(5):447–453, 2010 20403503

Kleinstäuber M, Witthöft M, Steffanowski A, et al: Pharmacological interventions for somatoform disorders in adults. Cochrane Database Syst Rev (11):CD010628, 2014 25379990

Maunder RG, Hunter JJ, Atkinson L, et al: An attachment-based model of the relationship between childhood adversity and somatization in children and adults. Psychosom Med 79(5):506–513, 2017 27941580

Rosendal M, Blankenstein AH, Morriss R, et al: Enhanced care by generalists for functional somatic symptoms and disorders in primary care. Cochrane Database Syst Rev (10):CD008142, 2013 24142886

Schäfert R, Hausteiner-Wiehle C, Häuser W, et al: Non-specific, functional, and somatoform bodily complaints. Dtsch Arztebl Int 109(47):803–813, 2012 23248710

Sunderland M, Newby JM, Andrews G: Health anxiety in Australia: prevalence, comorbidity, disability and service use. Br J Psychiatry 202(1):56–61, 2013 22500013

Tyrer P, Cooper S, Crawford M, et al: Prevalence of health anxiety problems in medical clinics. J Psychosom Res 71(6):392–394, 2011 22118381

van Dessel N, den Boeft M, van der Wouden JC, et al: Non-pharmacological interventions for somatoform disorders and medically unexplained physical symptoms (MUPS) in adults. Cochrane Database Syst Rev (11):CD011142, 2014 25362239

CHAPTER 12

Deception Syndromes: Factitious Disorders and Malingering

12.1 Which psychiatric condition is often associated with pseudologia fantastica?

A. Learning disability.
B. Adult trauma.
C. Superior intelligence.
D. Malingering.

The correct response is option A: Learning disability.

Frequently, patients with factitious disorders (option D is incorrect) will exhibit *pseudologia fantastica*, a form of pathological lying characterized by a matrix of fact and fiction, although this is not a diagnostic criterion. These stories, told repetitively, usually present the storyteller in a grandiose manner and/or as a victim. Pseudologia fantastica is often associated with cognitive dysfunction (option C is incorrect), learning disabilities (option A is correct), or childhood traumatic experiences (option B is incorrect) (King and Ford 1988). Neuropsychological testing is indicated for patients presenting with pseudologia fantastica or other forms of pathological lying. One middle-aged man with late-onset pathological lying was shown by neuropsychological testing to have developed behavior-variant frontotemporal dementia (Poletti et al. 2011). **Chapter 12 (p. 324)**

12.2 Which deception syndrome is *not* a psychiatric diagnosis?

A. Factitious disorder with physical symptoms.
B. Factitious disorder with psychological symptoms.
C. Factitious disorder imposed on another.
D. Malingering.

The correct response is option D: Malingering.

Malingering is not a psychiatric diagnosis (option D is correct). DSM-5 describes malingering as "the intentional production of false or grossly exaggerated physical or psychological problems" (American Psychiatric Association 2013, p. 726). Motivation for malingering is usually external (e.g., to avoid military duty, imprisonment, or work; to obtain financial compensation; to evade criminal prosecution; to obtain drugs). Malingering often must be considered in a differential diagnosis, but caution must be exercised in making such a "diagnosis." First, feigning of symptoms is most often dimensional and continuous rather than an absolute condition; thus, malingering often coexists with real symptoms or illness (as summarized in Bass and Halligan 2014 and Berry and Nelson 2010). Second, malingering is less a diagnosis than a socially unacceptable behavior with legal ramifications (Szasz 1956). Third, clinicians are not trained or skilled in detecting feigned illness. The large majority of published cases of factitious disorder describe physical symptoms alone (option A is incorrect). When factitious psychological symptoms are recognized, they are generally in association with either authentic or fabricated physical complaints (option B is incorrect). The introduction of a new diagnosis in DSM-5 (American Psychiatric Association 2013), factitious disorder imposed on another (FDIA), clarified the previous ambiguous and often misleading diagnosis "factitious disorder by proxy," which was more frequently called "Munchausen by proxy" syndrome (option C is incorrect). All three types of factitious disorder listed, including with physical symptoms, with psychological symptoms, and imposed on another, are all psychiatric diagnoses in the DSM-5. **Chapter 12 (pp. 326, 331, 334)**

12.3   Which patient phenotype is usually associated with common factitious disorder?

A. Single, male, age in the 40s, antisocial traits.
B. Single, female, age in the 30s, Cluster B traits.
C. Married, female, age in the 50s, Cluster B traits.
D. Married, male, age in the 20s, histrionic traits.

The correct response is option B: Single, female, age in the 30s, Cluster B traits.

Self-induced factitious disorders fit into two major syndromes. Unfortunately, the terminology in the general medical literature is inconsistent, and the terms *Munchausen syndrome* and *factitious disorder* are often used interchangeably (Fink and Jensen 1989). In this chapter, *Munchausen syndrome* refers specifically to the subtype of factitious disorders originally described by Richard Asher in 1951. Risk factors for factitious disorder vary according to the subtype of the clinical syndrome. The most common subtype is *common factitious disorder* (or *nonperegrinating factitious disorder*), in which the person does not use aliases or travel from hospital to hospital. In this syndrome, female gender, unmarried status, age in the 30s, prior work or experience in the health care professions (e.g., nursing), and Cluster B personality disorders with borderline features are frequently found (option B is correct; options C and D are incorrect). For *full-blown Munchausen syndrome*, in which the patient uses aliases and travels from hospital to hospital (and often from state to state), risk factors include male gender, single marital status, age often in the 40s, and a personality disorder of the Cluster B type with at least some antisocial features (option A is incorrect). In their review of 93 cases of factitious disorder diagnosed at the Mayo Clinic, Krahn et al. (2003) found that 72% were women, of whom 65.7% had some association with health-related occupations. The mean age for women was 30.7 years, and the mean age for men was 40.0 years. A recent systematic review of 455 published cases reported 66% female, a mean age of 34.2 years, 27% in a health care or laboratory profession, and depression more common than personality disorder, with more patients self-inducing illness or injury (58.7%) than simulating or falsely reporting it (Yates and Feldman 2016). The psychological data in this study must be interpreted with caution in that the majority of cases were reported by nonpsychiatrists and only 37% of case reports described comorbid psychiatric disorders. **Chapter 12 (pp. 324–326)**

12.4 Which feature occurs in classic Munchausen syndrome and distinguishes it from common factitious disorder?

 A. Simulation of disease.
 B. Self-induction of disease.
 C. Pseudologia fantastica.
 D. Peregrinating behavior.

The correct response is option D: Peregrinating behavior.

Munchausen syndrome refers specifically to the subtype of factitious disorders originally described by Richard Asher in 1951. The most common subtype is *common factitious disorder* (or *nonperegrinating factitious disorder*), in which the person does not use aliases or travel from hospital to hospital. In this syndrome, the patient tends to seek treatment repetitively with the same physician or within the same health system (option D is correct). These patients, although deceitful, are not as inclined to pseudologia fantastica as are patients with full-blown Munchausen syndrome. Classic Munchausen syndrome consists of three essential components: the simulation or self-induction of disease (options A and B are incorrect), pseudologia fantastica (option C is incorrect), and travel from hospital to hospital, often with the use of aliases to disguise identity. These patients frequently present in the emergency department with dramatic symptoms, such as hemoptysis, acute chest pain suggesting a myocardial infarction, or coma from self-induced hypoglycemia. **Chapter 12 (pp. 324–325)**

12.5 Which symptoms are most commonly reported in patients with factitious disorder with psychological symptoms?

 A. Depression and suicidal ideation.
 B. Dissociative identity disorder.
 C. Substance use disorder.
 D. Posttraumatic stress disorder.

The correct response is option A: Depression and suicidal ideation.

Patients with factitious psychological symptoms fabricate a wide range of symptoms. The most commonly reported include depression and suicidal thinking tied to claims of bereavement (Phillips et al. 1983; Snowdon et al. 1978) (option A is correct). The patient reports that his or her emotional distress is due to the death of someone close such as a parent or child. Distress appears genuine, is often accompanied by tears, and characteristically elicits sympathy from medical personnel. Later, staff members may discover that the mourned person is very much alive, that the circumstances of the death were less dramatic than the patient reported, or that the death was many years in the past. Case reports of factitious psychological symptoms also describe feigned dissociative identity disorder (multiple personality disorder) (option B is incorrect), substance use disorders (option C is incorrect), dissociative and conversion reactions, memory loss, and posttraumatic stress disorder (option D is incorrect). **Chapter 12 (p. 326)**

12.6   What treatment strategy is recommended for patients with factitious disorder?

A. Direct confrontation of the patient to "let them have it."
B. Invasive diagnostic testing to rule out "real" disease.
C. Indirect "interpretation" and therapy focused on acting-out behaviors.
D. Identify the patient on circulated "blacklists" for other hospitals.

The correct response is option C: Indirect "interpretation" and therapy focused on acting-out behaviors.

Circulated "blacklists" that identify these patients have found disfavor in the United States, largely because of legal and ethical concerns, and would be considered a violation of the Health Insurance Portability and Accountability Act of 1996 (P.L. 104-191) (best known as HIPAA) (option D is incorrect). No matter how understandable the anger at these deceptive patients might be, the temptation to "let them have it" must be resisted (option A is incorrect). To act out in an angry way plays into the patient's pathology by drawing the physician into a dramatized scene. A direct, accusative confrontation is likely to result in anger from the patient and in his or her subsequent departure from the hospital, often against medical advice, or with threats to bring a lawsuit for defamation. It has been suggested that the confrontation be more indirect, in a manner that allows face-saving for the patient or an opportunity for therapy. Treatment should be conceptualized essentially as being for a severe underlying personality disorder manifested by acting-out defenses (option C is correct). In the medical care of patients with any somatizing disorder (including factitious illness and malingering), the physician should proceed with invasive diagnostic and treatment procedures only when objective evidence of medical disorder is available (option B is incorrect). **Chapter 12 (pp. 329–330)**

12.7 When should a clinician entertain the diagnosis of factitious disorder imposed on another (FDIA)?

A. If the illness resolves when the child is separated from the caregiver.
B. In spite of the absence of a parental history of psychiatric treatment.
C. When an angry parent seems very comfortable with the child staying in the hospital.
D. When the mother adamantly denies a personal history of abuse as a child.

The correct response is option A: If the illness resolves when the child is separated from the caregiver.

Greiner et al. (2013) developed a screening instrument for early identification of medical child abuse in hospitalized children. The most important items were that the illness resolves when the child is separated from the caregiver (option A is correct) and the caregiver 1) has features of Munchausen syndrome; 2) has a history of counseling/psychiatric care (option B is incorrect); 3) has a history of child abuse (option D is incorrect); and 4) signs the child out of hospital against medical advice or insists on transfer to another facility (option C is incorrect). **Chapter 12 (p. 332)**

12.8 What is the feared outcome of FDIA?

A. Failure to meet developmental milestones.
B. False accusations.
C. High cost of medical care.
D. Death of a child.

The correct response is option D: Death of a child.

The first responsibility of clinicians involved in these cases is to ensure the safety of the child (option D is correct). A review of 451 cases of medical child abuse (Sheridan 2003) indicated that the mortality rate was 6.0% and that 25% of the known siblings were deceased. Separation of the child from the caregiver not only might result in resolution of the child's illness but also may be lifesaving. It is obvious, however, that decisions as to whether a child should be separated from the caregiver and when he or she, if ever, should be returned home are to be made by the court, with input from involved clinicians and child protective services. The diagnosis of FDIA in children is underrecognized, and accurate diagnosis often takes months to years. Failure to consider it in the differential diagnosis may result in unnecessary extensive testing and procedures (option C is incorrect). There are reported cases in which overzealous clinicians or child protective agencies have made accusations that were later proven to be inaccurate (Rand and Feldman 1999) (option B is incorrect). The child victim's medical care should be centralized to one treatment center and overseen by a primary physician or a specialist who can coordinate care. The child should be evaluated and monitored for the presence of psychological symptoms and/or failure to meet developmental milestones (option A is incorrect). For those cases that require child protective services and/or court involvement, monitoring should continue indefinitely until all concern for abuse or relapse of abusing behavior has abated. **Chapter 12 (pp. 332–333)**

12.9 When malingering is suspected, how should the psychiatric consultant approach the case?

A. Direct patient confrontation.
B. Diagnosis of antisocial personality disorder.
C. Careful written documentation.
D. Functional neuroimaging assessment.

The correct response is option C: Careful written documentation.

Preliminary evidence suggests some utility in functional neuroimaging to evaluate conscious symptom production (Jiang et al. 2015; Ofen et al. 2017); however, use of neuroimaging is fraught with legal implications (Moriarty 2008) (option D is incorrect). By definition, the etiology of malingering is to obtain external gain as a result of the symptoms. However, malingering does tend to be more common in persons who may have histrionic or antisocial personality features (option B is incorrect). Malingering is more a management problem than a therapeutic issue. With this in mind, the primary physician and psychiatric consultant must be circumspect in their approach to the patient. Every note must be written with the awareness that it may be read by the patient or even become a courtroom exhibit (option C is correct). Malingering is often listed among diagnostic possibilities but is rarely proven conclusively in medical settings. The person who is suspected of malingering, as a rule, should not be confronted with a direct accusation (option A is incorrect). Instead, subtle communication can indicate that the physician is "onto the game" (Kramer et al. 1979). **Chapter 12 (pp. 335–336)**

12.10 Who is a typical victim in angel of death syndrome?

A. The patient who intentionally feigns physical disease.
B. The patient who gives approximate answers.
C. The elderly patient resuscitated by a nurse on an evening shift.
D. The wealthy housewife seeking to evade arrest by feigning coma.

The correct response is option C: The elderly patient resuscitated by a nurse on an evening shift.

Persons who have factitious disorders intentionally feign, exaggerate, aggravate, or self-induce symptoms or disease. They are conscious of their behaviors, although the underlying motivation may be unconscious. By convention, this diagnosis is also characterized by the surreptitious nature of the behavior (option A is incorrect).

There have been multiple reports in which health care providers have been accused of causing epidemics of acute cardiac or pulmonary arrests and unusual patterns of deaths (Yorker 1996; Yorker et al. 2006), the so-called *angel of death syndrome* (Kalisch et al. 1980). Tragically, many of these epidemics have been shown to be caused by the very persons entrusted with the patients' care. In their detailed review of multiple hospital epidemics, Yorker et al. (2006) concluded that the perpetrators were usually nurses or nurse's aides and that the victims were physically compromised: critically ill, elderly, or very young (option C is correct). The epidemics tend to cluster on evening and night shifts and also involve numerous, often successful, resuscitations. Yorker et al. (2006) proposed that one motive of the perpetrators is the excitement and exhilaration derived from participating in "codes." This behavior constitutes serial murder, and prosecution has resulted in several convictions.

Ganser's syndrome is closely related to factitious disorder with predominantly psychological symptoms (Wirtz et al. 2008). This syndrome is characterized by the provision of approximate answers (*Vorbeireden*) to questions (e.g., the examiner asks, "What is the color of snow?" and the patient answers, "Green") (option B is incorrect). Complaints of amnesia, disorientation, and perceptual disturbance are generally present as well. Malingering is not a psychiatric diagnosis. Motivation for malingering is usually external (e.g., to avoid military duty, imprisonment, or work; to obtain financial compensation; to evade criminal prosecution; to obtain drugs) (option D is incorrect). **Chapter 12 (pp. 324, 328, 334)**

References

American Psychiatric Association: Diagnostic and Statistical Manual of Mental Disorders, 5th Edition. Arlington, VA, American Psychiatric Association, 2013

Asher R: Munchausen's syndrome. Lancet 1(6650):339–341, 1951 14805062

Bass C, Halligan P: Factitious disorders and malingering: challenges for clinical assessment and management. Lancet 383(9926):1422–1432, 2014 24612861

Berry TR, Nelson NW: DSM-5 and malingering: a modest proposal. Psychol Inj Law 3(4):295–303, 2010

Fink P, Jensen J: Clinical characteristics of the Munchausen syndrome. A review and 3 new case histories. Psychother Psychosom 52(1-3):164–171, 1989 2486395

Greiner MV, Palusci VJ, Keeshin BR, et al: A preliminary screening instrument for early detection of medical child abuse. Hosp Pediatr 3(1):39–44, 2013 24319834

Jiang W, Liu H, Zeng L, et al: Decoding the processing of lying using functional connectivity MRI. Behav Brain Funct 11:1, 2015 25595193

Kalisch PA, Kalisch BJ, Livesay E: The "Angel of Death": the anatomy of 1980's major news story about nursing. Nurs Forum 19(3):212–241, 1980 6909883

King BH, Ford CV: Pseudologia fantastica. Acta Psychiatr Scand 77(1):1–6, 1988 3279719

Krahn LE, Li H, O'Connor MK: Patients who strive to be ill: factitious disorder with physical symptoms. Am J Psychiatry 160(6):1163–1168, 2003 12777276

Kramer KK, La Piana FG, Appleton B: Ocular malingering and hysteria: diagnosis and management. Surv Ophthalmol 24(2):89–96, 1979 515946

Moriarty JC: Flickering admissibility: neuroimaging evidence in the U.S. courts. Behav Sci Law 26(1):29–49, 2008 18327830

Ofen N, Whitfield-Gabrieli S, Chai XJ, et al: Neural correlates of deception: lying about past events and personal beliefs. Soc Cogn Affect Neurosci 12(1):116–127, 2017 27798254

Phillips MR, Ward NG, Ries RK: Factitious mourning: painless patienthood. Am J Psychiatry 140(4):420–425, 1983 6837777

Poletti M, Borelli P, Bonuccelli U: The neuropsychological correlates of pathological lying: evidence from behavioral variant frontotemporal dementia. J Neurol 258(11):2009–2013, 2011 21512737

Rand DC, Feldman MD: Misdiagnosis of Munchausen syndrome by proxy: a literature review and four new cases. Harv Rev Psychiatry 7(2):94–101, 1999 10471247

Sheridan MS: The deceit continues: an updated literature review of Munchausen Syndrome by Proxy. Child Abuse Negl 27(4):431–451, 2003 12686328

Snowdon J, Solomons R, Druce H: Feigned bereavement: twelve cases. Br J Psychiatry 133:15–19, 1978 667502

Szasz TS: Malingering: diagnosis or social condemnation? Analysis of the meaning of diagnosis in the light of some interrelations of social structure, value judgment, and the physician's role. AMA Arch Neurol Psychiatry 76(4):432–443, 1956 13361605

Wirtz G, Baas U, Hofer H, et al: [Psychopathology of Ganser's syndrome. Literature review and case report]. Nervenarzt 79(5):543–557, 2008 18274720

Yates GP, Feldman MD: Factitious disorder: a systematic review of 455 cases in the professional literature. Gen Hosp Psychiatry 41:20–28, 2016 27302720

Yorker BC: Hospital epidemics of factitious disorder by proxy, in The Spectrum of Factitious Disorders. Edited by Feldman MD, Eisendrath SJ. Washington, DC, American Psychiatric Press, 1996, pp 157–174

Yorker BC, Kizer KW, Lampe P, et al: Serial murder by healthcare professionals. J Forensic Sci 51(6):1362–1371, 2006 17199622

CHAPTER 13

Eating Disorders

13.1 You evaluate a 4-year-old boy for significant weight loss who does not exhibit fear of weight gain, body image disturbance, or drive for thinness. His mother reports noticing that he avoids food with a certain bitter taste, will only eat foods that are crunchy, does not engage in recurrent regurgitation of food, and does not consume nonnutritive substances (e.g., dirt, clay, soap, paper). His day care teachers have requested an evaluation for suspected autism spectrum diagnoses. What is the most appropriate diagnosis given the aforementioned information from the evaluation?

A. Pica.
B. Avoidant/restrictive food intake disorder (ARFID).
C. Rumination disorder.
D. Anorexia nervosa (AN).

The correct response is option B: Avoidant/restrictive food intake disorder (ARFID).

Pica is characterized by developmentally inappropriate and culturally nonnormative consumption of nonnutritive substances (e.g., dirt, clay, soap, paper, paint chips) for at least 1 month (option A is incorrect). Rumination disorder is characterized by recurrent regurgitation of food, which may be re-chewed, re-swallowed, or spit out (option C is incorrect). The diagnostic category of ARFID captures children, adolescents, and adults with severe food restriction or avoidance and significant weight loss or compromised growth and nutritional deficiencies who do not exhibit fear of weight gain, body image disturbance, or drive for thinness. Some, including those with autism spectrum diagnoses, may reject foods with certain textures, consistencies, or tastes (option B is correct). The three primary features of AN in DSM-5 (American Psychiatric Association 2013) are 1) persistent food intake restriction and low body weight, 2) either intense fear of gaining weight or behavior that interferes with weight gain, and 3) either disturbance in self-perceived weight or shape or persistent lack of recognition of the seriousness of being in a starved state (option D is incorrect). **Chapter 13 (pp. 342–344)**

13.2 How do patients with eating disorder typically approach behavior change?

A. Ambivalence toward behavior change is the norm.
B. They exhibit overall comfort with engaging in weight-control behaviors.
C. Symptom concealment is uncommon.
D. Embarrassment and shame typically do not complicate patient engagement.

The correct response is option A: Ambivalence toward behavior change is the norm.

Symptom concealment and minimization are common (option C is incorrect) because patients are often anxious about changing their underlying eating and weight-control behaviors (option B is incorrect) and may even explicitly deny having an eating disorder. Ambivalence toward behavior change is therefore the norm (option A is correct), and feelings of shame, embarrassment (option D is incorrect), and stigma further complicate patient engagement. **Chapter 13 (p. 341)**

13.3 A 34-year-old woman discloses feeling depressed and guilty about weekly episodes of heavy consumption of food over a period of 6 months during a consultation regarding depression. She typically eats alone, even when not hungry, consumes food more rapidly than usual, and eats until physically full and uncomfortable. She does not vomit and experiences strong feelings of disgust. She denies any compensatory behaviors in order to lose weight and does not engage in restricting behaviors to limit caloric intake. She has metabolic syndrome and newly diagnosed hypertension. She is concerned about her obesity and has been considering weight-loss surgery. Given the aforementioned presentation, what is the most appropriate diagnosis?

A. Bulimia nervosa (BN).
B. Anorexia nervosa (AN).
C. Binge-eating disorder (BED).
D. Rumination disorder.

The correct response is option C: Binge-eating disorder (BED).

BED is characterized by recurrent weekly binge-eating episodes, accompanied by a sense of loss of control over eating, that extend over a period of 3 months or more (option C is correct). In contrast to BN, however, BED does not involve regular use of compensatory behaviors (Guerdjikova et al. 2017) (option A is incorrect). Moreover, binge-eating episodes in BED must be associated with at least three of the following additional symptoms: eating alone, eating when not physically hungry, eating more rapidly than usual, eating until physically full and uncomfortable, and feeling disgusted with oneself, depressed, or guilty after a binge. About 40% of patients with BED meet criteria for metabolic syndrome, and evidence suggests that BED represents an obesity-independent risk factor for hypertension, diabetes, and dyslipidemia (Barnes et al. 2011). BED is one of the most common psychiatric diagnoses in morbidly obese individuals seeking weight-loss surgery, with rates estimated to be as high as 17% (Dawes et al. 2016).

The defining features of BN are recurrent episodes of binge eating associated with a sense of loss of control over eating, use of compensatory behaviors to prevent weight gain or to promote weight loss, and self-evaluation that is unduly influenced by body weight and shape (option A is incorrect).

The three primary features of AN in DSM-5 are 1) persistent food intake restriction and low body weight, 2) either intense fear of gaining weight or behavior that interferes with weight gain, and 3) either disturbance in self-perceived weight or shape or persistent lack of recognition of the seriousness of being in a starved state (option B is incorrect).

Rumination disorder is characterized by recurrent regurgitation of food, which may be re-chewed, re-swallowed, or spit out (option D is incorrect)—behaviors which this patient does not exhibit. **Chapter 13 (pp. 342–346)**

13.4   Which of the following treatment plans is recommended for individuals with comorbid eating disorders and substance use disorders (SUDs)?

A. Both disorders should be addressed at the same time.
B. Patients with eating disorders do not have an elevated prevalence of SUDs and therefore SUDs are of little concern.
C. Addressing each disorder one at a time will result in symptomatic improvement of both disorders.
D. Comorbid SUDs have not been shown to increase mortality, medical complications, and psychopathology and are, therefore, of little concern.

The correct response is option A: Both disorders should be addressed at the same time.

Patients with eating disorders have an elevated prevalence of SUDs, with rates as high as 37% among patients with BN, 27% among patients with AN, and 23% among patients with BED (Hudson et al. 2007) (option B is incorrect). Comorbid SUDs contribute to increased mortality, medical complications, and psychopathology; poor functional outcomes; and high relapse rates (Munn-Chernoff and Baker 2016; option D is incorrect). The treatment of patients with comorbid eating disorders and SUDs is challenging. Ideally, both disorders should be addressed at the same time (option A is correct) because improvement in one behavioral disorder may be paralleled by worsening symptomatology in the other behavioral disorder (option C is incorrect). **Chapter 13 (p. 348)**

13.5   Which of the following phenomena should raise suspicion for an underlying eating disorder in patients with type 1 diabetes mellitus?

A. Frequent requests to be weighed during medical appointments.
B. Optimal glycemic control.

C. Requests for multiple medical appointments.
D. Skipping doses of insulin.

The correct response is option D: Skipping doses of insulin.

Perhaps the most significant comorbid medical condition with eating disorders is type 1 diabetes mellitus, because the co-occurrence of these two disorders is associated with elevated morbidity and mortality (Peveler et al. 2005). Individuals with type 1 diabetes mellitus may purge calories by intentionally skipping or reducing their prescribed doses of insulin, resulting in increased urinary excretion of glucose and weight loss (option D is correct). Overdosing of insulin to induce hypoglycemia and justify binge eating and consumption of high-carbohydrate foods have also been described (Scheuing et al. 2014). Unexplained weight loss, suboptimal glycemic control (option B is incorrect), and/or recurrent hypoglycemia or diabetic ketoacidosis, as well as missed appointments (option C is incorrect) and reluctance to be weighed (option A is incorrect), should raise suspicion for an underlying eating disorder (Pinhas-Hamiel et al. 2015). **Chapter 13 (p. 349)**

13.6   Signs and symptoms of starvation and purging include which of the following?

   A. Increase in energy.
   B. Sinus tachycardia.
   C. Parotid gland enlargement.
   D. Elevated mood.

The correct response is option C: Parotid gland enlargement.

Weakness, sinus bradycardia, and low mood are seen in starvation- and purging-related behaviors (options A, B, and D are incorrect). Parotid gland enlargement is seen in purging-related behaviors (option C is correct). See Table 13–1. **Chapter 13 (Table 13–1, p. 352)**

TABLE 13–1. Signs and symptoms of eating disorders

Starvation related	Purging related
Dry skin, lanugo, hair loss	Parotid gland enlargement
Cold intolerance, hypothermia	Dental caries and erosion
Weakness, fatigue	Perioral acne
Low mood, poor concentration, insomnia	Low mood, poor concentration
Hot flashes, diaphoresis	Orthostatic tachycardia, dehydration
Sinus bradycardia, orthostasis	Heartburn/reflux/abdominal pain
Early satiety, bloating, constipation	Hematemesis
Primary or secondary amenorrhea	Amenorrhea/oligomenorrhea
Low libido	Muscle cramps, paresthesias
Decreased bone density, fractures	Palpitations, cardiac arrhythmias
Muscle wasting/cachexia	Diarrhea/constipation
Nose bleeds, bruising	Hemorrhoids/rectal prolapse
Stress fractures	Presyncope or syncope
Presyncope or syncope	

13.7 Which of the following factors contributes to the sustaining behavior of eating disorders?

A. Cognitive rigidity.
B. Low self-directedness.
C. Alterations in satiety and hunger signaling.
D. Excessive exercise.

The correct response is option C: Alterations in satiety and hunger signaling.

A useful conceptual etiological framework separates risk factors into those that predispose to the condition, those that precipitate its onset, and those that come to maintain the self-sustaining nature of the behaviors over time.

Family studies have identified a number of inherited personality traits, including perfectionism, harm avoidance, cognitive rigidity (option A is incorrect), neuroticism, and low self-directedness (option B is incorrect), in individuals with eating disorders and in their first-degree relatives, suggesting that these may be predisposing traits.

Precipitating factors other than acute and chronic stressors in adolescents include dieting behavior (Evans et al. 2017); depressive symptoms and body dissatisfaction (Goldschmidt et al. 2015; Rohde et al. 2015); and excessive exercise (option D is incorrect), which is present in the majority of patients with AN and often precedes the onset of dieting behavior (Davis et al. 2005).

In AN, as the disorder progresses, the physiological consequences of starvation and purging behaviors lead to alterations in satiety and hunger signaling (Monteleone et al. 2008; option C is correct), neural reward circuitry (Bischoff-Grethe et al. 2013; Cha et al. 2016; Monteleone et al. 2017), and attention and decision-making processes (Foerde et al. 2015; Guillaume et al. 2015). Although these are consequences of the disorder, there is increasing evidence that some of these changes likely feed forward and come to sustain disordered eating and weight-control behaviors and eating disorder cognitions over time. **Chapter 13 (pp. 353–354)**

13.8   Which of the electrolyte abnormalities is seen in patients with AN?

A. Hypokalemia.
B. Hyperglycemia.
C. Hyperphosphatemia.
D. Hypernatremia.

The correct response is option A: Hypokalemia.

Electrolyte abnormalities and associated cardiac arrhythmia constitute one of the most common causes of death in patients with AN and BN (Williams et al. 2008; Winston 2008). Hypokalemia poses a major risk. Unexplained hypokalemia should raise suspicion for purging behaviors because it can be the consequence of frequent vomiting and laxative or diuretic abuse (option A is correct). Hyponatremia (option D is incorrect) may result from excessive water intake, a behavior often employed by patients with AN to suppress appetite, increase satiety, or artificially inflate weight. Hypophosphatemia (option C is incorrect) can be a manifesting symptom associated with starvation in AN. Starvation-related hypoglycemia (option B is incorrect) in patients with AN can present in the acute setting with altered mental status and/or coma (Rich et al. 1990). **Chapter 13 (pp. 354–355)**

13.9   A woman with a recent diagnosis of AN is contemplating becoming pregnant. What are the gynecological and obstetric complications associated with AN?

A. Patients with AN do not respond to fertility treatment.
B. AN is associated with high estrogen levels.
C. AN is associated with primary hypogonadotropic amenorrhea.
D. AN is associated with low follicle-stimulating hormone and luteinizing hormone.

The correct response is option D: AN is associated with low follicle-stimulating hormone and luteinizing hormone.

Low body mass index (BMI) in AN is associated with the onset of secondary hypogonadotropic amenorrhea and infertility (option C is incorrect), with low serum levels of estrogen (option B is incorrect), follicle-stimulating hormone, and luteinizing hormone (option D is correct). Anovulatory patients with AN who desire fertility respond to hormonal interventions and assisted reproductive technologies (option A is incorrect). **Chapter 13 (p. 355)**

13.10 Refeeding syndrome carries which of the following risks to patients?

A. High risk of hypophosphatemia.
B. High risk of hyperglycemia.
C. Rare risk of edema or congestive heart failure.
D. Higher risk from oral feeding than parenteral feeding.

The correct response is option A: High risk of hypophosphatemia.

Refeeding syndrome is a constellation of metabolic and clinical changes that may occur in malnourished patients during renourishment. The hallmark finding is hypophosphatemia (option A is correct) resulting from depleted whole-body stores of phosphate in starvation coupled with intracellular movement of phosphate for anabolic processes as refeeding is initiated. Refeeding can also be associated with hypoglycemia (option B is incorrect), which is thought to be related to depleted glycogen stores and increased insulin release, resulting in unpredictable blood glucose fluctuations. Congestive heart failure following intravenous hydration is especially a risk in older patients with chronic AN, who may have an occult starvation-related cardiomyopathy. Echocardiography is indicated to assess cardiac function in these cases or those that progress to severe edema. Edema is also common in patients with a history of laxative or diuretic abuse and results from activation of the renin–aldosterone system due to persistent fluid losses leading to fluid retention and edema when diuretic or laxative use is abruptly interrupted following hospitalization (Roerig et al. 2010) (option C is incorrect). Finally, it is important to note that refeeding syndrome is most common with parenteral or enteral feeding (option D is incorrect). Meal-based oral refeeding should therefore be prioritized whenever possible, in order to both minimize the risk of refeeding complications and help patients overcome anxiety about consuming a variety of foods of differing calorie densities in regular meals. **Chapter 13 (p. 358)**

13.11 Which of the following patient populations has been shown to benefit from outpatient interventions designed for weight restoration and symptom remission in medically stable patients diagnosed with AN?

A. Acutely ill patients.
B. Chronic cases.
C. Adults rather than adolescents.
D. Only inpatient treatments are indicated for patients with AN.

The correct response is option A: Acutely ill patients.

Outpatient interventions for AN are more effective at achieving weight restoration and symptom remission in adolescents than in adults (option C is incorrect) and for acutely ill patients (option A is correct) as opposed to chronic and severe cases (option B is incorrect). Inpatient treatment is indicated when patients are medically unstable or fail to gain weight (option D is incorrect). **Chapter 13 (p. 360)**

13.12 What medication is approved by the U.S. Food and Drug Administration (FDA) for the treatment of BN?

A. Topiramate.
B. Fluoxetine.
C. Ondansetron.
D. Bupropion.

The correct response is option B: Fluoxetine.

Fluoxetine is the only FDA-approved medication for BN (option B is correct). Although bupropion was found to be effective in reducing the frequency of bingeing and purging, it was associated with an increased risk of generalized tonic-clonic seizures, and its use is contraindicated in patients with BN (Horne et al. 1988; option D is incorrect). Among anticonvulsants studied in BN, topiramate seems to be the most effective in reducing the frequency of bingeing and purging and in decreasing food preoccupation and body weight. However, topiramate is not FDA approved for the treatment of BN (option A is incorrect). In one randomized controlled trial in patients with severe BN who had been engaging in binge-purge episodes at least seven times per week over a 6-month period, ondansetron, a selective antagonist of the type-3 serotonin receptor (5-HT3), was associated with a significant decrease in binge eating and vomiting and with normalization of eating behaviors and satiety cues, likely through its pharmacological effect on vagal nerve neurotransmission (Faris et al. 2000). However, ondansetron is not FDA approved for the treatment of BN (option C is incorrect). **Chapter 13 (pp. 363–364)**

13.13 A consultation-liaison psychiatrist is asked to evaluate a patient hospitalized after a syncopal episode, who was found to have a low BMI. The patient is a 20-year-old woman who presents with recent significant weight loss, persistent food intake restriction, and intense fear of gaining weight. She reluctantly admits to occasional laxative use in order to maintain low weight. The patient does not believe that she has an eating disorder despite her hospitalization in the setting of a syncopal episode due to prolonged starvation. After discussing the patient's diagnosis, the psychiatrist is considering pharmacological interventions. Which of the following is correct regarding pharmacological agents approved for the treatment of a diagnosis of AN?

A. To date, no pharmacological agent is approved for the treatment of AN.
B. Fluoxetine has been FDA approved for the treatment of AN.
C. Chlorpromazine has been FDA approved for the treatment of AN.
D. Alprazolam has been FDA approved for the treatment of AN.

The correct response is option A: To date, no pharmacological agent is approved for the treatment of AN.

This patient meets criteria for AN. The three primary features of AN in DSM-5 are 1) persistent food intake restriction and low body weight, 2) either intense fear of gaining weight or behavior that interferes with weight gain, and 3) either disturbance in self-perceived weight or shape or persistent lack of recognition of the seriousness of being in a starved state. To date, no pharmacological agent is approved for the treatment of AN (option A is correct). Fluoxetine has been studied in the treatment of AN primarily because of its known benefit in the treatment of BN, but it has shown no advantage over placebo (Attia et al. 1998; Barbarich et al. 2004; Ferguson et al. 1999; option B is incorrect). Chlorpromazine was the first antipsychotic to be studied in AN. Although patients showed initial weight gain and had shorter lengths of hospital stay, the side effect of seizures precluded its further use (Dally and Sargant 1960; option C is incorrect). Although benzodiazepines are frequently prescribed clinically for meal-related anxiety, a small randomized controlled trial of alprazolam in inpatients with AN demonstrated no effect on anxiety, food intake, or weight (Steinglass et al. 2014; option D is incorrect). **Chapter 13 (pp. 344, 362)**

13.14 Which of the following eating disorders meets all the criteria for AN except for low weight?

A. Night eating syndrome.
B. BED.
C. ARFID.
D. Atypical AN.

The correct response is option D: Atypical AN.

The three primary features of AN in DSM-5 are 1) persistent food intake restriction and low body weight, 2) either intense fear of gaining weight or behavior that interferes with weight gain, and 3) either disturbance in self-perceived weight or shape or persistent lack of recognition of the seriousness of being in a starved state. Low weight is defined as less than minimally normal or less than minimally expected in children and adolescents based on their weight trajectory (Call et al. 2013). Atypical AN is a syndrome that meets all of the criteria for AN, except low weight (option D is correct). The diagnostic category of ARFID captures children, adolescents, and adults with severe food restriction or avoidance and significant weight loss or compromised growth and nutritional deficiencies who do not exhibit fear of weight gain, body image disturbance, or drive for thinness (option C is incorrect). BED is one of the most common psychiatric diagnoses in morbidly obese individuals (option B is incorrect). BED is characterized by recurrent weekly binge-eating episodes, accompanied by a sense of loss of control over eating, that extend over a period of 3 months or more. This is in stark contrast to food intake restriction that characterizes AN. Night eating syndrome is defined as a circadian disturbance in both sleep-wake cycles and meal consumption, with excess calorie intake at night, often upon awakening from sleep, that is outside cultural norms and causes impairment of function (option A is incorrect). **Chapter 13 (pp. 343–346)**

References

American Psychiatric Association: Diagnostic and Statistical Manual of Mental Disorders, 5th Edition. Arlington, VA, American Psychiatric Association, 2013

Attia E, Haiman C, Walsh BT, Flater SR: Does fluoxetine augment the inpatient treatment of anorexia nervosa? Am J Psychiatry 155(4):548–551, 1998 9546003

Barbarich NC, McConaha CW, Halmi KA, et al: Use of nutritional supplements to increase the efficacy of fluoxetine in the treatment of anorexia nervosa. Int J Eat Disord 35(1):10–15, 2004 14705152

Barnes RD, Boeka AG, McKenzie KC, et al: Metabolic syndrome in obese patients with binge eating disorder in primary care clinics: a cross-sectional study. Prim Care Companion CNS Disord 13(2):pii, 2011

Bischoff-Grethe A, McCurdy D, Grenesko-Stevens E, et al: Altered brain response to reward and punishment in adolescents with anorexia nervosa. Psychiatry Res 214(3):331–340, 2013 24148909

Call C, Walsh BT, Attia E: From DSM-IV to DSM-5: changes to eating disorder diagnoses. Curr Opin Psychiatry 26(6):532–536, 2013 24064412

Cha J, Ide JS, Bowman FD, et al: Abnormal reward circuitry in anorexia nervosa: a longitudinal, multimodal MRI study. Hum Brain Mapp 37(11):3835–3846, 2016 27273474

Dally PJ, Sargant W: A new treatment of anorexia nervosa. BMJ 1(5188):1770–1773, 1960 13813846

Davis C, Blackmore E, Katzman DK, Fox J: Female adolescents with anorexia nervosa and their parents: a case-control study of exercise attitudes and behaviours. Psychol Med 35(3):377–386, 2005 15841873

Dawes AJ, Maggard-Gibbons M, Maher AR, et al: Mental health conditions among patients seeking and undergoing bariatric surgery: a meta-analysis. JAMA 315(2):150–163, 2016 26757464

Evans EH, Adamson AJ, Basterfield L, et al: Risk factors for eating disorder symptoms at 12 years of age: a 6-year longitudinal cohort study. Appetite 108:12–20, 2017 27612559

Faris PL, Kim SW, Meller WH, et al: Effect of decreasing afferent vagal activity with ondansetron on symptoms of bulimia nervosa: a randomised, double-blind trial. Lancet 355(9206):792–797, 2000 10711927

Ferguson CP, La Via MC, Crossan PJ, Kaye WH: Are serotonin selective reuptake inhibitors effective in underweight anorexia nervosa? Int J Eat Disord 25(1):11–17, 1999 9924648

Foerde K, Steinglass JE, Shohamy D, Walsh BT: Neural mechanisms supporting maladaptive food choices in anorexia nervosa. Nat Neurosci 18(11):1571–1573, 2015 26457555

Goldschmidt AB, Wall MM, Loth KA, Neumark-Sztainer D: Risk factors for disordered eating in overweight adolescents and young adults. J Pediatr Psychol 40(10):1048–1055, 2015 26050243

Guerdjikova AI, Mori N, Casuto LS, McElroy SL: Binge eating disorder. Psychiatr Clin North Am 40(2):255–266, 2017 28477651

Guillaume S, Gorwood P, Jollant F, et al: Impaired decision-making in symptomatic anorexia and bulimia nervosa patients: a meta-analysis. Psychol Med 45(16):3377–3391, 2015 26497047

Horne RL, Ferguson JM, Pope HG Jr, et al: Treatment of bulimia with bupropion: a multicenter controlled trial. J Clin Psychiatry 49(7):262–266, 1988 3134343

Hudson JI, Hiripi E, Pope HG Jr, Kessler RC: The prevalence and correlates of eating disorders in the National Comorbidity Survey Replication. Biol Psychiatry 61(3):348–358, 2007 16815322

Monteleone AM, Monteleone P, Esposito F, et al: Altered processing of rewarding and aversive basic taste stimuli in symptomatic women with anorexia nervosa and bulimia nervosa: an fMRI study. J Psychiatr Res 90:94–101, 2017 28249187

Monteleone P, Castaldo E, Maj M: Neuroendocrine dysregulation of food intake in eating disorders. Regul Pept 149(1-3):39–50, 2008 18582958

Munn-Chernoff MA, Baker JH: A primer on the genetics of comorbid eating disorders and substance use disorders. Eur Eat Disord Rev 24(2):91–100, 2016 26663753

Peveler RC, Bryden KS, Neil HA, et al: The relationship of disordered eating habits and attitudes to clinical outcomes in young adult females with type 1 diabetes. Diabetes Care 28(1):84–88, 2005 15616238

Pinhas-Hamiel O, Hamiel U, Levy-Shraga Y: Eating disorders in adolescents with type 1 diabetes: challenges in diagnosis and treatment. World J Diabetes 6(3):517–526, 2015 25897361

Rich LM, Caine MR, Findling JW, Shaker JL: Hypoglycemic coma in anorexia nervosa. Case report and review of the literature. Arch Intern Med 150(4):894–895, 1990 2183736

Roerig JL, Steffen KJ, Mitchell JE, et al: Laxative abuse: epidemiology, diagnosis and management. Drugs 70(12):1487–1503, 2010 20687617

Rohde P, Stice E, Marti CN: Development and predictive effects of eating disorder risk factors during adolescence: implications for prevention efforts. Int J Eat Disord 48(2):187–198, 2015 24599841

Scheuing N, Bartus B, Berger G, et al; DPV Initiative; German BMBF Competence Network Diabetes Mellitus: Clinical characteristics and outcome of 467 patients with a clinically recognized eating disorder identified among 52,215 patients with type 1 diabetes: a multicenter German/Austrian study. Diabetes Care 37(6):1581–1589, 2014 24623022

Steinglass JE, Kaplan SC, Liu Y, et al: The (lack of) effect of alprazolam on eating behavior in anorexia nervosa: a preliminary report. Int J Eat Disord 47(8):901–904, 2014 25139178

Williams PM, Goodie J, Motsinger CD: Treating eating disorders in primary care. Am Fam Physician 77(2):187–195, 2008 18246888

Winston AP: Management of physical aspects and complications of eating disorders. Psychiatry 7(4):174–178, 2008

C H A P T E R   1 4

Sleep Disorders

14.1   What characterizes rapid eye movement (REM) sleep?

A. Three distinct stages.
B. Decreased levels of cortical activation.
C. Reduced muscle tone.
D. Spindles and K complexes.

The correct response is option C: Reduced muscle tone.

Sleep can be subdivided into two major components: REM sleep, which is characterized by increased levels of cortical activation accompanied by reduced muscle tone to prevent corresponding movements, and non–rapid eye movement (NREM) sleep, which is separated into three distinct stages (option C is correct; options A and B are incorrect). Sleep spindles and K complexes are used to identify stage N2 NREM sleep (option D is incorrect). **Chapter 14 (pp. 377–378)**

14.2   Which of the following conditions is most likely to cause insomnia?

A. Hyperglycemia.
B. Hypothyroidism.
C. Psychostimulant withdrawal.
D. Gastrointestinal reflux.

The correct response is option D: Gastrointestinal reflux.

Causes of insomnia include primarily medical conditions, such as obstructive sleep apnea hypopnea (OSAH), chronic obstructive pulmonary disease, asthma, gastrointestinal reflux, angina, hypoglycemia, hyperthyroidism, and pain (option D is correct; options A and B are incorrect). Insomnia can also be caused by primarily psychiatric conditions, such as anxiety and mood disorders. It can be induced by medications, such as xanthines and psychostimulants (option C is incorrect). **Chapter 14 (Table 14–3, p. 381)**

14.3   For which sleep disorder is a portable sleep study appropriate?

   A. Obstructive sleep apnea hypopnea (OSAH).
   B. Central sleep apnea.
   C. Restless leg syndrome.
   D. Fatal familial insomnia.

The correct response is option A: Obstructive sleep apnea hypopnea (OSAH).

Until recently, most sleep studies were conducted in facilities using computerized equipment that monitor and store the multiple physiological measurements that compose a polysomnographic study (Table 14–6). Trained technologists attend the patient during the study, making adjustments or intervening as needed. Today, a variety of portable devices are increasingly in use for patients suspected to be at high risk of OSAH (Claman and Sunwoo 2017) (option A is correct). When the differential diagnosis includes sleep disorders other than obstructive sleep apnea or when a patient sleeps poorly, portable studies have not been demonstrated to be as reliable (options B, C, and D are incorrect). In these cases, the sleep study may need to be repeated in a laboratory setting. **Chapter 14 (p. 382; Table 14–6, p. 384)**

14.4   What is the most important part of an evaluation for narcolepsy?

   A. Decreased cerebrospinal fluid (CSF) hypocretin levels.
   B. Clinical interview.
   C. Presence of deep-tendon reflexes during cataplexy episode.
   D. Negative wrist actigraphy.

The correct response is option B: Clinical interview.

The most important part of an evaluation for narcolepsy is a careful interview to screen for long-standing excessive daytime sleepiness and spells triggered by emotions (option B is correct). The definitive bedside test for cataplexy is demonstrating the transient absence of deep-tendon reflexes during the episode (Krahn et al. 2000). This procedure also aids in differentiating cataplexy from pseudocataplexy (Krahn et al. 2001). However, cataplexy is difficult to provoke, and the episode is often too brief to allow for a physical exam (option C is incorrect). A polysomnogram is important for ruling out other causes of excessive daytime sleepiness. This study is ideally preceded by wrist actigraphy to confirm adequate sleep in the weeks before testing in order to eliminate sleep deprivation as the cause (option D is incorrect). Hypocretin testing in the CSF is not yet clinically available (option A is incorrect). **Chapter 14 (p. 386)**

14.5   What is the cardinal feature of hypersomnolence disorder?

   A. Sleep-onset REM episodes.
   B. Undetectable CSF hypocretin levels.

C. Excessive daytime sleepiness.

D. Short duration of nocturnal sleep.

The correct response is option C: Excessive daytime sleepiness.

Hypersomnolence disorder is a disorder of unknown etiology characterized by excessive daytime sleepiness in the absence of other specific symptoms (American Academy of Sleep Medicine 2014; American Psychiatric Association 2013) (option C is correct). Patients typically have a prolonged duration of nocturnal sleep and unrefreshing daytime naps (option D is incorrect). Unlike patients with narcolepsy, those with hypersomnolence disorder have no sleep-onset REM episodes and have normal levels of hypocretin in the CSF (options A and B are incorrect). **Chapter 14 (pp. 387–388)**

14.6   Which of the following is a risk factor for REM sleep behavior disorder?

A. Selective serotonin reuptake inhibitors (SSRIs).

B. Female gender.

C. Childhood age.

D. Alzheimer's dementia.

The correct response is option A: Selective serotonin reuptake inhibitors (SSRIs).

Patients with REM sleep behavior disorder appear to "act out their dreams" by yelling or gesturing during REM sleep (American Academy of Sleep Medicine 2014; American Psychiatric Association 2013). They lack the muscle atonia normally found in REM sleep and move in response to dream imagery. Risk factors for this sleep disorder are male sex (90% of patients described in the literature) and advanced age (most patients are age 50 or older) (Schenck 2016) (options B and C are incorrect). SSRIs and serotonin-norepinephrine reuptake inhibitors have been suggested as possible triggers (option A is correct). REM sleep behavior disorder is associated with several neurological disorders, including Parkinson's disease (15%–33% of patients), multiple system atrophy (69%–90%), and dementia with Lewy bodies (50%–80%) (option D is incorrect). **Chapter 14 (p. 388)**

14.7   Which of the following sleep disorders is treated with behavioral techniques, such as relaxation and exposure?

A. Non–rapid eye movement (NREM) sleep behavior disorder.

B. Hypersomnolence disorder.

C. Narcolepsy.

D. Nightmare disorder.

The correct response is option D: Nightmare disorder.

Treatment of NREM sleep arousal disorders includes modifying the sleeping environment to promote safety, adhering to a consistent sleep schedule, reducing nocturnal awakenings, and, if warranted, using medications such as hypnotics to prevent arousal (Pilon et al. 2008) (option A is incorrect).

There is less agreement regarding treatment of hypersomnolence disorder than that of other sleep disorders. Patient education regarding adequate sleep is critical. A common strategy is initially to request patients to extend sleep time by at least an hour, with the intent to aid patients whose sleepiness may be related to inadequate nocturnal sleep. Apart from sleep extension, treatment is otherwise similar to that for narcolepsy. In contrast to narcolepsy, however, daytime naps are not encouraged in hypersomnolence disorder because they are not refreshing (option B is incorrect).

Patient education should emphasize the importance of a consistent sleep-wake schedule, the need for adequate sleep, the value of brief daytime naps, and refraining from driving a car when sleepy. Pharmacological options for narcolepsy include methylphenidate or amphetamines. Modafinil and its R-enantiomer armodafinil are wake-promoting medications approved by the U.S. Food and Drug Administration (FDA) for the treatment of narcolepsy (option C is incorrect).

In DSM-5 (American Psychiatric Association 2013), the "Parasomnia" section includes nightmare disorder. Treatment includes behavioral techniques such as exposure, relaxation, and rescripting therapy in which the upsetting content is reframed (Pruiksma et al. 2016) (option D is correct). **Chapter 14 (pp. 387–389)**

14.8   What is an appropriate treatment for an obese patient with OSAH unable to tolerate continuous positive airway pressure (CPAP)?

A. Bilevel positive airway pressure.
B. Supplemental oxygen.
C. Tonsillectomy.
D. A 10-pound weight loss.

The correct response is option A: Bilevel positive airway pressure.

Another treatment of OSAH is bilevel positive airway pressure. This therapy represents a modification of CPAP whereby the positive pressure fluctuates depending on whether the airflow is inspiratory or expiratory. Bilevel pressure therapy is considerably more expensive than conventional CPAP and is reserved for patients who cannot tolerate CPAP (option A is correct). Supplemental oxygen alone is inadequate for OSAH because the oxygen cannot pass through the obstruction to reach the lungs (option B is incorrect). Weight loss through diet and exercise is a critical component of the treatment plan for any overweight patient with breathing-related sleep disorder (Koo et al. 2017). In general, a 20-pound weight loss can reduce the required CPAP pressure; however, many patients gain rather than lose weight, with the result that CPAP pressure needs to be increased (option D is incorrect). Patients with abnormalities of the soft tissue or skeletal structures surrounding the upper airway may consider surgery. Surgical procedures include laser-assisted uvulo-palato-pharyngoplasty, tonsillectomy, mandibular advancement, tracheostomy, and neuromuscular electrical stimulation of the hypoglossal nerve. Patients must be carefully selected. They must have upper airway obstructions that are resectable (e.g., large tonsils) and have no other comorbid conditions (e.g., a high body mass index that compromises upper airway patency at multiple points) (option C is incorrect). **Chapter 14 (pp. 392–393)**

14.9   How does central sleep apnea differ from OSAH?

A. Central sleep apnea is characterized by respiratory pauses with airway collapse.
B. Patient's airway is narrowed in central sleep apnea.
C. Patients with central sleep apnea present with insomnia.
D. Snoring is a typical warning sign in central sleep apnea.

The correct response is option C: Patients with central sleep apnea present with insomnia.

Central sleep apnea, a condition in which patients have respiratory pauses without any airway collapse, is more likely to be asymptomatic than is OSAH (option A is incorrect). Because the patient's airway is not narrowed and vibrating, snoring is not a typical warning sign (options B and D are incorrect). Patients often present with insomnia rather than excessive daytime sleepiness (option C is correct). Central sleep apnea can be differentiated from OSAH through the absence of snoring, this differentiation being confirmed by the presence of polysomnographic features of apnea (Quaranta et al. 1997). **Chapter 14 (p. 393)**

14.10 What is the treatment of choice for restless leg syndrome (RLS)?

A. Clonazepam.
B. Gabapentin.
C. Pramipexole.
D. Methadone.

The correct response is option B: Gabapentin.

Treatment of RLS primarily involves dopaminergic medications. Gabapentin has recently been recognized as the preferred agent for treatment of RLS because of its effectiveness and tolerability (Winkelman et al. 2016) (option B is correct). Initiation of dopamine receptor direct agonists, such as pramipexole and ropinirole, should be considered with caution because of the risk of exacerbating restless legs by augmenting the symptoms as well as triggering behaviors such as compulsive gambling (Garcia-Borreguero et al. 2016) (option C is incorrect). Long-acting benzodiazepines, such as clonazepam, and opioids, including codeine and methadone, also have been used, but they can lead to physical dependence. As a result, these drugs are not preferred treatment choices (options A and D are incorrect). **Chapter 14 (p. 395)**

References

American Academy of Sleep Medicine: International Classification of Sleep Disorders, 3rd Edition. Westchester, IL, American Academy of Sleep Medicine, 2014

American Psychiatric Association: Diagnostic and Statistical Manual of Mental Disorders, 5th Edition. Arlington, VA, American Psychiatric Association, 2013

Claman D, Sunwoo B: Improving accuracy of home sleep apnea testing. J Clin Sleep Med 13(1):9–10, 2017 27998372

Garcia-Borreguero D, Silber MH, Winkelman JW, et al: Guidelines for the first-line treatment of restless legs syndrome/Willis-Ekbom disease, prevention and treatment of dopaminergic augmentation: a combined task force of the IRLSSG, EURLSSG, and the RLS-foundation. Sleep Med 21:1–11, 2016 27448465

Koo SK, Kwon SB, Kim YJ, et al: Acoustic analysis of snoring sounds recorded with a smartphone according to obstruction site in OSAS patients. Eur Arch Otorhinolaryngol 274(3):1735–1740, 2017 27709292

Krahn LE, Boeve BF, Olson EJ, et al: A standardized test for cataplexy. Sleep Med 1(2):125–130, 2000 10767653

Krahn LE, Hansen MR, Shepard JW: Pseudocataplexy. Psychosomatics 42(4):356–358, 2001 11496028

Pilon M, Montplaisir J, Zadra A: Precipitating factors of somnambulism: impact of sleep deprivation and forced arousals. Neurology 70(24):2284–2290, 2008 18463368

Pruiksma KE, Cranston CC, Rhudy JL, et al: Randomized controlled trial to dismantle exposure, relaxation and rescripting therapy (ERRT) for trauma-related nightmares. Psychol Trauma 8:335–355, 2016 27977223

Quaranta AJ, D'Alonzo GE, Krachman SL: Cheyne-Stokes respiration during sleep in congestive heart failure. Chest 111(2):467–473, 1997 9041998

Schenck CH: Expanded insights into idiopathic REM sleep behavior disorder. Sleep (Basel) 39(1):7–9, 2016 26564130

Winkelman JW, Armstrong MJ, Allen RP, et al: Practice guideline summary: Treatment of restless legs syndrome in adults: Report of the Guideline Development, Dissemination, and Implementation Subcommittee of the American Academy of Neurology. Neurology 87(24):2585–2593, 2016 27856776

CHAPTER 15

Sexual Dysfunctions

15.1 What type of therapy for sexual dysfunction includes sensate focus therapy?

    A. Mindfulness-based cognitive therapy.
    B. Sex therapy.
    C. Hypnotherapy.
    D. Cognitive-behavioral therapy (CBT).

The correct response is option B: Sex therapy.

Standard therapies for sexual dysfunction include psychoeducation, CBT, mindfulness-based cognitive therapy, and sex therapy. The latter usually involves sensate focus therapy (option B is correct), whereby each partner is encouraged to take turns giving or receiving sensual and later sexual touches, caresses, and kisses. Initially, genital areas and breasts are off limits. Past goals and expectations are put aside. Encouragement to stay in the moment is needed. Couples plan 15- to 20-minute sessions two to three times per week for 3–4 weeks. The clinician guides as to when breast and genital areas are included and when ultimately intercourse (if still possible) is also "on the menu."

Mindfulness, although practiced for some 3,500 years, is a new addition to therapy for sexual dysfunction (Mize 2015). Early studies show benefit for sexual dysfunction in health and after pelvic cancer (Brotto et al. 2008a, 2008b) (option A is incorrect). CBT can be very helpful in challenging a distorted self-view or catastrophic thinking from the changes imposed by the illness (option D is incorrect). Chronically unwell persons may view their sexual disability as so unattractive to their partner that they do not deserve care and attention. Some may even stay in a relationship in which they experience emotional, physical, or sexual abuse.

Hypnotherapy involves the induction of a hypnotic trance using progressive relaxation and other induction procedures to deepen the hypnotic state. This is followed by suggestions, imagery, and other individualized techniques directed toward control and improvement of bodily function or pain (option C is incorrect). **Chapter 15 (p. 411), Chapter 37 (p. 1264)**

15.2   Which of the following disease categories is considered high risk and would defer sexual dysfunction treatment?

A. Moderate or severe valve disease.
B. Stable angina.
C. History of uncomplicated myocardial infarction (MI).
D. Left ventricular dysfunction/congestive heart failure (LVD/CHF) (New York Heart Association [NYHA] Class II).

The correct response is option A: Moderate or severe valve disease.

Cardiac conditions that are high risk and require stabilization prior to sexual dysfunction treatment include unstable refractory angina, uncontrolled hypertension, LVD/CHF (NYHA Class III/IV), recent MI (<2 weeks), cerebrovascular accident, high-risk arrhythmias, moderate or severe valve disease (option A is correct), hypertrophic obstructive, and other cardiomyopathies.

Intermediate risk cardiac conditions should be evaluated by a cardiologist prior to initiation of any therapy for erectile dysfunction (ED) because of risk of myocardial ischemia during sexual activity and orgasm. Intermediate risk conditions include three or more risk factors for coronary artery disease excluding gender, moderate stable angina (option B is incorrect), recent MI (>2, <6 weeks), LVD/CHF (NYHA Class II) (option D is incorrect), and noncardiac sequelae of atherosclerotic disease (e.g., cerebrovascular accident, peripheral vascular disease).

Low-risk cardiac conditions can be managed by primary care providers, and all first-line sexual dysfunction treatment should be considered and reassessed at regular intervals (6–12 months). Low-risk cardiac categories include asymptomatic, fewer than three major risk factors for coronary artery disease, excluding gender and age; controlled hypertension; mild stable angina (option B is incorrect); after successful coronary revascularization; uncomplicated past MI (>6–8 weeks) (option C is incorrect); mild valve disease; and LVD/CHF (NYHA Class I). **Chapter 15 (Table 15–5, p. 415)**

15.3   Which of the following medications would be safe to use with vardenafil?

A. Cimetidine.
B. Amiodarone.
C. Nitroglycerin.
D. Sertraline.

The correct response is option D: Sertraline.

The phosphodiesterase type 5 (PDE-5) inhibitors can be used in men with cardiac disease provided that there is no risk of hypotension from concomitant prescription of nitrates or nonselective alpha-adrenergic blockers (option C is incorrect). Inhibitors of cytochrome P450 (CYP) 3A4 (e.g., cimetidine, efavirenz, erythromycin, ketoconazole, itraconazole, ritonavir) can significantly decrease metabolism of PDE-5 inhibitors to cause unwanted accumulation (option A is incorrect). Vardenafil may prolong the duration of ST depression; the clinical significance of this is unclear. Vardenafil should not be prescribed to persons with the long QT syndrome, nor should it be prescribed to persons taking quinidine, procainamide, amiodarone (option B is incorrect), or sotalol because of further increase in the QT interval.

More than 50% of patients with coronary artery disease are depressed. The mutually reinforcing triad of depression, ischemic heart disease, and ED (Goldstein 2000) should encourage screening for the other two conditions if one is present. Sildenafil can improve sexual function in depression in men with heart failure (Freitas et al. 2006). Antidepressant-induced ED can be ameliorated with PDE-5 inhibitors (Nurnberg et al. 2007) (option D is correct). **Chapter 15 (p. 414)**

15.4   What is a predictor of sexual dysfunction in patients with rheumatic disease?

A. Genital tissue changes.
B. Impaired mobility.
C. Comorbid anxiety disorder.
D. Pain.

The correct response is option C: Comorbid anxiety disorder.

The sexual lives of men and women with rheumatic disease are frequently negatively affected by pain, debility, loss of mobility, comorbid depression, and genital tissue changes in some of the disorders. In a study examining 509 consecutive patients (men and women) with rheumatic disease, depression and anxiety were identified as the only predictors of sexual dysfunction, and this association remained even after adjustment for physical factors (Anyfanti et al. 2014) (option C is correct; options A, B, and D are incorrect). **Chapter 15 (p. 416)**

15.5   The treatment of which neurological condition puts male patients at risk for hypersexuality?

A. Seizure disorder.
B. Stroke.
C. Spinal cord injury.
D. Parkinson's disease.

The correct response is option D: Parkinson's disease.

No clear relation has been found between the site of stroke or the duration of coma and the degree of sexual impairment (Boller et al. 2015). In some studies, close to 60% of stroke patients report sexual dysfunction. When their sexual partners are also assessed, a similar number report also having sexual dysfunction subsequent to all the changes in both of their lives, medical and psychological, since the partner's stroke (Boller et al. 2015). The most common dysfunctions are low desire, ED, premature or delayed ejaculation, and dyspareunia secondary to loss of lubrication. Antidepressant and antipsychotic medications can further add to the incidence of low desire and delayed/absent orgasm (option B is incorrect).

Dopamine agonist drugs may increase sexual function and motivation through direct stimulation of the dopamine type 2 (D_2) receptors in the medial preoptic area and may also facilitate erections by inhibiting prolactin production and increasing oxytocin activity at the lumbosacral spinal cord. These effects help to explain why dopaminergic therapy may allow resumption of sexual activity in some patients with Parkinson's disease but may lead to hypersexuality in others (option D is correct).

With strong stimulation (vibrator), many men with lesions above the lumbosacral level can ejaculate. This may occur extremely quickly, and the ability to delay ejaculation, if desired, may not be present (Courtois and Charvier 2015). Reflex ejaculation is accompanied by cardiac, muscle, and autonomic sensations similar to orgasm and similar to autonomic hyperreflexia. This hyperreflexia generally affects patients with lesions above T6 because signals to inhibit sympathetic outflow are interrupted. Sustained genital stimulation, whether sexual or painful, travels through the somatic and visceral afferents to the thoracic segments of the spinal cord and can reflexively trigger sudden generalized vasoconstriction, thereby increasing blood pressure. There may be a pounding headache, flushing of the neck and face, increased skin temperature, and even blurred vision. Hypotensive treatment may be necessary; nifedipine is the usual choice, although it is not ideal (Courtois et al. 2012) (option C is incorrect).

Treatment of seizure disorders with enzyme-inducing antiepileptic drugs increases the level of sex hormone–binding globulin by an unknown mechanism. Although the total (free plus bound) serum concentration of testosterone is generally unchanged by these anticonvulsants, the increase in sex hormone–binding globulin raises the proportion of bound testosterone and reduces the level of free or bioavailable testosterone. These older antiepileptic drugs impair male sexuality, but data on women are inconclusive (option A is incorrect). The CYP enzyme-inhibiting antiepileptic drug valproic acid may increase the serum androgen levels and estradiol level in both men and women. **Chapter 15 (pp. 417–418, 420–421)**

15.6   Erectile dysfunction (ED) in a patient with uncomplicated type 2 diabetes could be an indicator of which of the following conditions?

A. Cardiac ischemia.
B. Neuropathy.
C. Hypertension.
D. Hypoglycemia.

The correct response is option A: Cardiac ischemia.

In uncomplicated type 2 diabetes without other risk factors for coronary artery disease, ED can signal silent cardiac ischemia (Gazzaruso et al. 2004) (option A is correct), yet some 63% of diabetic patients report never having been questioned about sexual dysfunction (Peak et al. 2016). Etiologies of diabetes-induced ED are multifactorial and can include endothelial and smooth muscle dysfunction, autonomic and somatic neuropathy, and interpersonal or psychological issues. Men with both diabetes and ED tend to have a history of poor metabolic control, untreated hypertension, peripheral neuropathy, microalbuminuria and macroalbuminuria, retinopathy, cardiovascular disease, diuretic treatment, obesity-related testosterone decline, and psychological vulnerability (options B, C, and D are incorrect) (Bhasin et al. 2007). **Chapter 15 (p. 422)**

15.7 Which of the following anticonvulsants has the lowest profile of sexual side effects in men?

A. Lamotrigine.
B. Carbamazepine.
C. Phenytoin.
D. Barbiturates.

The correct response is option A: Lamotrigine.

Enzyme-inducing antiepileptic drugs, including phenytoin, barbiturates, and carbamazepine (but not oxcarbazepine), increase the level of sex hormone–binding globulin by an unknown mechanism. Although the total (free plus bound) serum concentration of testosterone is generally unchanged by these anticonvulsants, the increase in sex hormone–binding globulin raises the proportion of bound testosterone and reduces the level of free or bioavailable testosterone. These older antiepileptic drugs impair male sexuality (options B, C, and D are incorrect), but data on women are inconclusive. The CYP enzyme-*inhibiting* antiepileptic drug valproic acid may increase serum androgen levels and estradiol level in both men and women. At least in theory, enzyme-*neutral* antiepileptic drugs are less likely to cause sexual side effects. The latter include oxcarbazepine, gabapentin, pregabalin, levetiracetam, and lamotrigine. Some evidence indicates that lamotrigine has the lowest profile of sexual side effects (Devinsky 2005) (option A is correct). **Chapter 15 (p. 421)**

15.8 Which of the following factors is directly involved in sexual dysfunction associated with chronic disease?

A. Reduction of self-image.
B. Fear of sexual activity worsening medical condition.
C. Disruption of sexual desire and response because of nonhormonal medications.
D. Partnership difficulties.

The correct response is option C: Disruption of sexual desire and response because of nonhormonal medications.

Chronic medical illness can affect sexual function both directly and indirectly. Disease-related interruption of the neurovascular pathways and the hormonal milieu may not be the major determinant of dissatisfaction. Direct effects of chronic medical illness include disruption of sexual desire and response because of nonhormonal medications (option C is correct). Indirect impacts on sexual function include reduction of self-image, fear of sexual activity worsening medical condition, and partnership difficulties (options A, B, and D are incorrect). **Chapter 15 (p. 405; Table 15–1, pp. 406–407)**

15.9   Which of the following has evidence to support its use in reversing ejaculatory dysfunction?

A. Improving glycemic control.
B. Narcotics.
C. Anabolic steroids.
D. Diuretics.

The correct response is option A: Improving glycemic control.

Narcotics have been shown to cause low desire in men via suppression of GnRH; there is limited evidence in women (option B is incorrect). Chronic use of anabolic steroids is associated with low desire, ED, anejaculation, and testicular atrophy (option C is incorrect). ED has been seen in diuretic treatment with thiazides, chlorthalidone, and spironolactone (Düsing 2005) (option D is incorrect). Improving glycemic control may reverse ejaculatory dysfunction. In men, poor glycemic control and diabetic complications are the main predictors of sexual dysfunction (option A is correct). **Chapter 15 (Table 15–4, pp. 412–413; p. 422)**

15.10 Which of the following combinations are predictors of sexual dysfunction in diabetes?

A. Depression and being married, in women.
B. Depression and being married, in men.
C. Depression and poor glycemic control, in women.
D. Depression and poor glycemic control, in men.

The correct response is option A: Depression and being married, in women.

A meta-analysis of 26 studies found an increased risk of sexual dysfunction in women with diabetes (odds ratio=2.27 and 2.49 for type 1 and 2, respectively) compared with the healthy women control subjects (Pontiroli et al. 2013). Meta-regression indicated that sexual dysfunction may be related to increased body weight. In some but not all series, reduced lubrication from hyperglycemia-induced vaginal mucosal dehydration, dyspareunia, orgasmic difficulty, and sexual dissatisfaction were about twice as common in women with diabetes compared with control subjects. Of note, both in studies limited to type 1 or to type 2 and in prospective studies (Enzlin et al. 2009), the only predictors of sexual dysfunction in women were having depression and being married (option A is correct; option C is incorrect). This finding is in marked contrast to findings in men, in whom poor glycemic control and diabetic complications are the main predictors of sexual dysfunction (options B and D are incorrect). **Chapter 15 (p. 422)**

References

Anyfanti P, Pyrpasopoulou A, Triantafyllou A, et al: Association between mental health disorders and sexual dysfunction in patients suffering from rheumatic diseases. J Sex Med 11(11):2653–2660, 2014 25124339

Bhasin S, Enzlin P, Coviello A, Basson R: Sexual dysfunction in men and women with endocrine disorders. Lancet 369(9561):597–611, 2007 17307107

Boller F, Agrawal K, Romano A: Sexual function after strokes. Handb Clin Neurol 130:289–295, 2015 26003250

Brotto LA, Basson R, Luria M: A mindfulness-based group psychoeducational intervention targeting sexual arousal disorder in women. J Sex Med 5(7):1646–1659, 2008a 18507718

Brotto LA, Heiman JR, Goff B, et al: A psychoeducational intervention for sexual dysfunction in women with gynecologic cancer. Arch Sex Behav 37(2):317–329, 2008b 17680353

Courtois F, Charvier K: Sexual dysfunction in patients with spinal cord lesions. Handb Clin Neurol 130:225–245, 2015 26003247

Courtois F, Rodrigue X, Côté I, et al: Sexual function and autonomic dysreflexia in men with spinal cord injuries: how should we treat? Spinal Cord 50(12):869–877, 2012 22869221

Devinsky O: Neurologist-induced sexual dysfunction: enzyme-inducing antiepileptic drugs. Neurology 65(7):980–981, 2005 16217046

Düsing R: Sexual dysfunction in male patients with hypertension: influence of antihypertensive drugs. Drugs 65(6):773–786, 2005 15819590

Enzlin P, Rosen R, Wiegel M, et al; DCCT/EDIC Research Group: Sexual dysfunction in women with type 1 diabetes: long-term findings from the DCCT/ EDIC study cohort. Diabetes Care 32(5):780–785, 2009 19407075

Freitas D, Athanazio R, Almeida D, et al: Sildenafil improves quality of life in men with heart failure and erectile dysfunction. Int J Impot Res 18(2):210–212, 2006 16121207

Gazzaruso C, Giordanetti S, De Amici E, et al: Relationship between erectile dysfunction and silent myocardial ischemia in apparently uncomplicated type 2 diabetic patients. Circulation 110(1):22–26, 2004 15210604

Goldstein I: The mutually reinforcing triad of depressive symptoms, cardiovascular disease, and erectile dysfunction. Am J Cardiol 86(2A)(suppl):41F–45F, 2000 10899278

Mize SJS: A review of mindfulness-based sex therapy interventions for sexual desire and arousal difficulties: from research to practice. Curr Sex Health Rep 7(2):89–97, 2015, https://link.springer.com/article/10.1007/s11930-015-0048-8. Accessed May 28, 2017.

Nurnberg HG, Fava M, Gelenberg AJ, et al: Open-label sildenafil treatment of partial and non-responders to double-blind treatment in men with antidepressant-associated sexual dysfunction. Int J Impot Res 19(2):167–175, 2007 16871270

Peak TC, Gur S, Hellstrom WJG: Diabetes and sexual function. Curr Sex Health Rep 8(1):9–18, 2016, https://link.springer.com/article/10.1007/s11930-016-0065-2. Accessed May 28, 2017.

Pontiroli AE, Cortelazzi D, Morabito A: Female sexual dysfunction and diabetes: a systematic review and meta-analysis. J Sex Med 10(4):1044–1051, 2013 23347454

CHAPTER 16

Substance-Related Disorders

16.1   You are called to help manage severe alcohol withdrawal in a 64-year-old patient who is extremely agitated and aggressive. Which of the following is appropriate as a single-agent treatment for moderate to severe alcohol withdrawal?

A. Propranolol.
B. Phenobarbital.
C. Carbamazepine.
D. Clonidine.

The correct response is option B: Phenobarbital.

Pharmacotherapy is indicated for management of moderate to severe withdrawal, and any cross-tolerant medication may be used; both benzodiazepines and barbiturates effectively treat alcohol withdrawal (Mayo-Smith and American Society of Addiction Medicine Working Group on Pharmacological Management of Alcohol Withdrawal 1997). In the United States, alcohol withdrawal is most often managed with benzodiazepines, but barbiturates also have been used successfully to treat acute alcohol withdrawal syndrome in general medical inpatients, with phenobarbital the most common choice (option B is correct). Severe alcohol withdrawal that is refractory to high-dose benzodiazepines has been treated successfully with the addition of phenobarbital (Gold et al. 2007). The long half-life of phenobarbital provides some protection if the patient leaves the hospital prematurely. Phenobarbital is safe to use in patients with liver disease who are not at risk for hepatic encephalopathy; this is an advantage over most long-acting benzodiazepines (e.g., chlordiazepoxide, diazepam), which undergo extensive liver metabolism to additional active metabolites (Olkkola and Ahonen 2008). Beta-adrenergic blockers (atenolol, propranolol), clonidine, and anticonvulsant agents (carbamazepine, valproate) decrease alcohol withdrawal symptoms and have been used successfully in treatment of mild withdrawal. However, they are not cross-tolerant with alcohol and may result in progression of the withdrawal syndrome. These alternative medications are not appropriate as single agents to treat moderate or severe withdrawal (options A, C, and D are incorrect). **Chapter 16 (pp. 441–442)**

16.2   A 56-year-old diabetic man is brought to the emergency room for altered mental status and receives IV glucose. Shortly after his admission, he becomes confused and displays difficulty with coordination with an abnormal gait. Immediate treatment with which of the following IV medications is most appropriate for this patient?

A. Flumazenil.
B. Magnesium.
C. Ethanol.
D. Thiamine.

The correct response is option D. Thiamine.

Wernicke's encephalopathy results from thiamine deficiency and consists of ophthalmoplegia, ataxia, and altered mental status; this may be difficult to differentiate from acute alcohol intoxication, as the ophthalmoplegia may be difficult to observe, especially if a patient is uncooperative. Wernicke's encephalopathy is a medical emergency requiring immediate treatment with parenteral thiamine to prevent development of *Korsakoff's syndrome*, the irreversible form of thiamine deficiency, consisting of chronic loss of working memory accompanied by confabulation (Sechi and Serra 2007) (option D is correct). Thiamine must be given before or concurrently with intravenous glucose because giving glucose alone to a thiamine-deficient patient can precipitate Wernicke's encephalopathy due to thalamic neuronal damage (Thomson et al. 2002). In addition to pharmacotherapy for alcohol withdrawal, some patients need intravenous glucose, because many individuals with alcohol use disorder (AUD) are hypoglycemic as a result of poor diet and hepatic dysfunction. It is essential to administer thiamine and folate, as well as magnesium and phosphate, before or concurrently with glucose. While magnesium would have some benefit for alcohol withdrawal delirium, it is not the treatment for Wernicke's encephalopathy (option B is incorrect). Flumazenil is a benzodiazepine antagonist available for the treatment of acute benzodiazepine intoxication (option A is incorrect). It is inappropriate to give beverage alcohol to prevent or treat alcohol withdrawal; use of intravenous alcohol infusion is reserved for poisoning with methanol, isopropanol, or ethylene glycol and should not be given for treatment of acute alcohol withdrawal because of complications such as intoxication with delirium or development of gastritis (Weaver 2007) (option C is incorrect). **Chapter 16 (pp. 439, 441, 443)**

16.3   You are called to see a 35-year-old woman who takes oral naltrexone 50 mg daily for alcohol use disorder (AUD). Two days ago, she began taking a prescription medication for a newly diagnosed condition. Earlier today, she consumed several mixed drinks at a wedding reception. On presentation to the emergency room, she had palpitations, nausea, vomiting, headache, hypotension, shortness of breath, and flushing. Which of the following medications is the most likely cause of the patient's symptoms?

A. Metronidazole.
B. Meperidine.

C. Diazepam.

D. Naltrexone.

The correct response is option A: Metronidazole.

Metronidazole has been reported to cause a disulfiram-like effect including nausea and vomiting, flushing, palpitations, dyspnea, hypotension, headache, and sympathetic overactivity when alcohol is consumed while taking it (option A is correct). Although the disulfiram-like effect associated with metronidazole has been disputed, it is recommended that patients avoid alcohol while taking metronidazole and for at least 48 hours after stopping it (Williams and Woodcock 2000). Meperidine is an opioid that can cause an agitated delirium due to accumulation of normeperidine, which is a neuroexcitatory toxic metabolite; this is most prevalent in patients with acute or chronic renal impairment (Adunsky et al. 2002) (option B is incorrect). Clinical features of acute intoxication with diazepam, a benzodiazepine, include slurred speech, incoordination, unsteady gait, and impaired attention or memory; physical signs include nystagmus and decreased reflexes (option C is incorrect). Naltrexone reduces the pleasurable effects of alcohol through blockade of opioid receptors (option D is incorrect). **Chapter 16 (pp. 439, 443, 445)**

16.4 A 49-year-old man, maintained on methadone 80 mg daily, is hit by a car and suffers compound fractures of both femurs. Which of the following is the most appropriate approach to managing the patient's acute pain in the hospital?

A. Continue the methadone maintenance dosage and use only nonsteroidal analgesics because the methadone maintenance doses will produce sufficient analgesia.

B. Divide the patient's daily methadone maintenance dosage into four equal amounts to be given orally every 6 hours.

C. Continue the patient's methadone maintenance dosage once daily by the intravenous route.

D. Continue the methadone maintenance dosage and treat with additional opioid analgesics, as well as other analgesics, as needed.

The correct response is option D: Continue the methadone maintenance dosage and treat with additional opioid analgesics, as well as other analgesics, as needed.

Patients receiving methadone maintenance (MM) with acute pain should be treated for pain with opioid or nonopioid medications, as would be appropriate if they were not receiving MM. Higher-than-usual opioid analgesic doses may be required because of opioid cross-tolerance (option D is correct). Acutely ill or injured MM patients experience the same pain despite receiving methadone because methadone reaches steady-state levels and does not provide additional analgesia (option A is incorrect). The patient's usual MM dose should be continued, and additional short-acting opioid analgesics should be administered (option B is incorrect). If the patient cannot take oral medication, methadone can be given by the intramuscular or subcutaneous route. The parenteral dose should be given as one-half to two-thirds of the maintenance dose, divided into two to four equal doses per day (option C is incorrect). **Chapter 16 (p. 447)**

16.5   A 58-year-old homeless man with AUD and opioid use disorder, maintained on methadone 100 mg daily, is treated with rifampicin for tuberculosis. His physicians should monitor for which of the following potential adverse reactions due to the antibiotic?

A. Opioid intoxication due to inhibition of cytochrome P450 3A4.
B. Opioid withdrawal due to induction of cytochrome P450 3A4.
C. Development of torsades de pointes due to prolongation of the QTc interval.
D. Emergence of hypomagnesemia and/or hypokalemia.

The correct response is option B: Opioid withdrawal due to induction of cytochrome P450 3A4.

Many different medications affect methadone metabolism, primarily because it is metabolized by cytochrome P450 3A4. Risperidone, carbamazepine, rifampicin, and many antiretrovirals can lower serum methadone levels, resulting in opioid withdrawal symptoms (option B is correct). These interactions usually do not have life-threatening consequences for patients, other than acute discomfort and risk of relapse to opioid use disorder (Ferrari et al. 2004). Diazepam, fluoxetine, and erythromycin can elevate methadone serum levels and increase the risk of opioid intoxication (option A is incorrect). Methadone can prolong the QTc interval; torsades de pointes has been reported with very high doses of methadone in outpatient settings, occurring in a few patients who had risk factors for arrhythmias (option C is incorrect). The risk of QTc prolongation is increased when methadone is given intravenously; is used in conjunction with other QTc-prolonging drugs (e.g., antipsychotics, amiodarone, erythromycin) or drugs that inhibit cytochrome P450 3A4; and is administered to patients with hypokalemia, hypocalcemia, hypomagnesemia, or impaired liver function (Vieweg et al. 2013) (option D is incorrect). **Chapter 16 (p. 448)**

16.6   You are asked to help manage a 34-year-old woman at 22 weeks gestation who presents with vaginal bleeding in the setting of heroin withdrawal; the patient's Clinical Opiate Withdrawal Scale (COWS) score is 8 points. Which of the following is the most appropriate next step in management?

A. Treat symptoms with nonopioid medications only until the opioid withdrawal syndrome resolves.
B. Administer naloxone 1 mg intravenously to reduce the opioid-induced uterine bleeding.
C. Induct the patient onto buprenorphine for maintenance treatment of opioid use disorder during pregnancy.
D. Begin intramuscular naltrexone for maintenance treatment of opioid use disorder during pregnancy and to protect the fetus from the effects of opioids.

The correct response is option C: Induct the patient onto buprenorphine for maintenance treatment of opioid use disorder during pregnancy.

Opioid withdrawal syndrome during pregnancy can lead to fetal distress and premature labor as a result of increased oxygen consumption by both the mother and the fetus (Cooper et al. 1983). Even minimal symptoms in the mother may indicate fetal distress because the fetus may be more susceptible to withdrawal symptoms. Buprenorphine has now emerged as a first-line medication alongside methadone (World Health Organization 2014) (option C is correct). Naloxone should not be administered to a pregnant woman except as a last resort for severe opioid overdose because withdrawal precipitated by an opioid antagonist can result in spontaneous abortion, premature labor, or stillbirth (option B is incorrect). Illicitly bought heroin is adulterated with other compounds that may be harmful to the fetus, so elimination of heroin use and provision of adequate doses of methadone or buprenorphine are needed to prevent harm to the fetus from exposure to these other compounds (option A is incorrect). Pregnant women who use opioids should be referred for prenatal care as well as for maintenance treatment from a local MM or buprenorphine program, if available, because (as for option B above) administration of an opioid antagonist (naltrexone) can result in spontaneous abortion, premature labor, or stillbirth (option D is incorrect). **Chapter 16 (pp. 446, 449)**

16.7   A 23-year-old man is brought to the emergency room after developing grandiosity, auditory hallucinations, paranoia, and agitation. Vitals signs are notable for blood pressure of 160/105 mmHg and heart rate of 125 beats per minute. Friends report he has been compulsively using a new drug and may have accidentally overdosed. Which of the following is the most likely causative agent of this patient's presentation?

A. Methcathinone (a synthetic cathinone compound).
B. Gamma-hydroxybutyrate (GHB).
C. NBOMe ("N-bomb").
D. Nitrous oxide ("laughing gas").

The correct response is option A: Methcathinone (a synthetic cathinone compound).

Stimulant intoxication includes behavior changes such as hypervigilance, psychomotor agitation, grandiosity, and impaired judgment. Cathinone is a psychostimulant found in the leaves of the khat plant, which is chemically altered into much more potent stimulant designer drugs known collectively as "bath salts." Young adults are the primary users of synthetic cathinone compounds (Paillet-Loilier et al. 2014; Weaver et al. 2015) (option A is correct). GHB is a sedative that is both a precursor and a metabolite of gamma-aminobutyric acid (GABA), with effects likened to those of alcohol, with mild euphoria, mild numbing, and pleasant disinhibition (option B is incorrect). NBOMe ("N-bomb") is a designer drug considered a hallucinogen, a group of drugs that produce perceptual distortions and cognitive changes with a clear sensorium, without impairment in level of consciousness or attention (Abraham et al. 1996) (option C is incorrect). Examples of illicitly used inhalants include glue, dry-cleaning fluids (carbon tetrachloride), gasoline, aerosol propellants from whipped cream cans or deodorant sprays, amyl nitrite, butyl nitrite, nitrous oxide ("laughing gas"), and some industrial solvents. Many of the inhalants are similar to general anesthetics and sensitize the myocardium to catecholamines; fatal arrhythmias have been reported resulting from inhalant abuse (Shepherd 1989) (option D is incorrect). Chronic complications from abuse of inhalants usually clear if the patient remains abstinent, but impairment of working memory and executive cognitive function may persist. **Chapter 16 (pp. 449–450, 455–456)**

16.8   A daily marijuana smoker for many years, a 25-year-old man is hospitalized for several weeks for treatment of pneumonia. He develops the following symptoms: insomnia with strange dreams, nausea, tremor, elevated mood, decreased appetite, and marked irritability. Which of this patient's symptoms is uncharacteristic of cannabis withdrawal?

A. Nausea.
B. Irritability.
C. Tremor.
D. Elevated mood.

The correct response is option D: Elevated mood.

Heavy cannabis use for more than 3 weeks results in a withdrawal syndrome after abrupt cessation (American Psychiatric Association 2013). Cannabis withdrawal begins within 10 hours of the last dose and consists of irritability, agitation, depression, insomnia, nausea, anorexia, and tremor (option D is correct; options A, B, and C are incorrect). Most symptoms peak in 48 hours and last for 5–7 days. Some symptoms, such as unusual dreams and irritability, can persist for weeks (Budney et al. 2004). Cannabis withdrawal is uncomfortable but not life-threatening. Thus, treatment is entirely supportive and nearly always accomplished without the need for adjunctive medications. **Chapter 16 (p. 454)**

16.9   You are called to evaluate a patient who was admitted a week ago for abdominal pain and vomiting, for which no immediate cause is identified. Symptoms have been refractory to usual antiemetics. The patient frequently insists upon using the bathroom and takes multiple long showers each day, which, according to nursing staff, is both highly unusual and often disruptive to the patient sharing the room. Chronic use of which of the following drugs can lead to cycles of abdominal pain and vomiting, often relieved by bathing or showering with hot water?

A. Cathinone (khat).
B. Meperidine.
C. Cannabis.
D. GHB.

The correct response is option C: Cannabis.

Cannabinoid hyperemesis syndrome, a disorder originally characterized in chronic cannabis users, involves cycles of vomiting and abdominal pain that are relieved by bathing or showering with hot water, an unusual feature that helps to confirm the diagnosis (Sorensen et al. 2017) (option C is correct). Cathinone is the primary psychoactive compound in khat leaves; it is chemically altered into much more potent stimulant designer drugs. Chronic stimulant use can lead to paranoid psychosis that is clinically indistinguishable from schizophrenia, but this effect usually abates after a prolonged period of abstinence (option A is incorrect). Meperidine is an opioid that can cause seizures in overdose and an agitated delirium due to accumulation of a neuroexcitatory toxic metabolite. Meperidine is also a weak serotonin reuptake inhibitor, which can cause serotonin syndrome if given—especially at high doses—with monoamine oxidase inhibitors or other serotonergic drugs (option B is incorrect). GHB is a sedative that has been used as a sleep aid and for treatment of narcolepsy; it also increases episodic secretion of growth hormone, so some bodybuilders use it to promote muscle growth. The dose-response curve for GHB is exceedingly steep, so small increases in the amount ingested may lead to significant intensification of effects and onset of central nervous system depression (option D is incorrect). **Chapter 16 (pp. 445, 447, 450, 454, 455)**

16.10 A 19-year-old patient with a severe daily substance use disorder presents to the emergency room with severe gastrointestinal cramping. The patient is fully oriented and remains alert, with an unremarkable mental status examination. Review of systems is notable for abdominal pain but is otherwise negative, with no nausea, diarrhea, or constipation. Use of which substance most likely caused this presentation?

A. Heroin.
B. Ketamine.
C. PCP (phencyclidine).
D. Cannabis.

The correct response is option B: Ketamine.

Ketamine is a hallucinogen, which may produce perceptual distortions and cognitive changes with a clear sensorium, without impairment in level of consciousness or attention. Hallucinogen use may result in long-term psychiatric consequences and may result in medical consequences. Up to a third of frequent ketamine users experience severe gastrointestinal cramping known as "k-cramps," but the cause is unknown, and no treatment exists currently (Muetzelfeldt et al. 2008) (option B is correct). Narcotic bowel syndrome is a form of bowel hyperalgesia with chronic or recurring abdominal pain that is worsened with continued or escalating dosages of opioids (Drossman and Szigethy 2014) (option A is incorrect). Intoxication with phencyclidine (PCP) causes a characteristic vertical nystagmus (it can also cause horizontal or rotatory nystagmus); PCP may cause hypertensive encephalopathy or life-threatening hyperthermia (Weaver and Schnoll 2008) (option C is incorrect). Cannabinoid hyperemesis syndrome, a disorder originally characterized in chronic cannabis users, involves cycles of vomiting and abdominal pain that are relieved by bathing or showering with hot water, an unusual feature that helps to confirm the diagnosis (Sorensen et al. 2017). Adverse psychological effects, especially acute psychosis, are common and more severe with synthetic cannabinoids than with cannabis. These acute psychological effects may persist for up to several months (option D is incorrect). **Chapter 16 (pp. 447, 454, 455)**

References

Abraham HD, Aldridge AM, Gogia P: The psychopharmacology of hallucinogens. Neuropsychopharmacology 14(4):285–298, 1996 8924196

Adunsky A, Levy R, Heim M, et al: Meperidine analgesia and delirium in aged hip fracture patients. Arch Gerontol Geriatr 35(3):253–259, 2002 14764364

American Psychiatric Association: Diagnostic and Statistical Manual of Mental Disorders, 5th Edition. Arlington, VA, American Psychiatric Association, 2013

Budney AJ, Hughes JR, Moore BA, Vandrey R: Review of the validity and significance of cannabis withdrawal syndrome. Am J Psychiatry 161(11):1967–1977, 2004 15514394

Cooper JR, Altman F, Brown BS, et al: Research on the Treatment of Narcotic Addiction—State of the Art (NIDA Treatment Research Monograph Series). Rockville, MD, U.S. Department of Health and Human Services, 1983

Drossman D, Szigethy E: The narcotic bowel syndrome: a recent update. Am J Gastroenterol Suppl 2(1):22–30, 2014 25207609

Ferrari A, Coccia CP, Bertolini A, Sternieri E: Methadone--metabolism, pharmacokinetics and interactions. Pharmacol Res 50(6):551–559, 2004 15501692

Gold JA, Rimal B, Nolan A, Nelson LS: A strategy of escalating doses of benzodiazepines and phenobarbital administration reduces the need for mechanical ventilation in delirium tremens. Crit Care Med 35(3):724–730, 2007 17255852

Mayo-Smith MF; American Society of Addiction Medicine Working Group on Pharmacological Management of Alcohol Withdrawal: Pharmacological management of alcohol withdrawal. A meta-analysis and evidence-based practice guideline. JAMA 278(2):144–151, 1997 9214531

Muetzelfeldt L, Kamboj SK, Rees H, et al: Journey through the K-hole: phenomenological aspects of ketamine use. Drug Alcohol Depend 95(3):219–229, 2008 18355990

Olkkola KT, Ahonen J: Midazolam and other benzodiazepines. Handb Exp Pharmacol 182(182):335–360, 2008 18175099

Paillet-Loilier M, Cesbron A, Le Boisselier R, et al: Emerging drugs of abuse: current perspectives on substituted cathinones. Subst Abuse Rehabil 5:37–52, 2014 24966713

Sechi G, Serra A: Wernicke's encephalopathy: new clinical settings and recent advances in diagnosis and management. Lancet Neurol 6(5):442–455, 2007 17434099

Shepherd RT: Mechanism of sudden death associated with volatile substance abuse. Hum Toxicol 8(4):287–291, 1989 2777268

Sorensen CJ, DeSanto K, Borgelt L, et al: Cannabinoid hyperemesis syndrome: diagnosis, pathophysiology, and treatment—a systematic review. J Med Toxicol 13(1):71–87, 2017 28000146

Thomson AD, Cook CCH, Touquet R, et al: Royal College of Physicians, London: The Royal College of Physicians report on alcohol: guidelines for managing Wernicke's encephalopathy in the accident and Emergency Department. Alcohol Alcohol 37(6)(suppl):513–521, 2002 12414541

Vieweg WV, Hasnain M, Howland RH, et al: Methadone, QTc interval prolongation and torsade de pointes: case reports offer the best understanding of this problem. Ther Adv Psychopharmacol 3(4):219–232, 2013 24167694

Weaver MF: Dealing with the DTs: managing alcohol withdrawal in hospitalized patients. Hospitalist 11:22–25, 2007

Weaver MF, Schnoll SH: Hallucinogens and club drugs, in The American Psychiatric Publishing Textbook of Substance Abuse Treatment, 4th Edition. Edited by Galanter M, Kleber HD. Washington, DC, American Psychiatric Publishing, 2008, pp 191–200

Weaver MF, Hopper JA, Gunderson EW: Designer drugs 2015: assessment and management. Addict Sci Clin Pract 10:8, 2015 25928069

Williams CS, Woodcock KR: Do ethanol and metronidazole interact to produce a disulfiram-like reaction? Ann Pharmacother 34(2):255–257, 2000 10676835

World Health Organization: Guidelines for the identification and management of substance use and substance use disorders in pregnancy. Geneva, Switzerland, WHO Press, 2014, pp 10–14. Available at: http://apps.who.int/iris/bitstream/10665/107130/1/9789241548731_eng.pdf. Accessed June 7, 2017.

CHAPTER 17

Heart Disease

17.1   Which of the following is true regarding the relationship between congenital heart disease and psychiatric illness?

A. The lifetime rates of mood and anxiety disorders in survivors of congenital heart disease may be as high as 90%.
B. Subtle neuropsychological deficits are common in persons with congenital heart disease.
C. In cyanotic conditions, the time of surgical repair does not seem to have an impact on intellectual function.
D. Low rates of posttraumatic stress disorder (PTSD) are found in parents of children with critical congenital heart disease.

The correct response is option B: Subtle neuropsychological deficits are common in persons with congenital heart disease.

Psychological maladjustment is common in children after surgery for congenital heart disease (Latal et al. 2009), and lifetime rates of mood and anxiety disorders in survivors of congenital heart disease may be as high as 50% (Kovacs et al. 2009) (option A is incorrect). Overall IQ scores are typically in the normal range in persons with congenital heart disease but lower than those of healthy control subjects, and subtle neuropsychological deficits are common (Forbess et al. 2002; Miatton et al. 2007) (option B is correct). For cyanotic conditions, delayed repair appears to exacerbate intellectual impairment (Newburger et al. 1984) (option C is incorrect). Parents of children with critical congenital heart disease frequently have anxiety and depression symptoms as well as high rates of PTSD and psychological distress (option D is incorrect). The period after cardiac surgery is a time of heightened risk (Woolf-King et al. 2017). Parental anxiety and overprotectiveness may play a role in the development of anxiety in congenital heart disease patients (Ong et al. 2011). **Chapter 17 (p. 469)**

17.2   Which of the following statements is true regarding coronary artery disease (CAD)–associated depression?

A. Depression is the most common psychiatric disorder in patients with CAD.
B. It is not recommended to screen for depression in patients with CAD.

C. There is no association between social support and the likelihood of persistent depression after an acute coronary event.

D. Depression is a normal reaction to illness; subsyndromal depression in CAD patients rarely evolves into major depressive disorder.

The correct response is option A: Depression is the most common psychiatric disorder in patients with CAD.

Depression appears to be the most common psychiatric disorder in patients with CAD (Barth et al. 2004; Glassman and Shapiro 1998; Rugulies 2002; van Melle et al. 2004; Wulsin and Singal 2003) (option A is correct). Numerous surveys of patients with established CAD, acute myocardial infarction, and unstable angina consistently indicate a point prevalence of depression in the range of 15%–20% (Barth et al. 2004; van Melle et al. 2004). Depression can be persistent, and subsyndromal depression in CAD patients often evolves into major depressive disorder (MDD) (Hance et al.1996), belying the notion that depression is a "normal" reaction to illness that does not deserve attention (option D is incorrect). The availability of good social support reduces the likelihood of persistent depression after an acute coronary event (Frasure-Smith et al. 2000) (option C is incorrect). Guidelines (Davidson et al. 2006; Lichtman et al. 2008) recommend screening for depression in patients with CAD, but the added value of screening is not established (Thombs et al. 2013) (option B is incorrect). **Chapter 17 (p. 470)**

17.3   Which of the following is a proposed risk factor for PTSD in patients with cardiac disease?

A. Male gender.
B. Older age.
C. Delayed acute stress reaction following cardiac event.
D. Personality traits such as repressive coping, alexithymia, and neuroticism.

The correct response is option D: Personality traits such as repressive coping, alexithymia, and neuroticism.

Proposed risk factors for PTSD in cardiac disease include personality traits such as repressive coping, alexithymia, and neuroticism; history of depression or of previous trauma; younger age; female gender; limited social support; dissociative symptoms during, and acute stress reactions immediately following, index cardiac events; and subjective factors related to the experience of the event (option D is correct; options A, B, and C are incorrect). **Chapter 17 (p. 472)**

17.4   Which of the following is considered a risk factor for delirium after cardiac surgery?

A. Short time on ventilator support.
B. Preoperative atrial fibrillation.
C. Preoperative or postoperative blood product transfusions.
D. Absence of history of psychiatric illness.

The correct response is option C: Preoperative or postoperative blood product transfusions.

Strong risk factors for delirium include older age, previous cerebrovascular disease, previous psychiatric illness, postoperative atrial fibrillation, preoperative or postoperative blood product transfusions, and longer time on ventilator support (option C is correct; options A, B, and D are incorrect). Prolonged sedation with opiates, renal failure, and metabolic derangement have also been identified as delirium factors. In patients older than 70 years, diabetes, hyponatremia, fever, and fluid overload during surgery are additional risk factors (Gosselt et al. 2015; Kazmierski et al. 2008; Smulter et al. 2013). **Chapter 17 (p. 473)**

17.5   What is the correct pairing regarding cardiac medications and their most likely neuropsychiatric side effects?

A. Beta-blockers/increased energy.
B. Digoxin/visual hallucinations.
C. Reserpine/mania.
D. Diuretics/hypernatremia resulting in weakness.

The correct response is option B: Digoxin/visual hallucinations.

Digoxin is known to cause visual hallucinations (classically yellow rings around objects), delirium, and depression (option B is correct). Beta-blockers may cause fatigue and sexual dysfunction (option A is incorrect). Reserpine causes depression (option C is incorrect). Diuretics may cause hyponatremia resulting in anorexia, weakness, and apathy (option D is incorrect). **Chapter 17 (Table 17–1, p. 474)**

17.6   Which of the following symptoms is the best indicator of depression in a patient with advanced heart failure?

A. Anhedonia.
B. Appetite loss.
C. Cachexia.
D. Fatigue.

The correct response is option A: Anhedonia.

Most psychiatric diagnoses are reached in a straightforward fashion in patients with heart disease; however, confusion may arise because of the overlap of symptoms of heart disease with symptoms of psychiatric disorders and because treatments for heart disease may cause psychiatric side effects. A depression diagnosis should never be based solely on a positive score on a depression screening measure (Thombs et al. 2013). The most frequent problem in psychiatric diagnosis is attribution of symptoms of depression to the underlying cardiac disease to a "normal" reaction to the illness, with a resultant underdiagnosis of depression. Generally, in practice, however, an inclusive approach is appropriate, with symptoms such as fatigue and poor sleep counted toward a diagnosis of depression even if those symptoms might also be attributable to the patient's cardiac condition (see Chapter 7, "Depression"). Patients who report somatic symptoms of depression should be evaluated for the presence of the cardinal mood and interest symptoms, and they should be considered to be depressed if these symptoms are present. Patients with advanced heart failure often develop appetite loss and cachexia, but in the absence of loss of self-esteem, loss of interest in ordinarily enjoyable events, or depressed mood, these patients should not be diagnosed with a depressive disorder (option A is correct; options B, C, and D are incorrect). **Chapter 17 (p. 482)**

17.7   In the absence of CAD, which of the following characteristics of patients with chest pain is predictive of panic disorder?

A. Male sex.
B. Older age.
C. Higher education and income.
D. Atypical chest pain quality.

The correct response is option D: Atypical chest pain quality.

In the absence of CAD, the characteristics of patients with chest pain that predict panic disorder include female sex, atypical chest pain quality, younger age, lower education and income, and high self-reported anxiety (Dammen et al. 1999; Huffman and Pollack 2003) (option D is correct; options A, B, and C are incorrect). **Chapter 17 (p. 483)**

17.8   Which of the following drugs has the *least* potential for causing cardiac conduction side effects?

A. Sertraline.
B. Desipramine.
C. Nortriptyline.
D. Carbamazepine.

The correct response is option A: Sertraline.

Tricyclic antidepressants have quinidine-like effects on cardiac conduction and are classified as type IA antiarrhythmics (options B and C are incorrect). Carbamazepine resembles tricyclic antidepressants in having quinidine-like class IA antiarrhythmic effects and may cause atrioventricular conduction disturbances (option D is incorrect). Sertraline is not a type IA antiarrhythmic (option A is correct). **Chapter 17 (Table 17–2, p. 485; p. 490)**

17.9   What selective serotonin reuptake inhibitor (SSRI) has a black box warning against its use at dosages greater than 40 mg/day because it causes dose-dependent QT interval prolongation?

A. Fluoxetine.
B. Sertraline.
C. Paroxetine.
D. Citalopram.

The correct response is option D: Citalopram.

Dose-dependent QT interval prolongation occurs with citalopram treatment and to a lesser degree with other SSRIs (Castro et al. 2013) (options A, B, and C are incorrect). Although the U.S. Food and Drug Administration has imposed a boxed warning against use of citalopram dosages greater than 40 mg/day because of concerns about ventricular arrhythmias (option D is correct), there is little evidence that higher dosages of citalopram are associated with an increased risk of sudden cardiac death (Zivin et al. 2013). **Chapter 17 (p. 487)**

17.10   Which cytochrome P450 (CYP) isoenzyme is responsible for the caution when beta-blockers are coadministered with known inhibitors of this isoenzyme, such as haloperidol or paroxetine?

A. CYP2D6.
B. CYP3A4.
C. CYP1A2.
D. CYP2B6.

The correct response is option A: CYP2D6.

CYP2D6 is responsible for the metabolism of many beta-blockers, carvedilol, and antiarrhythmics; this metabolic pathway is inhibited by haloperidol, fluoxetine, and paroxetine, with resulting elevation of blood levels of CYP2D6 substrates. Conversely, amiodarone is a 2D6 inhibitor and can elevate blood levels of tricyclic antidepressants, fluoxetine, and risperidone (option A is correct; options B, C, and D are incorrect). **Chapter 17 (p. 491)**

17.11   You are asked to counsel a 50-year-old man regarding resumption of sexual activity following a myocardial infarction. Which of the following statements regarding energy equivalence is true regarding the safety of resuming sexual activity?

A. The energy requirement necessary increases the chance of a recurrence five-fold following sexual activity.
B. The risk of further cardiac damage is very high following sexual activity.
C. The patient should be able to walk up one flight of stairs.
D. The patient should be able to walk up three flights of stairs.

The correct response is option C: The patient should be able to walk up one flight of stairs.

Most patients report reduced frequency of sexual activity after myocardial infarction, and 10%–54% do not resume sexual activity at all (Drory et al. 2000). It is important to advise patients that risk of further cardiac damage is low and short-lived (option B is incorrect). Energy requirements for sexual stimulation, intercourse, and orgasm are estimated to be 3–4 metabolic equivalents—similar to climbing a flight of stairs (option C is correct; option D is incorrect). For a 50-year-old patient with a previous myocardial infarction, the risk of a recurrence during the 2-hour period after sexual activity has been calculated to increase from 10 chances to 20 chances in a million per hour (Muller et al. 1996) (option A is incorrect). **Chapter 15 (p. 414)**

References

Barth J, Schumacher M, Herrmann-Lingen C: Depression as a risk factor for mortality in patients with coronary heart disease: a meta-analysis. Psychosom Med 66(6):802–813, 2004 15564343

Castro VM, Clements CC, Murphy SN, et al: QT interval and antidepressant use: a cross sectional study of electronic health records. BMJ 346:f288, 2013 23360890

Dammen T, Ekeberg O, Arnesen H, Friis S: The detection of panic disorder in chest pain patients. Gen Hosp Psychiatry 21(5):323–332, 1999 10572773

Davidson KW, Kupfer DJ, Bigger JT, et al; National Heart, Lung, and Blood Institute Working Group: Assessment and treatment of depression in patients with cardiovascular disease: National Heart, Lung, and Blood Institute Working Group Report. Psychosom Med 68(5):645–650, 2006 17012516

Drory Y, Kravetz S, Weingarten M: Comparison of sexual activity of women and men after a first acute myocardial infarction. Am J Cardiol 85(11):1283–1287, 2000 10831940

Forbess JM, Visconti KJ, Hancock-Friesen C, et al: Neurodevelopmental outcome after congenital heart surgery: results from an institutional registry. Circulation 106(12)(Suppl 1):I95–I102, 2002 12354716

Frasure-Smith N, Lespérance F, Gravel G, et al: Social support, depression, and mortality during the first year after myocardial infarction. Circulation 101(16):1919–1924, 2000 10779457

Glassman AH, Shapiro PA: Depression and the course of coronary artery disease. Am J Psychiatry 155(1):4–11, 1998 9433332

Gosselt AN, Slooter AJ, Boere PR, Zaal IJ: Risk factors for delirium after on-pump cardiac surgery: a systematic review. Crit Care 19:346, 2015 26395253

Hance M, Carney RM, Freedland KE, Skala J: Depression in patients with coronary heart disease. A 12-month follow-up. Gen Hosp Psychiatry 18(1):61–65, 1996 8666215

Huffman JC, Pollack MH: Predicting panic disorder among patients with chest pain: an analysis of the literature. Psychosomatics 44(3):222–236, 2003 12724504

Kazmierski J, Kowman M, Banach M, et al: Clinical utility and use of DSM-IV and ICD-10 Criteria and The Memorial Delirium Assessment Scale in establishing a diagnosis of delirium after cardiac surgery. Psychosomatics 49(1):73–76, 2008 18212180

Kovacs AH, Saidi AS, Kuhl EA, et al: Depression and anxiety in adult congenital heart disease: predictors and prevalence. Int J Cardiol 137(2):158–164, 2009 18707776

Latal B, Helfricht S, Fischer JE, et al: Psychological adjustment and quality of life in children and adolescents following open-heart surgery for congenital heart disease: a systematic review. BMC Pediatr 9:6, 2009 19161602

Lichtman JH, Bigger JT Jr, Blumenthal JA, et al; American Heart Association Prevention Committee of the Council on Cardiovascular Nursing; American Heart Association Council on Clinical Cardiology; American Heart Association Council on Epidemiology and Prevention; American Heart Association Interdisciplinary Council on Quality of Care and Outcomes Research; American Psychiatric Association: Depression and coronary heart disease: recommendations for screening, referral, and treatment: a science advisory from the American Heart Association Prevention Committee of the Council on Cardiovascular Nursing, Council on Clinical Cardiology, Council on Epidemiology and Prevention, and Interdisciplinary Council on Quality of Care and Outcomes Research: endorsed by the American Psychiatric Association. Circulation 118(17):1768–1775, 2008 18824640

Miatton M, De Wolf D, François K, et al: Neuropsychological performance in school-aged children with surgically corrected congenital heart disease. J Pediatr 151(1):73–78, 78.e1, 2007

Muller JE, Mittleman MA, Maclure M, et al; Determinants of Myocardial Infarction Onset Study Investigators: Triggering myocardial infarction by sexual activity. Low absolute risk and prevention by regular physical exertion. JAMA 275(18):1405–1409, 1996 8618365

Newburger JW, Silbert AR, Buckley LP, Fyler DC: Cognitive function and age at repair of transposition of the great arteries in children. N Engl J Med 310(23):1495–1499, 1984 6717539

Ong L, Nolan RP, Irvine J, Kovacs AH: Parental overprotection and heart-focused anxiety in adults with congenital heart disease. Int J Behav Med 18(3):260–267, 2011 20842471

Rugulies R: Depression as a predictor for coronary heart disease: a review and meta-analysis. Am J Prev Med 23(1):51–61, 2002 12093424

Smulter N, Lingehall HC, Gustafson Y, et al: Delirium after cardiac surgery: incidence and risk factors. Interact Cardiovasc Thorac Surg 17(5):790–796, 2013 23887126

Thombs BD, Roseman M, Coyne JC, et al: Does evidence support the American Heart Association's recommendation to screen patients for depression in cardiovascular care? An updated systematic review. PLoS One 8(1):e52654, 2013 23308116

van Melle JP, de Jonge P, Spijkerman TA, et al: Prognostic association of depression following myocardial infarction with mortality and cardiovascular events: a meta-analysis. Psychosom Med 66(6):814–822, 2004 15564344

Woolf-King SE, Anger A, Arnold EA, et al: Mental health among parents of children with critical congenital heart defects: a systematic review. J Am Heart Assoc 6(2):e004862, 2017 28151402

Wulsin LR, Singal BM: Do depressive symptoms increase the risk for the onset of coronary disease? A systematic quantitative review. Psychosom Med 65(2):201–210, 2003 12651987

Zivin K, Pfeiffer PN, Bohnert AS, et al: Evaluation of the FDA warning against prescribing citalopram at doses exceeding 40 mg. Am J Psychiatry 170(6):642–650, 2013 23640689

CHAPTER 18

Lung Disease

18.1   Which of the following diagnoses is most appropriate for a patient who has a psychogenic cough consisting of single dry coughs that are suppressible, distractible, suggestible, and variable?

A. Hyperventilation syndrome.
B. Somatic cough disorder.
C. Tic cough.
D. Vocal cord dysfunction.

The correct response is option C: Tic cough.

Tic cough is a type of psychogenic cough with single dry coughs (tics) that are suppressible, distractible, suggestible, and variable (option C is correct). *Somatic cough disorder* (previously psychogenic cough) is broadly indicated by core features, including chronic persistence, nonresponsiveness to medical treatment, daytime occurrence, absence at night, and the potential of a barking or honking sound (Vertigan 2017) (option B is incorrect). *Hyperventilation* arises when breathing occurs in excess of metabolic demand (Wilhelm et al. 2001) (option A is incorrect). Vocal cord dysfunction occurs when abnormal adduction of the vocal cords during the inspiratory phase of the respiratory cycle produces airflow obstruction at the level of the larynx (Dunn et al. 2015) (option D is incorrect). **Chapter 18 (pp. 517–518)**

18.2   Which of the following is a factor predictive of vocal cord dysfunction?

A. Female sex.
B. Older age.
C. Low body mass index.
D. Absence of psychiatric illness.

The correct response is option A: Female sex.

Vocal cord dysfunction occurs when abnormal adduction of the vocal cords during the inspiratory phase of the respiratory cycle produces airflow obstruction at the level of the larynx (Dunn et al. 2015). Factors predictive of vocal cord dysfunction include younger age (option B is incorrect), female sex (option A is correct), high body mass index (option C is incorrect), history of childhood sexual trauma, and presence of anxiety and depression (Goldberg and Kaplan 2000; Idrees and Fitz-Gerald 2015; Li et al. 2016) (option D is incorrect). **Chapter 18 (pp. 518–519)**

18.3 What is the *most* definitively established risk factor for psychiatric side effects of corticosteroids?

    A. Dose of corticosteroid.
    B. Inhaled route of administration.
    C. Duration of exposure to corticosteroid.
    D. Recurrent treatment with corticosteroid.

The correct response is option A: Dose of corticosteroid.

Corticosteroids are associated with an increased risk of depression, mania, and mixed episodes (Judd et al. 2014). Psychotic symptoms also can occur. Diffuse cognitive changes, including delirium, are also reported during corticosteroid therapy (Fardet et al. 2012). Dose is the most definitively established risk factor for psychiatric side effects (option A is correct). Even inhaled corticosteroids can cause hypothalamic-pituitary-adrenal axis suppression at higher doses, as well as psychiatric side effects (option B is incorrect). Acute, high-dose corticosteroid therapy appears to be more strongly associated with mania or hypomania, whereas chronic, lower-dose therapy may be more associated with depression (options C and D are incorrect). **Chapter 18 (p. 519)**

18.4 A pulmonologist colleague asks you about managing the psychiatric side effects of theophylline. Which of the following is the most appropriate response?

    A. Theophylline has been linked to completed suicide.
    B. Theophylline is sometimes associated with anxiety.
    C. There are several established treatments for psychiatric side effects of theophylline.
    D. Dose reduction does not impact psychiatric side effects.

The correct response is option B: Theophylline is sometimes associated with anxiety.

Theophylline is sometimes associated with anxiety, insomnia, restlessness, agitation, and depression (option B is correct). Theophylline use may even be associated with an increased risk of suicidal ideation, although more recent analyses do not suggest a link with completed suicide (Gibbons and Mann 2011) (option A is incorrect). Other than dose reduction or discontinuation, no known treatments have been established for psychiatric side effects of these medications (options C and D are incorrect). **Chapter 18 (p. 519)**

18.5   Which class of medications has *most* strongly demonstrated improved respiratory outcomes in patients with asthma as evidenced by decreased corticosteroid use?

A. Antipsychotics.
B. Benzodiazepines.
C. Opioids.
D. Antidepressants.

The correct response is option D: Antidepressants.

There is evidence suggesting potential benefits of pharmacotherapy in managing adult respiratory asthma and its psychiatric comorbidities. A randomized 12-week clinical trial of citalopram in 82 adults with both asthma and major depressive disorder (MDD) showed reductions in oral corticosteroid use and depression symptom scores in patients receiving citalopram versus placebo (Brown et al. 2005) (option D is correct). Additionally, trends toward reduction in depression scores, as well as a correlation between changes in asthma and changes in depressive symptoms, have been observed in small proof-of-concept randomized trials of escitalopram and bupropion in outpatients with asthma and MDD (Brown et al. 2007, 2012). Antipsychotic use has been associated with an acute and dose-dependent increased risk of acute respiratory failure in patients with COPD (Wang et al. 2017). Chronic antipsychotic use uncommonly causes laryngeal and other respiratory dyskinesias (option A is incorrect). A recent meta-analysis concluded that benzodiazepines are safe and effective as hypnotics in less severe COPD (Lu et al. 2016); however, they also have a higher rate of adverse respiratory events (Chung et al. 2015; Ekström et al. 2014). Benzodiazepines have not been shown to be effective in relieving breathlessness in advanced COPD (Simon et al. 2016) (option B is incorrect); low-dose opioids are suggested as a safer and more effective alternative (Ekström et al. 2014) (option C is incorrect). **Chapter 18 (p. 520)**

18.6   Which psychiatric comorbidity has been shown to be *most* common in patients with sarcoidosis?

A. Panic disorder.
B. Major depressive disorder (MDD).
C. Bipolar disorder.
D. Generalized anxiety disorder.

The correct response is option B: Major depressive disorder (MDD).

Sarcoidosis, a chronic disease characterized by noncaseating granulomatous involvement of lymph nodes, lymphatic channels in the lung, and other tissues, rarely has been investigated from a psychological standpoint. A large study of members of the Dutch Sarcoidosis Society found that perceived stress was high and was related to depressive symptoms (De Vries and Drent 2004). In addition, psychiatric comorbidity was reported in 44% of Italian sarcoidosis patients, with

MDD in 25% (option B is correct), panic disorder in 6.3% (option A is incorrect), bipolar disorder in 6.3% (option C is incorrect), generalized anxiety disorder in 5% (option D is incorrect), and obsessive-compulsive disorder in 1.3% (Goracci et al. 2008). **Chapter 18 (pp. 516, 517)**

18.7 Which behavioral intervention for asthma patients has shown the *most* beneficial impact on quality of life and respiratory symptoms?

A. Meditation.
B. Yoga.
C. Breathing training.
D. Relaxation training.

The correct response is option C: Breathing training.

A range of behavioral interventions with varying support by psychophysiological rationales have been tested for asthma management. Studies of meditation, yoga, and relaxation training have produced mixed results (Lahmann et al. 2009; Pbert et al. 2012; Posadzki and Ernst 2011) (options A, B, and D are incorrect), which is not surprising, given that physical activation, rather than deactivation, dilates the airways. By contrast, various forms of breathing training show more promise (option C is correct), with clinical trial evidence supporting slow abdominal breathing (Thomas et al. 2009), slow breathing with heart rate variability feedback (Lehrer et al. 2004), and hypoventilation training with (Ritz et al. 2014) or without (Bruton and Lewith 2005) feedback of end-tidal carbon dioxide levels. Benefits are seen mostly for asthma symptoms, quality of life, and bronchodilator or maintenance medication needs. **Chapter 18 (p. 513)**

18.8 The symptoms of which psychiatric disorder show the *greatest* relative increase in prevalence in patients with chronic obstructive pulmonary disease (COPD) compared with the general population?

A. Generalized anxiety.
B. Panic disorder.
C. Depression.
D. Alcohol use disorder.

The correct response is option B: Panic disorder.

The prevalence of comorbid psychiatric symptoms, in particular mood and anxiety disorders, is generally high in COPD, with panic-related symptoms or panic disorder being up to 10 times more prevalent in patients with COPD than the general population (option B is correct). Clinically significant anxiety is estimated to be two times more prevalent in patients with COPD than in the general population. Approximately one-fourth of COPD patients experience clinically significant depression. Depression, generalized anxiety disorder, and alcohol use disorder are also more common among individuals who subsequently develop

COPD than among those who do not (Rapsey et al. 2015) (options A, C, and D are incorrect). **Chapter 18 (p. 514)**

18.9 Which individual component of rehabilitation programs for COPD has been found to yield substantial effects on physical activity levels?

A. Exercise training.
B. Smoking cessation.
C. Nutrition counseling.
D. Psychosocial support.

The correct response is option A: Exercise training.

A review of rehabilitation programs found that components of rehabilitation programs for COPD have variably included optimization of medical treatment, exercise training, smoking cessation, patient education and self-management training, nutrition counseling, relaxation, breathing and respiratory muscle training, and psychosocial support (von Leupoldt et al. 2012). However, the effectiveness of individual components has often been difficult to determine. The exercise training component alone has been shown to yield substantial effects on physical activity levels (Lahham et al. 2016) (option A is correct; options B, C, and D are incorrect). **Chapter 18 (p. 515)**

References

Brown ES, Vigil L, Khan DA, et al: A randomized trial of citalopram versus placebo in outpatients with asthma and major depressive disorder: a proof of concept study. Biol Psychiatry 58(11):865–870, 2005 15993860

Brown ES, Vornik LA, Khan DA, Rush AJ: Bupropion in the treatment of outpatients with asthma and major depressive disorder. Int J Psychiatry Med 37(1):23–28, 2007 17645195

Brown ES, Howard C, Khan DA, Carmody TJ: Escitalopram for severe asthma and major depressive disorder: a randomized, double-blind, placebo-controlled proof-of-concept study. Psychosomatics 53(1):75–80, 2012 22221724

Bruton A, Lewith GT: The Buteyko breathing technique for asthma: a review. Complement Ther Med 13(1):41–46, 2005 15907677

Chung WS, Lai CY, Lin CL, Kao CH: Adverse respiratory events associated with hypnotics use in patients of chronic obstructive pulmonary disease: a population-based case-control study. Medicine (Baltimore) 94(27):e1110, 2015 26166105

De Vries J, Drent M: Relationship between perceived stress and sarcoidosis in a Dutch patient population. Sarcoidosis Vasc Diffuse Lung Dis 21(1):57–63, 2004 15127976

Dunn NM, Katial RK, Hoyte FCL: Vocal cord dysfunction: a review. Asthma Res Pract 1:9, 2015 27965763

Ekström MP, Bornefalk-Hermansson A, Abernethy AP, Currow DC: Safety of benzodiazepines and opioids in very severe respiratory disease: national prospective study. BMJ 348:g445, 2014 24482539

Fardet L, Petersen I, Nazareth I: Suicidal behavior and severe neuropsychiatric disorders following glucocorticoid therapy in primary care. Am J Psychiatry 169(5):491–497, 2012 22764363

Gibbons RD, Mann JJ: Strategies for quantifying the relationship between medications and suicidal behaviour: what has been learned? Drug Saf 34(5):375–395, 2011 21513361

Goldberg BJ, Kaplan MS: Non-asthmatic respiratory symptomatology. Curr Opin Pulm Med 6(1):26–30, 2000 10608422

Goracci A, Fagiolini A, Martinucci M, et al: Quality of life, anxiety and depression in sarcoidosis. Gen Hosp Psychiatry 30(5):441–445, 2008 18774427

Idrees M, FitzGerald JM: Vocal cord dysfunction in bronchial asthma. A review article. J Asthma 52(4):327–335, 2015 25365113

Judd LL, Schettler PJ, Brown ES, et al: Adverse consequences of glucocorticoid medication: psychological, cognitive, and behavioral effects. Am J Psychiatry 171(10):1045–1051, 2014 25272344

Lahham A, McDonald CF, Holland AE: Exercise training alone or with the addition of activity counseling improves physical activity levels in COPD: a systematic review and meta-analysis of randomized controlled trials. Int J Chron Obstruct Pulmon Dis 11:3121–3136, 2016 27994451

Lahmann C, Nickel M, Schuster T, et al: Functional relaxation and guided imagery as complementary therapy in asthma: a randomized controlled clinical trial. Psychother Psychosom 78(4):233–239, 2009 19401624

Lehrer PM, Vaschillo E, Vaschillo B, et al: Biofeedback treatment for asthma. Chest 126(2):352–361, 2004 15302717

Li RC, Singh U, Windom HP, et al: Clinical associations in the diagnosis of vocal cord dysfunction. Ann Allergy Asthma Immunol 117(4):354–358, 2016 27590638

Lu XM, Zhu JP, Zhou XM: The effect of benzodiazepines on insomnia in patients with chronic obstructive pulmonary disease: a meta-analysis of treatment efficacy and safety. Int J Chron Obstruct Pulmon Dis 11:675–685, 2016 27110106

Pbert L, Madison JM, Druker S, et al: Effect of mindfulness training on asthma quality of life and lung function: a randomised controlled trial. Thorax 67(9):769–776, 2012 22544892

Posadzki P, Ernst E: Yoga for asthma? A systematic review of randomized clinical trials. J Asthma 48(6):632–639, 2011 21627405

Rapsey CM, Lim CC, Al-Hamzawi A, et al: Associations between DSM-IV mental disorders and subsequent COPD diagnosis. J Psychosom Res 79(5):333–339, 2015 26526305

Ritz T, Rosenfield D, Steele AM, et al: Controlling asthma by training of Capnometry-Assisted Hypoventilation (CATCH) vs slow breathing: a randomized controlled trial. Chest 146(5):1237–1247, 2014 25122497

Simon ST, Higginson IJ, Booth S, et al: Benzodiazepines for the relief of breathlessness in advanced malignant and non-malignant diseases in adults. Cochrane Database Syst Rev 10(10):CD007354, 2016 27764523

Thomas M, McKinley RK, Mellor S, et al: Breathing exercises for asthma: a randomised controlled trial. Thorax 64(1):55–61, 2009 19052047

Vertigan AE: Somatic cough syndrome or psychogenic cough-what is the difference? J Thorac Dis 9(3):831–838, 2017 28449492

von Leupoldt A, Fritzsche A, Trueba AF, et al: Behavioral medicine approaches to chronic obstructive pulmonary disease. Ann Behav Med 44(1):52–65, 2012 22351032

Wang MT, Tsai CL, Lin CW, et al: Association between antipsychotic agents and risk of acute respiratory failure in patients with chronic obstructive pulmonary disease. JAMA Psychiatry 74(3):252–260, 2017 28055066

Wilhelm FH, Gerlach AL, Roth WT: Slow recovery from voluntary hyperventilation in panic disorder. Psychosom Med 63(4):638–649, 2001 11485118

CHAPTER 19

Gastrointestinal Disorders

19.1   What should a patient taking daily ibuprofen as well as fluoxetine be informed about regarding the risk for an upper gastrointestinal (GI) bleed?

    A. The risk is unaffected by fluoxetine.
    B. The patient should immediately stop fluoxetine and start sertraline, given the extremely high risk of upper-GI bleed.
    C. The patient's absolute risk is more than twice as high as a healthy control subject not taking fluoxetine and ibuprofen.
    D. Evidence demonstrates that venlafaxine would have a similar effect on his risk for upper-GI bleed.

The correct response is option C: The patient's absolute risk is more than twice as high as a healthy control subject not taking fluoxetine and ibuprofen.

Despite their relatively robust tolerability and safe side-effect profiles, selective serotonin reuptake inhibitors (SSRIs) have been associated with an increased risk of upper-GI bleeding (Wee 2017) (option A is incorrect). Normally, serotonin is released from platelets, promoting platelet aggregation and hemostasis. However, because serotonin is not synthesized by platelets de novo, adequate platelet serotonin requires receptor reuptake of serotonin from plasma. This process is blocked by SSRIs, and platelet aggregation is thereby impaired (Anglin et al. 2014; Cheng et al. 2015; Patel et al. 2015; Wee 2017). Despite differences in research design and antidepressants investigated, most studies suggest that there is about double the risk of GI hemorrhage in patients who are taking SSRIs (odds ratio=2.36) (Anglin et al. 2014) compared with control subjects (Cheng et al. 2015; Dalton et al. 2006; Laporte et al. 2017; Loke et al. 2008) (option B is incorrect). Furthermore, patients taking a combination of SSRIs and nonsteroidal anti-inflammatory drugs (NSAIDs) have more than two times the risk of upper-GI bleeding compared with patients taking SSRIs alone (Oka et al. 2014) (option C is correct). Serotonin-norepinephrine reuptake inhibitors do not appear to carry this risk (Cheng et al. 2015) (option D is incorrect). **Chapter 19 (pp. 538–539)**

19.2 What psychopharmacological intervention is best supported for treatment of poorly controlled irritable bowel syndrome (IBS)–diarrhea symptoms in a patient with comorbid depression and anxiety?

A. Duloxetine.
B. Desipramine.
C. Paroxetine.
D. Sertraline.

The correct response is option B: Desipramine.

Antidepressants, specifically tricyclic antidepressants (TCAs) and SSRIs, have been used for IBS in many clinical trials. The estimated number needed to treat to prevent persistent IBS symptoms was four for both TCAs and SSRIs; however, significant heterogeneity among SSRI studies was noted (Ford et al. 2014). Another meta-analysis (Xie et al. 2015) concluded that patients receiving SSRIs showed no statistically significant differences in symptoms compared with the control groups. A third meta-analysis concluded that insufficient evidence exists to support use of SSRIs to treat individuals with IBS who do not have a comorbid psychiatric condition (Bundeff and Woodis 2014) (options C and D are incorrect). Although the evidence for SSRIs is less positive and less consistent than the evidence for TCAs (option B is correct), SSRIs do offer greater tolerability than TCAs and can be used if other treatment has not proven efficacious. Small open-label studies of serotonin-norepinephrine reuptake inhibitors have shown encouraging but not conclusive evidence of benefit in IBS (Brennan et al. 2009; Kaplan et al. 2014; Lewis-Fernández et al. 2016) (option A is incorrect). **Chapter 19 (pp. 545–546)**

19.3 Which of the following is the reason for caution in the use of direct-acting antiviral agents (DAAs) for hepatitis C treatment in patients with comorbid psychiatric illness?

A. DAAs are not effective in patients with active substance use.
B. DAAs carry a significant risk of drug-induced depression and suicidality.
C. Given longer duration of DAA therapy, "high-risk" patients are less likely to remain adherent to DAA versus interferon (IFN).
D. DAA regimens containing ritonavir may have significant drug-drug interactions with psychotropic medications.

The correct response is option D: DAA regimens containing ritonavir may have significant drug-drug interactions with psychotropic medications.

Currently, IFN-based therapy has fallen out of favor with the introduction of DAAs (e.g., protease inhibitors, nonstructural protein 5B [NS5B] and 5A [NS5A] inhibitors), which offer marked advancements in treatment tolerability, length of therapy, and sustained virological response (option C is incorrect). DAAs have not been found to cause significant psychiatric side effects, and treatment discontinuation rates have been minimal (option B is incorrect). Studies including "high-risk" patients receiving opioid substitution therapy (i.e., methadone, buprenorphine) have also shown optimal treatment adherence and clinical responsiveness, even among subjects who continued to use illicit drugs (Dore et al. 2016; Grebely et al. 2016; Rowan and Bhulani 2015) (option A is incorrect). Side effects of DAAs are usually mild and consist of fatigue, headache, insomnia, and nausea. Compared with IFN-based regimens, DAAs impose a greater need for caution because of the risk of clinically relevant drug-drug interactions (Dick et al. 2016; Menon et al. 2015; Smolders et al. 2016; Soriano et al. 2015). This risk is primarily an issue with the three-drug regimen (paritaprevir/ritonavir, ombitasvir, and dasabuvir) due to the presence of ritonavir (option D is correct). **Chapter 19 (p. 549)**

19.4   What abnormality seen in patients with liver disease necessitates cautious interpretation of therapeutic drug-monitoring results?

A. Disruption of phase II glucuronidation metabolism.
B. Prolongation of elimination half-life.
C. Altered plasma protein binding.
D. Impaired renal function and fluctuations in fluid balance.

The correct response is option C: Altered plasma protein binding.

When prescribing psychotropic medications for patients with liver disease, clinicians should take into account the severity of the disease, the medication being considered, the margin between therapeutic and toxic plasma levels, and whether the patient has or is at high risk of hepatic encephalopathy. Therapeutic drug monitoring may be helpful, but results should be interpreted with caution in the face of altered protein binding (Crone et al. 2017) (option C is correct). Generally, drugs with a narrow therapeutic window (e.g., lithium) should be avoided when possible. Hepatic dysfunction alters the absorption, distribution, metabolism, and elimination of most psychotropic medications. Although no specific biochemical test directly conveys the degree of pharmacokinetic disturbance present, the Child-Pugh Scale (CPS) provides a rough estimate to guide dosing in liver disease (Albers et al. 1989). Prolongation of the elimination half-life will delay the time required for drug levels to reach steady state; thus, smaller incremental dosing increases are recommended (option B is incorrect). Glucuronidation is generally preserved in cirrhosis (option A is incorrect). Even when drugs do not depend on hepatic metabolism, some (e.g., gabapentin, lithium) should be used cautiously because impaired renal function and fluctuations in fluid balance (option D is incorrect) may be present (e.g., as a result of diuretics prescribed for ascites). **Chapter 19 (pp. 551–552)**

19.5   A healthy 31-year-old man who recently started taking duloxetine develops abnormal liver function test results thought to be secondary to a drug-induced liver injury (DILI). His alanine aminotransferase is elevated more than his alkaline phosphatase. Which statement about DILI in this patient is correct?

A. The patient's liver function tests are most consistent with cholestatic DILI.
B. The patient's liver function tests should have been monitored more closely during initiation of duloxetine.
C. The patient's liver injury is likely to resolve with discontinuation of duloxetine.
D. The risk of DILI would have been significantly reduced by maintaining duloxetine at 30 mg.

The correct response is option C: The patient's liver injury is likely to resolve with discontinuation of duloxetine.

DILI ranges from mild asymptomatic transaminase elevations to rare cases of fulminant hepatic failure. Most reactions are idiosyncratic (and therefore unpredictable), are not dose dependent (option D is incorrect), and develop after a variable time taking the drug in question. Fortunately, liver injury usually resolves after the drug is discontinued (option C is correct), although full recovery may take up to a year. There are three classes of DILI: hepatocellular, cholestatic, and mixed. Hepatocellular damage causes significant elevation in alanine aminotransferase relative to alkaline phosphatase, whereas alkaline phosphatase is increased more with cholestatic injury (option A is incorrect). Although most psychotropic medications carry some risk of hepatotoxicity, overall risks are very low (Au and Pockros 2013; Marwick et al. 2012; Sarges et al. 2016; Sedky et al. 2012; Voican et al. 2014). For most patients, evidence does not support ordering of repeated liver function tests during treatment with a particular drug (except for valproate) because of the idiosyncratic nature of DILI (Crone et al. 2017; Senior 2009) (option B is incorrect). **Chapter 19 (pp. 552–553)**

19.6   Which of the following medications is the most common cause of psychotropic-induced pancreatitis?

A. Valproic acid.
B. Ziprasidone.
C. Haloperidol.
D. Sertraline.

The correct response is option A: Valproic acid.

Drug-induced pancreatitis is an infrequent cause of acute pancreatitis, accounting for approximately 5% of cases (Vinklerová et al. 2010). Although most cases are mild, prompt recognition is necessary to reduce the risk of serious complications (e.g., chronic pancreatitis, multiorgan failure) (Kaurich 2008). Accurate diagnosis is difficult because clinical presentations often are not readily distinguishable from other causes of acute pancreatitis (Nitsche et al. 2010). Most cases develop within a few weeks to months of starting a particular drug and are not dose dependent. Certain populations—women, children, elderly persons, and persons with advanced HIV infection or inflammatory bowel disease (IBD)—are at greater risk of drug-induced pancreatitis (Nitsche et al. 2010). Valproic acid is the most common cause of psychotropic-induced pancreatitis, with the majority of cases involving children (Gerstner et al. 2007) (option A is correct). Among antipsychotics, clozapine, olanzapine, quetiapine, and risperidone have been associated with the greatest number of cases, and haloperidol, ziprasidone, and aripiprazole with the fewest (Silva et al. 2016) (options B and C are incorrect). However, population-based studies have yielded conflicting results as to whether antipsychotics cause pancreatitis (Bodén et al. 2012; Gasse et al. 2008). Mirtazapine has been linked to cases, whereas cases associated with bupropion, venlafaxine, and SSRIs have been infrequently reported (Hussain and Burke 2008) (option D is incorrect). **Chapter 19 (p. 553)**

19.7   Which of the following statements most accurately describes the relationship between inflammatory bowel disease (IBD) and anxiety and depression?

A. Patients with active IBD symptoms have similar rates of anxiety and depression as do patients whose IBD symptoms are well controlled.
B. Antidepressants improve both psychological well-being and IBD disease activity in most patients with IBD.
C. Levels of anxiety and depression are lower among patients with IBD with comorbid IBS.
D. Evidence suggests that there is a significant relationship between the presence of depressive and anxiety symptoms and risk for clinical recurrence of IBD.

The correct response is option D: Evidence suggests that there is a significant relationship between the presence of depressive and anxiety symptoms and risk for clinical recurrence of IBD.

Given that IBD is a chronic disorder often involving significant morbidity, impaired functioning, and reduced quality of life (QoL), the presence of anxiety and depression is not surprising. A recent systematic review reported pooled incidence rates of 19% and 21% for anxiety and depressive symptoms, respectively. In the face of active IBD, these rates rise to 28% and 66% (Mikocka-Walus et al. 2016a) (option A is incorrect).

   Anxiety and/or depressive symptoms among IBD patients are associated with lower health-related QoL, medication nonadherence, increased risk of hospital readmission and surgery, greater perceived stress, increased disease activity, and poor response to IBD treatment across most, but not all, studies (Allegretti et al. 2015; Luo et al. 2016; Mikocka-Walus et al. 2016b). For example, a large prospective cohort study using clinical and treatment data from more than 2,000 IBD patients found significant relationships between the presence of depressive and anxiety symptoms and risk for clinical recurrences (Mikocka-Walus et al. 2016b) (option D is correct).

The presence of comorbid IBS symptoms significantly affects health-related QoL, as noted in a cross-sectional study of 378 patients with IBD (Gracie et al. 2017). The subgroup with true IBS symptoms and no active IBD had significantly worse QoL, with QoL levels comparable to those of patients with active IBD with intestinal mucosal inflammation. Levels of anxiety, depression, and somatization were also greater among the IBS-IBD patients (option C is incorrect).

Limited data are available on the role of psychopharmacological agents in IBD, despite the fact that nearly one-third of patients either are taking or have taken antidepressants (Mikocka-Walus et al. 2012). IBD patients are usually prescribed antidepressants to treat anxiety and/or depression rather than functional symptoms. Most patients report improvement in psychological well-being, and a small portion report improvements in IBD disease activity (Mikocka-Walus and Andrews 2014) (option B is incorrect). **Chapter 19 (pp. 540–542)**

19.8   Which of the following is *not* a mechanism through which psychiatric medications may contribute to gastroesophageal reflux disease (GERD) symptoms?

A. Clonazepam may increase lower esophageal sphincter pressure.
B. Amitriptyline may lead to decreased gastric transit or impaired GI peristalsis.
C. Sertraline may increase gastric acidity via increased vagal tone.
D. Psychotropic medications with anticholinergic effects may decrease salivary secretions.

The correct response is option A: Clonazepam may increase lower esophageal sphincter pressure.

The relationship of GERD to psychiatric syndromes such as major depressive disorder is complex. Possible mechanisms underlying this relationship may include reflux leading to depression; psychological issues leading to increased perception of GERD symptoms; stress leading to decreased lower esophageal sphincter pressure, altered esophageal motility, increased gastric acid secretion, and/or delayed gastric acid clearance from the esophagus; depression that is comorbid with unhealthy behaviors (e.g., smoking, overeating, alcohol consumption, sedentary lifestyle); and *psychiatric medications themselves* contributing to GERD symptoms (Chou et al. 2014; Martín-Merino et al. 2010). Medication effects can include benzodiazepines leading to decreased lower esophageal sphincter pressure (option A is correct), and anticholinergic medications, such as TCAs, leading to decreased gastric transit, impaired GI peristalsis (option B is incorrect), and/or decreased salivary secretions (option D is incorrect). SSRIs also may contribute to GERD by increasing gastric acidity via increased vagal tone (Andrade and Sharma 2016; Anglin et al. 2014; Bahuva et al. 2015) (option C is incorrect). **Chapter 19 (p. 531)**

19.9   What is the *best* treatment for dysphagia in a patient with haloperidol-induced parkinsonism and chronic complaints of difficulty swallowing?

A. Intravenous diphenhydramine.
B. Discontinuation of haloperidol.
C. Intravenous benztropine.
D. Oral clonazepam.

The correct response is option B: Discontinuation of haloperidol.

Case reports frequently cite antipsychotic medications as a cause of dysphagia, particularly secondary to acute dystonia, parkinsonism, or tardive dyskinesia/ dystonia (Dziewas et al. 2007; Nieves et al. 2007; O'Neill and Remington 2003). Whereas acute dystonia responds to intravenous diphenhydramine or benztropine (options A and C are incorrect), dysphagia from drug-induced parkinsonism requires reduction of antipsychotic dosing, switching of agents, or discontinuation of therapy (Dziewas et al. 2007; Nieves et al. 2007; O'Neill and Remington 2003) (option B is correct). Tardive dyskinesia/dystonia–associated dysphagia may respond to similar measures, with additional benefits from clonazepam (Nieves et al. 2007; O'Neill and Remington 2003) (option D is incorrect). **Chapter 19 (pp. 529–530)**

19.10   A 37-year-old woman recently diagnosed with peptic ulcer disease (PUD) is concerned that work-related stress and anxiety may have contributed to her condition. What should the patient be counseled regarding the relationship between stress and PUD?

A. Stress is the definitive cause of most cases of PUD.
B. *Helicobacter pylori* or nonsteroidal anti-inflammatory drug (NSAID) use are now recognized as the causes of PUD, and stress has no bearing on the development of PUD.
C. Studies suggest that high levels of stress may more than double the chances of developing an ulcer.
D. Given that her high levels of stress and anxiety are contributing to her GI illness, the patient should be started on a tricyclic antidepressant (TCA) for PUD.

The correct response is option C: Studies suggest that high levels of stress may more than double the chances of developing an ulcer.

Peptic ulcers traditionally are linked to infection with *H. pylori* and chronic use of NSAIDs, with an estimated 50% of peptic ulcers attributable to *H. pylori*, 25% to NSAIDs, and 25% to other sources (option A is incorrect). Additional causes include other infections and substance use (e.g., potassium chloride, bisphosphonates, crack cocaine, amphetamine, heavy alcohol use) (Jones 2006; Levenstein 2000). A significant body of research has demonstrated that stressful life events, and perhaps personality characteristics, play a role in PUD (option B is incorrect).

One recent study noted that a high "stress index" more than doubled the chances of developing an ulcer (Levenstein et al. 2015) (option C is correct); other researchers have noted increased ulcer incidence in people experiencing intense stressors, natural disasters, and refugee status (Lanas and Chan 2017). As in other upper-GI disorders, patient with PUD symptoms also often have comorbid psychiatric symptoms. One recent study of more than 900 patients found that anxiety symptoms were independently associated with GI ulcers (Niles et al. 2015). However, correlation does not imply causation. Several small randomized controlled trials in the 1980s (Andersen et al. 1984; Ries et al. 1984) demonstrated benefits from TCAs (doxepin, trimipramine)—perhaps via these agents' antihistaminic and anticholinergic effects—in the treatment and prevention of duodenal ulcers. However, because of their side effects (e.g., weight gain, constipation, dry mouth), TCAs are no longer used for PUD (option D is incorrect). **Chapter 19 (p. 537)**

References

Albers I, Hartmann H, Bircher J, Creutzfeldt W: Superiority of the Child-Pugh classification to quantitative liver function tests for assessing prognosis of liver cirrhosis. Scand J Gastroenterol 24(3):269–276, 1989 2734585

Allegretti JR, Borges L, Lucci M, et al: Risk factors for rehospitalization within 90 days in patients with inflammatory bowel disease. Inflamm Bowel Dis 21(11):2583–2589, 2015 26244647

Andersen OK, Bergsåker-Aspøy J, Halvorsen L, Giercksky KE: Doxepin in the treatment of duodenal ulcer. A double-blind clinical study comparing doxepin and placebo. Scand J Gastroenterol 19(7):923–925, 1984 6397849

Andrade C, Sharma E: Serotonin reuptake inhibitors and risk of abnormal bleeding. Psychiatr Clin North Am 39(3):413–426, 2016 27514297

Anglin R, Yuan Y, Moayyedi P, et al: Risk of upper gastrointestinal bleeding with selective serotonin reuptake inhibitors with or without concurrent nonsteroidal anti-inflammatory use: a systematic review and meta-analysis. Am J Gastroenterol 109(6):811–819, 2014 24777151

Au JS, Pockros PJ: Drug-induced liver injury from antiepileptic drugs. Clin Liver Dis 17(4):687–697, 2013

Bahuva R, Yee J, Gupta S, Atreja A: SSRI and the risk of gastrointestinal bleed: more than what meets the eye. Am J Gastroenterol 110(2):346, 2015 25646912

Bodén R, Bexelius TS, Mattsson F, et al: Antidopaminergic drugs and acute pancreatitis: a population-based study. BMJ Open 2(3):e000914, 2012 22581796

Brennan BP, Fogarty KV, Roberts JL, et al: Duloxetine in the treatment of irritable bowel syndrome: an open-label pilot study. Hum Psychopharmacol 24(5):423–428, 2009 19548294

Bundeff AW, Woodis CB: Selective serotonin reuptake inhibitors for the treatment of irritable bowel syndrome. Ann Pharmacother 48(6):777–784, 2014 24651166

Cheng YL, Hu HY, Lin XH, et al: Use of SSRI, but not SNRI, increased upper and lower gastrointestinal bleeding: a nationwide population-based cohort study in Taiwan. Medicine (Baltimore) 94(46):e2022, 2015 26579809

Chou PH, Lin CC, Lin CH, et al: Prevalence of gastroesophageal reflux disease in major depressive disorder: a population-based study. Psychosomatics 55(2):155–162, 2014 23953172

Crone CC, Marcangelo M, Lackamp J, et al: Gastrointestinal disorders, in Clinical Manual of Psychopharmacology in the Medically Ill, 2nd Edition. Edited by Levenson JL, Ferrando SJ. Arlington, VA, American Psychiatric Association Publishing, 2017, pp 129–193

Dalton SO, Sørensen HT, Johansen C: SSRIs and upper gastrointestinal bleeding: what is known and how should it influence prescribing? CNS Drugs 20(2):143–151, 2006 16478289

Dick TB, Lindberg LS, Ramirez DD, Charlton MR: A clinician's guide to drug-drug interactions with direct-acting antiviral agents for the treatment of hepatitis C viral infection. Hepatology 63(2):634–643, 2016 26033675

Dore GJ, Altice F, Litwin AH, et al; C-EDGE CO-STAR Study Group: C-EDGE CO-STAR Study Group: Elbasvir-grazoprevir to treat hepatitis C virus infection in persons receiving opioid agonist therapy: a randomized trial. Ann Intern Med 165(9):625–634, 2016 27537841

Dziewas R, Warnecke T, Schnabel M, et al: Neuroleptic-induced dysphagia: case report and literature review. Dysphagia 22(1):63–67, 2007 17024549

Ford AC, Quigley EM, Lacy BE, et al: Effect of antidepressants and psychological therapies, including hypnotherapy, in irritable bowel syndrome: systematic review and meta-analysis. Am J Gastroenterol 109(9):1350–1365, quiz 1366, 2014

Gasse C, Jacobsen J, Pedersen L, et al: Risk of hospitalization for acute pancreatitis associated with conventional and atypical antipsychotics: a population-based case-control study. Pharmacotherapy 28(1):27–34, 2008 18154471

Gerstner T, Büsing D, Bell N, et al: Valproic acid-induced pancreatitis: 16 new cases and a review of the literature. J Gastroenterol 42(1):39–48, 2007 17322992

Gracie DJ, Williams CJ, Sood R, et al: Negative effects on psychological health and quality of life of genuine irritable bowel syndrome-type symptoms in patients with inflammatory bowel disease. Clin Gastroenterol Hepatol 15(3):376–384.e5, 2017 27189912

Grebely J, Mauss S, Brown A, et al: Efficacy and safety of ledipasvir/sofosbuvir with and without ribavirin in patients with chronic HCV genotype 1 infection receiving opioid substitution therapy: analysis of phase 3 ION trials. Clin Infect Dis 63(11):1405–1411, 2016 27553375

Hussain A, Burke J: Mirtazapine associated with recurrent pancreatitis - a case report. J Psychopharmacol 22(3):336–337, 2008 18208920

Jones MP: The role of psychosocial factors in peptic ulcer disease: beyond Helicobacter pylori and NSAIDs. J Psychosom Res 60(4):407–412, 2006 16581366

Kaplan A, Franzen MD, Nickell PV, et al: An open-label trial of duloxetine in patients with irritable bowel syndrome and comorbid generalized anxiety disorder. Int J Psychiatry Clin Pract 18(1):11–15, 2014 23980534

Kaurich T: Drug-induced acute pancreatitis. Proc Bayl Univ Med Cent 21(1):77–81, 2008 18209761

Lanas A, Chan FKL: Peptic ulcer disease. Lancet 390(10094):613–624, 2017 28242110

Laporte S, Chapelle C, Caillet P, et al: Bleeding risk under selective serotonin reuptake inhibitor (SSRI) antidepressants: a meta-analysis of observational studies. Pharmacol Res 118:19–32, 2017 27521835

Levenstein S: The very model of a modern etiology: a biopsychosocial view of peptic ulcer. Psychosom Med 62(2):176–185, 2000 10772394

Levenstein S, Rosenstock S, Jacobsen RK, Jorgensen T: Psychological stress increases risk for peptic ulcer, regardless of Helicobacter pylori infection or use of nonsteroidal anti-inflammatory drugs. Clin Gastroenterol Hepatol 13(3):498–506.e1, 2015 25111233

Lewis-Fernández R, Lam P, Lucak S, et al: An open-label pilot study of duloxetine in patients with irritable bowel syndrome and comorbid major depressive disorder. J Clin Psychopharmacol 36(6):710–715, 2016 27755218

Loke YK, Trivedi AN, Singh S: Meta-analysis: gastrointestinal bleeding due to interaction between selective serotonin uptake inhibitors and non-steroidal anti-inflammatory drugs. Aliment Pharmacol Ther 27(1):31–40, 2008 17919277

Luo XP, Mao R, Chen BL, et al: Over-reaching beyond disease activity: the influence of anxiety and medical economic burden on health-related quality of life in patients with inflammatory bowel disease. Patient Prefer Adherence 11:23–31, 2016 28053510

Martín-Merino E, Ruigómez A, García Rodríguez LA, et al: Depression and treatment with antidepressants are associated with the development of gastro-oesophageal reflux disease. Aliment Pharmacol Ther 31(10):1132–1140, 2010 20199498

Marwick KFM, Taylor M, Walker SW: Antipsychotics and abnormal liver function tests: systematic review. Clin Neuropharmacol 35(5):244–253, 2012 22986798

Menon RM, Badri PS, Wang T, et al: Drug-drug interaction profile of the all-oral anti-hepatitis C virus regimen of paritaprevir/ritonavir, ombitasvir, and dasabuvir. J Hepatol 63(1):20–29, 2015 25646891

Mikocka-Walus A, Andrews JM: Attitudes towards antidepressants among people living with inflammatory bowel disease: an online Australia-wide survey. J Crohn's Colitis 8(4):296–303, 2014 24074632

Mikocka-Walus AA, Gordon AL, Stewart BJ, Andrews JM: The role of antidepressants in the management of inflammatory bowel disease (IBD): a short report on a clinical case-note audit. J Psychosom Res 72(2):165–167, 2012 22281460

Mikocka-Walus A, Knowles SR, Keefer L, Graff L: Controversies revisited: a systematic review of the comorbidity of depression and anxiety with inflammatory bowel diseases. Inflamm Bowel Dis 22(3):752–762, 2016a 26841224

Mikocka-Walus A, Pittet V, Rossel JB, von Känel R; Swiss IBD Cohort Study Group: Symptoms of depression and anxiety are independently associated with clinical recurrence of inflammatory bowel disease. Clin Gastroenterol Hepatol 14(6):829–835.e1, 2016b 26820402

Nieves JE, Stack KM, Harrison ME, Gorman JM: Dysphagia: a rare form of dyskinesia? J Psychiatr Pract 13(3):199–201, 2007 17522565

Niles AN, Dour HJ, Stanton AL, et al: Anxiety and depressive symptoms and medical illness among adults with anxiety disorders. J Psychosom Res 78(2):109–115, 2015 25510186

Nitsche CJ, Jamieson N, Lerch MM, Mayerle JV: Drug induced pancreatitis. Best Pract Res Clin Gastroenterol 24(2):143–155, 2010 20227028

Oka Y, Okamoto K, Kawashita N, et al: Meta-analysis of the risk of upper gastrointestinal hemorrhage with combination therapy of selective serotonin reuptake inhibitors and non-steroidal anti-inflammatory drugs. Biol Pharm Bull 37(6):947–953, 2014 24681541

O'Neill JL, Remington TL: Drug-induced esophageal injuries and dysphagia. Ann Pharmacother 37(11):1675–1684, 2003 14565800

Patel H, Gaduputi V, Sakam S, et al: Serotonin reuptake inhibitors and post-gastrostomy bleeding: reevaluating the link. Ther Clin Risk Manag 11:1283–1289, 2015 26346885

Ries RK, Gilbert DA, Katon W: Tricyclic antidepressant therapy for peptic ulcer disease. Arch Intern Med 144(3):566–569, 1984 6367680

Rowan PJ, Bhulani N: Psychosocial assessment and monitoring in the new era of non-interferon-alpha hepatitis C virus treatments. World J Hepatol 7(19):2209–2213, 2015 26380046

Sarges P, Steinberg JM, Lewis JH: Drug-induced liver injury: highlights from a review of the 2015 literature. Drug Saf 39(9):801–821, 2016 27142208

Sedky K, Nazir R, Joshi A, et al: Which psychotropic medications induce hepatotoxicity? Gen Hosp Psychiatry 34(1):53–61, 2012 22133982

Senior JR: Monitoring for hepatotoxicity: what is the predictive value of liver "function" tests? Clin Pharmacol Ther 85(3):331–334, 2009 19129750

Silva MA, Key S, Han E, Malloy MJ: Acute pancreatitis associated with antipsychotic medication: evaluation of clinical features, treatment, and polypharmacy in a series of cases. J Clin Psychopharmacol 36(2):169–172, 2016 26859276

Smolders EJ, de Kanter CTMM, de Knegt RJ, et al: Drug-drug interactions between direct-acting antivirals and psychoactive medications. Clin Pharmacokinet 55(12):1471–1494, 2016 27317413

Soriano V, Labarga P, Barreiro P, et al: Drug interactions with new hepatitis C oral drugs. Expert Opin Drug Metab Toxicol 11(3):333–341, 2015 25553890

Vinklerová I, Procházka M, Procházka V, Urbánek K: Incidence, severity, and etiology of drug-induced acute pancreatitis. Dig Dis Sci 55(10):2977–2981, 2010 20499176

Voican CS, Corruble E, Naveau S, Perlemuter G: Antidepressant-induced liver injury: a review for clinicians. Am J Psychiatry 171(4):404–415, 2014 24362450

Wee TC: Gastrointestinal hemorrhage related to fluoxetine in a patient with stroke. Am J Phys Med Rehabil 96(11):e201–e203, 2017 28141599

Xie C, Tang Y, Wang Y, et al: Efficacy and safety of antidepressants for the treatment of irritable bowel syndrome: a meta-analysis. PLoS One 10(8):e0127815, 2015 26252008

CHAPTER 20

Renal Disease

20.1 What is the *most* common psychiatric diagnosis in dialysis patients?

A. Delirium.
B. Dementia.
C. Depression.
D. Substance abuse.

The correct response is option C: Depression.

In a study of 200,000 adult U.S. dialysis patients, almost 9% had been hospitalized with a comorbid psychiatric diagnosis (Kimmel et al. 1998). Depression and other mood disorders were the most common diagnoses (option C is correct), followed by delirium and dementia (options A and B are incorrect). In a smaller study in an urban hemodialysis population, roughly 70% of the sample had at least one current DSM-IV (American Psychiatric Association 1994) Axis I diagnosis, as determined by the Structured Clinical Interview for DSM-IV Axis I Disorders (SCID-I) (Cukor et al. 2007). Depression and anxiety were the two most prevalent psychiatric disorders, followed by substance abuse (option D is incorrect) and psychosis. **Chapter 20 (pp. 572–573)**

20.2 Withdrawal from dialysis is most common in which of the following patient groups in the United States?

A. Younger patients.
B. Women.
C. African American patients.
D. Asian patients.

The correct response is option B: Women.

In the United States, dialysis withdrawal has been more common among women (option B is correct) and older patients (option A is incorrect) and less common among African American (option C is incorrect) and Asian patients (option D is incorrect), with significant regional variation (Gessert et al. 2013; Kurella Tamura et al. 2010; Munshi et al. 2001). **Chapter 20 (p. 579)**

20.3 Which anxiety- or stressor-related disorder has been shown to be *much* higher in end-stage renal disease (ESRD) patients than in community samples?

A. Anxiety disorders are equally prevalent in community and ESRD samples.
B. Phobias.
C. Posttraumatic stress disorder (PTSD).
D. Panic disorder.

The correct response is option D: Panic disorder.

In a study that assessed psychiatric diagnoses in a sample of 70 predominantly African American ESRD patients, about 45% had at least one anxiety disorder. The most common diagnoses identified were phobias and panic disorder (Cukor et al. 2008). The prevalence of panic disorder was much higher in ESRD patients than in community samples, a finding that may be related to hypervigilance to bodily sensations associated with hemodialysis or fears about the outcome of ESRD treatment (option D is correct; option A is incorrect). Posttraumatic stress symptoms are also common among hemodialysis patients (Tagay et al. 2007) (option C is incorrect). Phobias for needles or the sight of blood are common in the general population (see Chapter 10, "Anxiety Disorders"), and such phobias are among the most frequently reported reasons that hemodialysis patients choose self-care treatment instead of in-center dialysis (McLaughlin et al. 2003) (option B is incorrect). **Chapter 20 (p. 574)**

20.4 How does a disruptive patient *most* commonly interfere with the dialysis unit and staff?

A. Verbal aggression.
B. Noncompliance with treatment.
C. Coming late to appointments.
D. Physical abuse.

The correct response is option A: Verbal aggression.

There has been an increase in the number of reported disruptive patients within dialysis units (Hashmi and Moss 2008), with verbal aggression being the most prevalent behavior (Jones et al. 2014) (option A is correct). Disruption on the unit may affect the individual, for example, in the case of noncompliance with treatment (option B is incorrect). A patient's disruptive behavior may also affect other patients receiving dialysis therapy. A disruptive patient may harm others by coming late to appointments, thus disrupting dialysis scheduling for others, or by threatening the staff (Hashmi and Moss 2008) (option C is incorrect). Although all patients should be treated equally and with respect, the welfare of a disruptive patient must be balanced against the welfare of health care personnel and other patients. Verbal or physical abuse that occurs on the unit should not be tolerated, and the welfare of staff and other patients should not be compromised (option D is incorrect). **Chapter 20 (p. 575)**

20.5 Which of the following is associated with dialysis termination?

A. Pain.
B. Median time to death of 14 days.
C. Lethargy.
D. Increased suffering at the end of life.

The correct response is option C: Lethargy.

Withdrawal from dialysis may often be appropriate for a dialysis patient who is failing to thrive or is suffering. Many patients choose this option because it allows for a quicker death and the end of suffering (Cohen and Germain 2005; Cohen et al. 2003). The median time to death after stopping dialysis is 7–8 days (O'Connor et al. 2013) (option B is incorrect), and dialysis termination usually does not cause pain or discomfort (Cohen et al. 2000) (options A and D are incorrect). Withdrawal typically results in lethargy (option C is correct) progressing to coma and death. **Chapter 20 (p. 579)**

20.6 Which selective serotonin reuptake inhibitor (SSRI) would be expected to have the fewest potential interactions with other medications *and* may not need dose adjustment in patients with renal insufficiency?

A. Paroxetine.
B. Fluoxetine.
C. Citalopram.
D. Escitalopram.

The correct response is option C: Citalopram.

Among the SSRIs, citalopram, escitalopram, and sertraline would be expected to have the fewest potential interactions with other medications taken by patients with renal impairment. Some evidence suggests that dosage adjustments may not be needed for citalopram (Spigset et al. 2000) (option C is correct) and fluoxetine (Finkelstein and Finkelstein 2000) in patients with renal insufficiency (options B and D are incorrect). Paroxetine clearance is reduced in patients with renal insufficiency (Doyle et al. 1989) (option A is incorrect). **Chapter 20 (pp. 580–581)**

20.7 Which antipsychotic medication depends on renal elimination?

A. Haloperidol.
B. Paliperidone.
C. Prolixin.
D. Chlorpromazine.

The correct response is option B: Paliperidone.

Antipsychotics typically do not depend on renal elimination, with the exception of paliperidone, which is largely excreted unchanged in urine and thus requires dosage reduction in patients with renal insufficiency (Vermeir et al. 2008) (option B is correct; options A, C, and D are incorrect). **Chapter 20 (p. 581)**

20.8   Which diuretics reduce lithium excretion?

   A. Carbonic anhydrase inhibitors.
   B. Thiazide diuretics.
   C. Potassium-sparing diuretics.
   D. Loop diuretics.

The correct response is option B: Thiazide diuretics.

Diuretics variably affect lithium excretion, depending on the type of diuretic and the volume status of the patient. Thiazide diuretics may reduce lithium excretion, resulting in increased lithium levels (option B is correct). Acute administration of loop diuretics (e.g., furosemide, ethacrynic acid, bumetanide) increases lithium excretion (option D is incorrect), causing a drop in lithium levels, but with chronic use, compensatory changes leave lithium levels somewhat unpredictable but usually not significantly changed. Carbonic anhydrase inhibitors (e.g., acetazolamide) and osmotic diuretics (e.g., mannitol) reduce lithium levels (Levenson and Owen 2017) (option A is incorrect). Potassium-sparing diuretics (e.g., amiloride, triamterene, spironolactone) may increase lithium excretion (option C is incorrect). **Chapter 20 (p. 584)**

20.9   Which of the following medications may cause hypernatremia due to nephrogenic diabetes insipidus?

   A. Amiloride.
   B. Thiazides.
   C. Nonsteroidal anti-inflammatory drugs (NSAIDs).
   D. Lithium.

The correct response is option D: Lithium.

Hypernatremia due to nephrogenic diabetes insipidus (NDI) may be caused by lithium through inhibition of renal tubular water reabsorption (option D is correct). Amiloride is considered the treatment of choice for lithium-induced NDI, but NDI also has been treated with NSAIDs, thiazides, and sodium restriction (Grünfeld and Rossier 2009) (options A, B, and C are incorrect). **Chapter 20 (p. 582)**

20.10 Which of the following medications is removed during dialysis?

A. Valproate.
B. Carbamazepine.
C. Paroxetine.
D. Lorazepam.

The correct response is option A: Valproate.

Lithium is completely dialyzed and may be given safely as a single oral dose (300–600 mg) following hemodialysis treatment. Lithium levels should not be checked until at least 2–3 hours after dialysis because reequilibration from tissue stores occurs in the immediate postdialysis period. The dose of gabapentin, pregabalin, lithium, and topiramate should be modified on the basis of creatinine clearance (Levenson and Owen 2017). Because most psychotropics are lipophilic compounds with large volumes of distribution, they are not dialyzable. Only lithium, gabapentin, pregabalin, valproate, topiramate, and levetiracetam are removed by dialysis (option A is correct; options B, C, and D are incorrect). Significant fluid shifts occur during and several hours after each hemodialysis treatment, making dialysis patients more prone to orthostasis. Hence, drugs that frequently cause orthostatic hypotension should ideally be avoided. **Chapter 20 (p. 582), Chapter 36 (p. 1233)**

References

American Psychiatric Association: Diagnostic and Statistical Manual of Mental Disorders, 4th Edition. Washington, DC, American Psychiatric Association, 1994

Cohen LM, Germain MJ: The psychiatric landscape of withdrawal. Semin Dial 18(2):147–153, 2005 15771660

Cohen LM, Germain M, Poppel DM, et al: Dialysis discontinuation and palliative care. Am J Kidney Dis 36(1):140–144, 2000 10873883

Cohen LM, Germain MJ, Poppel DM: Practical considerations in dialysis withdrawal: "to have that option is a blessing." JAMA 289(16):2113–2119, 2003 12709469

Cukor D, Coplan J, Brown C, et al: Depression and anxiety in urban hemodialysis patients. Clin J Am Soc Nephrol 2(3):484–490, 2007 17699455

Cukor D, Coplan J, Brown C, et al: Anxiety disorders in adults treated by hemodialysis: a single-center study. Am J Kidney Dis 52(1):128–136, 2008 18440682

Doyle GD, Laher M, Kelly JG, et al: The pharmacokinetics of paroxetine in renal impairment. Acta Psychiatr Scand Suppl 350:89–90, 1989 2530798

Finkelstein FO, Finkelstein SH: Depression in chronic dialysis patients: assessment and treatment. Nephrol Dial Transplant 15(12):1911–1913, 2000 11096130

Gessert CE, Haller IV, Johnson BP: Regional variation in care at the end of life: discontinuation of dialysis. BMC Geriatr 13:39, 2013 23635315

Grünfeld JP, Rossier BC: Lithium nephrotoxicity revisited. Nat Rev Nephrol 5(5):270–276, 2009 19384328

Hashmi A, Moss AH: Treating difficult or disruptive dialysis patients: practical strategies based on ethical principles. Nat Clin Pract Nephrol 4(9):515–520, 2008 18612329

Jones J, Nijman H, Ross J, et al: Aggression on haemodialysis units: a mixed method study. J Ren Care 40(3):180–193, 2014 25042357

Kimmel PL, Thamer M, Richard CM, Ray NF: Psychiatric illness in patients with end-stage renal disease. Am J Med 105(3):214–221, 1998 9753024

Kurella Tamura M, Goldstein MK, Pérez-Stable EJ: Preferences for dialysis withdrawal and engagement in advance care planning within a diverse sample of dialysis patients. Nephrol Dial Transplant 25(1):237–242, 2010 19734137

Levenson JL, Owen JA: Renal and urological disorders, in Clinical Manual of Psychopharmacology in the Medically Ill, 2nd Edition. Edited by Levenson JL, Ferrando SJ. Arlington, VA, American Psychiatric Publishing, 2017, pp 195–232

McLaughlin K, Manns B, Mortis G, et al: Why patients with ESRD do not select self-care dialysis as a treatment option. Am J Kidney Dis 41(2):380–385, 2003 12552500

Munshi SK, Vijayakumar N, Taub NA, et al: Outcome of renal replacement therapy in the very elderly. Nephrol Dial Transplant 16(1):128–133, 2001 11209006

O'Connor NR, Dougherty M, Harris PS, Casarett DJ: Survival after dialysis discontinuation and hospice enrollment for ESRD. Clin J Am Soc Nephrol 8(12):2117–2122, 2013 24202133

Spigset O, Hägg S, Stegmayr B, Dahlqvist R: Citalopram pharmacokinetics in patients with chronic renal failure and the effect of haemodialysis. Eur J Clin Pharmacol 56(9-10):699–703, 2000 11214779

Tagay S, Kribben A, Hohenstein A, et al: Posttraumatic stress disorder in hemodialysis patients. Am J Kidney Dis 50(4):594–601, 2007 17900459

Vermeir M, Naessens I, Remmerie B, et al: Absorption, metabolism, and excretion of paliperidone, a new monoaminergic antagonist, in humans. Drug Metab Dispos 36(4):769–779, 2008 18227146

CHAPTER 21

Endocrine and Metabolic Disorders

21.1   Which of the following describes the impact of stress on patients with diabetes?

A. Those with an active lifestyle have high levels of stress.
B. Repeated stress leads to inhibition of the hypothalamic-pituitary-adrenal (HPA) axis.
C. Repeated stress leads to overstimulation of the HPA axis.
D. Glycemic control is poorer in people with diabetes who report less stress.

The correct response is option C: Repeated stress leads to overstimulation of the HPA axis.

The association between stress and diabetes is rooted in biological and behavioral causes (Pouwer et al. 2010). Those with high levels of stress tend to have a sedentary lifestyle (option A is incorrect) and poor dietary habits. Repeated stress leads to overstimulation (option C is correct), not inhibition (option B is incorrect), of the HPA axis. This leads to increases in the cortisol and inflammatory cytokines that play a role in insulin resistance (Golden 2007; Kan et al. 2013). Several studies have shown that glycemic control is poorer in people with diabetes who report more stress (Garay-Sevilla et al. 2000; Lloyd et al. 1999) (option D is incorrect). **Chapter 21 (p. 594)**

21.2   Which antipsychotic is the *least* likely to cause weight gain and glucose intolerance?

A. Clozapine.
B. Olanzapine.
C. Aripiprazole.
D. Quetiapine.

The correct response is option C: Aripiprazole.

Antipsychotics have been implicated in insulin resistance and weight gain. Carbohydrate cravings and antagonism of histamine and serotonin$_{2A}$ and serotonin$_{2C}$ receptors have been proposed as mechanisms for metabolic changes (Calkin et al. 2013). In patients with known diabetes, antipsychotics with lower propensities to cause weight gain and glucose intolerance, such as perphenazine, molindone, aripiprazole (option C is correct), and ziprasidone, should be favored (Meyer et al. 2008). Clozapine, olanzapine, and quetiapine have all been linked to high rates of weight gain and glucose intolerance (options A, B, and D are incorrect). A U.S. consensus statement concluded that hyperglycemia is associated with all marketed second-generation antipsychotics but is less common with aripiprazole and ziprasidone (American Diabetes Association et al. 2004). All currently marketed antipsychotics (with the possible exceptions of haloperidol, ziprasidone, lurasidone, and aripiprazole) are associated with weight gain. Among the second-generation antipsychotics, the relative propensity to cause weight gain (from greatest to least) is as follows: olanzapine > clozapine >> iloperidone > quetiapine > risperidone, paliperidone >> asenapine > amisulpride >> aripiprazole > lurasidone > ziprasidone (Citrome 2011; Leucht et al. 2013; Murray et al. 2017). **Chapter 21 (pp. 598–599), Chapter 36 (p. 1206)**

21.3   Which of the following is the *most* common manifesting symptom of hyperthyroidism in younger patients?

A. Paranoia.
B. Apathy.
C. Confusion.
D. Anxious dysphoria.

The correct response is option D: Anxious dysphoria.

In younger patients, hyperthyroidism typically manifests as hyperactivity or anxious dysphoria (option D is correct), whereas in the elderly, hyperthyroidism can manifest as apathy or depression (option B is incorrect). Paranoia and confusion can also occur but are not the most common symptoms (option A and C are incorrect). **Chapter 21 (p. 602)**

21.4   For a patient with rapid-cycling bipolar disorder and abnormal thyroid function tests, what is the most appropriate next step in management?

A. Discontinue lithium and switch to a different mood stabilizer.
B. Begin treatment with T_4 if thyroid-stimulating hormone (TSH) levels are elevated.
C. Begin treatment with T_4 only if TSH and T_4 levels are abnormal.
D. Begin treatment with T_4 only if patient has psychotic symptoms.

The correct response is option B: Begin treatment with T_4 if thyroid-stimulating hormone (TSH) levels are elevated.

Although lithium-induced thyroid dysfunction may be the cause in some cases, subclinical hypothyroidism is common in bipolar patients receiving other mood stabilizers (option A is incorrect). Every patient with rapid-cycling bipolar disorder should be evaluated for (subclinical) hypothyroidism and should receive T_4 if TSH levels are elevated (option B is correct). Patients with bipolar disorder with either rapid-cycling or mixed episodes have particularly high rates of subclinical hypothyroidism, almost 40% in one study. High-dose thyroid supplementation has been advocated in the treatment of bipolar disorder, even if patients are euthyroid, and studies have found that this treatment does not increase the risk of adverse cardiac effects or osteoporosis (option C is incorrect). Untreated hypothyroidism can result in psychosis, so-called myxedema madness; psychotic symptoms typically remit when TSH and T_4 levels return to normal (option D is incorrect). **Chapter 21 (p. 604)**

21.5 A 50-year-old man with a history of bipolar disorder, who has been stable for many years, presents with new onset of inattention, confusion, and belief that his coworker has planted a camera in his office to spy on him. He also complains of feeling thirsty, needing to urinate frequently, and pain in his joints. His wife mentions that about 1 year ago he became indifferent to events at home and work. Which of the following is the most likely explanation?

A. Valproate treatment for bipolar disorder caused hyperparathyroidism and severe hypercalcemia.
B. Lithium treatment for bipolar disorder caused hyperparathyroidism and severe hypercalcemia.
C. Lamotrigine treatment for bipolar disorder caused hyperparathyroidism and severe hypercalcemia.
D. Olanzapine treatment for bipolar disorder caused hyperparathyroidism and severe hypercalcemia.

The correct response is option B. Lithium treatment for bipolar disorder caused hyperparathyroidism and severe hypercalcemia.

The patient has hypercalcemia, which can be caused by hyperparathyroidism. Hyperparathyroidism is an underrecognized side effect of long-term lithium therapy (option B is correct). Symptoms of hypercalcemia include anorexia, thirst, frequent urination, lethargy, fatigue, muscle weakness, joint pain, and constipation. With mild hypercalcemia, patients may show personality changes and lack of initiative. Moderate hypercalcemia (serum calcium concentration=10–14 mg/dL) may cause dysphoria, anhedonia, apathy, anxiety, irritability, and cognitive impairment. In severe hypercalcemia (serum calcium concentration >14 mg/dL), confusion, disorientation, catatonia, agitation, paranoid ideation, delusions, hallucinations, and lethargy progressing to coma may occur. Valproate does not cause hypercalcemia (option A is incorrect) but is associated with weight gain, tremor, and thrombocytopenia. Lamotrigine does not cause hypercalcemia (option C is incorrect) but is associated with serious and potentially life-threatening immune reaction. Olanzapine does not cause hypercalcemia (option D is incorrect) but is associated with metabolic syndrome. **Chapter 17 (p. 489), Chapter 21 (p. 605), Chapter 36 (pp. 1199, 1200)**

21.6   Which of the following best characterizes the relationship between psychiatric disorders and osteoporosis?

A. Depression is a risk factor for osteoporosis in women but not men.
B. Osteoporosis in uncommon in patients with schizophrenia.
C. Depression is a risk factor for osteoporosis in both women and men.
D. Depression is a risk factor for osteoporosis in men but not women.

The correct response is option C: Depression is a risk factor for osteoporosis in both women and men.

Depression and osteoporosis commonly co-occur. The association between depression and osteoporosis is bidirectional; there is evidence that depression is a risk factor for osteoporosis in both women and men (Lee et al. 2015) (option C is correct; options A and D are incorrect). Some of the association between depression and osteoporosis may be due to antidepressants, especially selective serotonin reuptake inhibitors (SSRIs), which as a class are associated with reduced bone mineral density and increased fracture risk (Bruyère and Reginster 2015). Osteoporosis is common in people with schizophrenia, although the extent to which osteoporosis is due to antipsychotic-induced hyperprolactinemia is unclear (De Hert et al. 2016) (option B is incorrect). **Chapter 21 (pp. 605–606)**

21.7   Which neuropsychiatric symptom is *most* prevalent in Cushing's syndrome?

A. Psychosis.
B. Mania.
C. Anxiety.
D. Depression.

The correct response is option D: Depression.

Patients with Cushing's syndrome experience a variety of psychiatric symptoms including depression, anxiety, mania, psychosis, and cognitive dysfunction (Pivonello et al. 2015; Starkman 2013). Depression is the most prevalent psychiatric disturbance in Cushing's syndrome (option D is correct; options A, B, and C are incorrect). A full depressive syndrome has been reported in 50%–80% of cases, accompanied by irritability, insomnia, crying, decreased energy and libido, poor concentration and memory, and suicidal ideation (Pivonello et al. 2015). **Chapter 21 (p. 606)**

21.8   Which of the following tests can be used to definitively diagnose adrenal insufficiency?

A. Morning serum cortisol level.
B. Corticotropin stimulation test.
C. Adrenocorticotropic hormone (ACTH) level.
D. Fasting plasma glucose.

The correct response is option B: Corticotropin stimulation test.

Although the diagnosis of adrenal insufficiency may be suspected on the basis of a low morning serum cortisol level, further confirmatory testing is necessary (option A is incorrect). Definitive diagnosis requires a corticotropin stimulation test (option B is correct). A corticotropin stimulation test is typically performed with cosyntropin, a synthetic ACTH analogue. An increase in the serum cortisol concentration to >20 ng/dL following cosyntropin injection excludes the diagnosis of adrenal insufficiency. ACTH levels can be useful in distinguishing primary adrenal insufficiency from secondary adrenal insufficiency rather than definitively diagnosing the presence of adrenal insufficiency (option C is incorrect). In primary adrenal insufficiency (Addison's disease), ACTH levels are high; in secondary adrenal insufficiency, ACTH levels are low. Fasting plasma glucose is one of the tests used to diagnose diabetes mellitus, not adrenal insufficiency (option D is incorrect). **Chapter 21 (p. 607)**

21.9 Which antipsychotic can be used to treat medication-induced prolactinemia?

A. Aripiprazole.
B. Haloperidol.
C. Risperidone.
D. Paliperidone.

The correct response is option A: Aripiprazole.

Aripiprazole may reduce prolactin levels, and several clinical trials have demonstrated that switching from risperidone to aripiprazole, or adding it adjunctively, reduced previously elevated prolactin levels (Chen et al. 2015) (option A is correct). Haloperidol, risperidone, and paliperidone are all known to cause prolactinemia (options B, C, and D are incorrect). **Chapter 21 (p. 609)**

21.10 Polycystic ovarian syndrome (PCOS) is associated with which of the following adverse psychiatric consequences?

A. Psychosis.
B. Cognitive impairment.
C. Depression.
D. Mania.

The correct response is option C: Depression.

There are adverse psychosocial consequences of PCOS. Elevated rates of clinically significant anxiety and depression in women with PCOS have been noted in many studies (Barry et al. 2011; Blay et al. 2016; Dokras et al. 2012) (option C is correct). Psychosis, cognitive impairment, and mania are not thought to be adverse consequences of PCOS (options A, B, and D are incorrect). Of note, women with bipolar disorder treated with valproate were more likely than non-valproate-treated patients with bipolar disorder to have PCOS (Zhang et al. 2016). **Chapter 21 (p. 610), Chapter 36 (p. 1200)**

References

American Diabetes Association, American Psychiatric Association, American Association of Clinical Endocrinologists, et al: Consensus development conference on antipsychotics and obesity and diabetes. Diabetes Care 27:596–601, 2004

Barry JA, Kuczmierczyk AR, Hardiman PJ: Anxiety and depression in polycystic ovary syndrome: a systematic review and meta-analysis. Hum Reprod 26(9):2442–2451, 2011 21725075

Blay SL, Aguiar JV, Passos IC: Polycystic ovary syndrome and mental disorders: a systematic review and exploratory meta-analysis. Neuropsychiatr Dis Treat 12:2895–2903, 2016 27877043

Bruyère O, Reginster JY: Osteoporosis in patients taking selective serotonin reuptake inhibitors: a focus on fracture outcome. Endocrine 48(1):65–68, 2015 25091520

Calkin CV, Gardner DM, Ransom T, Alda M: The relationship between bipolar disorder and type 2 diabetes: more than just co-morbid disorders. Ann Med 45(2):171–181, 2013 22621171

Chen JX, Su YA, Bian QT, et al: Adjunctive aripiprazole in the treatment of risperidone-induced hyperprolactinemia: a randomized, double-blind, placebo-controlled, dose-response study. Psychoneuroendocrinology 58:130–140, 2015 25981348

Citrome L: Iloperidone, asenapine, and lurasidone: a brief overview of 3 new second-generation antipsychotics. Postgrad Med 123(2):153–162, 2011 21474903

De Hert M, Detraux J, Stubbs B: Relationship between antipsychotic medication, serum prolactin levels and osteoporosis/osteoporotic fractures in patients with schizophrenia: a critical literature review. Expert Opin Drug Saf 15(6):809–823, 2016 26986209

Dokras A, Clifton S, Futterweit W, Wild R: Increased prevalence of anxiety symptoms in women with polycystic ovary syndrome: systematic review and meta-analysis. Fertil Steril 97(1):225–30.e2, 2012 22127370

Garay-Sevilla ME, Malacara JM, González-Contreras E, et al: Perceived psychological stress in diabetes mellitus type 2. Rev Invest Clin 52(3):241–245, 2000 10953606

Golden SH: A review of the evidence for a neuroendocrine link between stress, depression and diabetes mellitus. Curr Diabetes Rev 3(4):252–259, 2007 18220683

Kan C, Silva N, Golden SH, et al: A systematic review and meta-analysis of the association between depression and insulin resistance. Diabetes Care 36(2):480–489, 2013 23349152

Lee CW, Liao CH, Lin CL, et al: Increased risk of osteoporosis in patients with depression: a population-based retrospective cohort study. Mayo Clin Proc 90(1):63–70, 2015 25572194

Leucht S, Cipriani A, Spineli L, et al: Comparative efficacy and tolerability of 15 antipsychotic drugs in schizophrenia: a multiple-treatments meta-analysis. Lancet 382(9896):951–962, 2013 23810019

Lloyd CE, Dyer PH, Lancashire RJ, et al: Association between stress and glycemic control in adults with type 1 (insulin-dependent) diabetes. Diabetes Care 22(8):1278–1283, 1999 10480771

Meyer JM, Davis VG, Goff DC, et al: Change in metabolic syndrome parameters with antipsychotic treatment in the CATIE Schizophrenia Trial: prospective data from phase 1. Schizophr Res 101(1-3):273–286, 2008 18258416

Murray R, Correll CU, Reynolds GP, Taylor D: Atypical antipsychotics: recent research findings and applications to clinical practice: Proceedings of a symposium presented at the 29th Annual European College of Neuropsychopharmacology Congress, 19 September 2016, Vienna, Austria. Ther Adv Psychopharmacol 7(1)(suppl):1–14, 2017 28344764

Pivonello R, Simeoli C, De Martino MC, et al: Neuropsychiatric disorders in Cushing's syndrome. Front Neurosci 9:129, 2015 25941467

Pouwer F, Kupper N, Adriaanse MC: Does emotional stress cause type 2 diabetes mellitus? A review from the European Depression in Diabetes (EDID) Research Consortium. Discov Med 9(45):112–118, 2010 20193636

Starkman MN: Neuropsychiatric findings in Cushing syndrome and exogenous glucocorticoid administration. Endocrinol Metab Clin North Am 42(3):477–488, 2013 24011881

Zhang L, Li H, Li S, Zou X: Reproductive and metabolic abnormalities in women taking valproate for bipolar disorder: a meta-analysis. Eur J Obstet Gynecol Reprod Biol 202:26–31, 2016 27160812

C H A P T E R   2 2

Oncology

22.1 Which of the following is a risk factor for the development of depression in cancer patients?

A. Older age.
B. Early stage of disease.
C. Female sex.
D. Insecure attachment style.

The correct response is option D: Insecure attachment style.

Established risk factors for the development of depression in cancer patients include younger age (option A is incorrect), advanced disease (option B is incorrect), inadequate social support, and insecure attachment style (option D is correct). The female predominance in major depressive disorder found in the general population is not consistently found in the oncology setting (Pirl 2004; Rodin et al. 2007; Strong et al. 2007) (option C is incorrect). **Chapter 22 (p. 628)**

22.2 Which of the following events is associated with a high risk of suicide in cancer patients?

A. Referral to palliative care.
B. Initial cancer diagnosis.
C. Completing chemotherapy treatment.
D. Undergoing surgery.

The correct response is option B: Initial cancer diagnosis.

The relative risk of suicide has been found to be highest, at 12.6, within the first week of receiving a cancer diagnosis (option B is correct). The relative risk drops to 3.1 during the first year (Fang et al. 2012) and is not correlated with referral to palliative care, completion of chemotherapy treatment, or undergoing surgery (options A, C, and D are incorrect). **Chapter 22 (pp. 628–630)**

22.3   Paroxetine affects which cytochrome P450 (CYP) enzyme important in the metabolism of tamoxifen?

A. CYP2D6.
B. CYP2C19.
C. CYP3A4.
D. CYP1A2.

The correct response is option A: CYP2D6.

Tamoxifen is a prodrug that requires metabolism by CYP2D6 to endoxifen, the active form. There is concern that coadministration of antidepressants that inhibit CYP2D6 may block the therapeutic effects of tamoxifen, although data are mixed regarding how serious a risk this presents (Leon-Ferre et al. 2017). It is recommended to avoid strong CYP2D6 inhibitors (e.g., paroxetine, fluoxetine, high-dosage sertraline, bupropion, duloxetine) in breast cancer patients (Haque et al. 2016) (option A is correct; options B, C, and D are incorrect). **Chapter 22 (pp. 640–641)**

22.4   In breast cancer patients, which of the following is associated with development of cancer-related fatigue?

A. Having a partner.
B. Being treated with surgery.
C. Being treated with surgery plus radiation.
D. Being treated with chemotherapy.

The correct response is option D: Being treated with chemotherapy.

In a meta-analysis involving more than 12,000 breast cancer patients, risk factors for development of cancer-related fatigue included having a more advanced disease stage, being treated with chemotherapy (option D is correct), and being treated with a combination of surgery, radiation, and chemotherapy. Having a partner, being treated with surgery, and being treated with surgery plus radiation reduced the risk of cancer-related fatigue (Abrahams et al. 2016) (options A, B, and C are incorrect). **Chapter 22 (p. 636)**

22.5   What is the *most* common motivation cited by patients for requesting physician-assisted suicide?

A. Loss of autonomy/dignity and the ability to enjoy life's activities.
B. Fears of increased pain and symptoms.
C. A sense of being a burden on loved ones.
D. Economic hardship associated with the costs of health care.

The correct response is option A: Loss of autonomy/dignity and the ability to enjoy life's activities.

The primary motivation cited by patients seeking physician-assisted suicide is loss of autonomy/dignity and the ability to enjoy life's activities (option A is correct). Other less commonly cited factors include fears of increased pain and symptoms, a sense of being a burden on loved ones, and economic hardship associated with the costs of health care (options B, C, and D are incorrect). **Chapter 22 (p. 631)**

22.6   Which of the following cancer types has been linked to the development of depression prior to the cancer diagnosis?

A. Esophageal cancer.
B. Gastric cancer.
C. Pancreatic cancer.
D. Colorectal cancer.

The correct response is option C: Pancreatic cancer.

Several studies have suggested there is a link between the development of depression and subsequent pancreatic cancer diagnosis (option C is correct). Two small studies found that up to 50% of pancreatic cancer patients manifested psychiatric symptoms at least 6 months prior to their cancer diagnosis (Green and Austin 1993; Joffe et al. 1986). Another study found that depression preceded pancreatic cancer more often than it preceded other gastrointestinal malignancies (Carney et al. 2003) (options A, B, and D are incorrect). **Chapter 22 (p. 643)**

22.7   What is the *most* common cause of hypomania or mania in cancer patients?

A. Interferon-alpha.
B. Methotrexate.
C. Corticosteroids.
D. Tamoxifen.

The correct response is option C: Corticosteroids.

In cancer patients, corticosteroids are the most common reason for hypomania or mania (option C is correct). Other neuropsychiatric side effects of steroids include mild to severe insomnia, anxiety, depression, and psychosis. Neuropsychiatric side effects of interferon-alpha include mania, depression, suicidality, psychosis, delirium, akathisia, and seizures. Although interferon-alpha is associated with mania, it is not the most common cause of hypomania or mania in cancer patients (option A is incorrect). Methotrexate, especially when given intrathecally, is associated with delirium and leukoencephalopathy (both acute and delayed-onset forms). Methotrexate is not associated with hypomania or mania (option B is incorrect). Neuropsychiatric side effects of tamoxifen include sleep disorders and irritability. Tamoxifen is not associated with hypomania or mania (option D is incorrect). **Chapter 22 (Table 22–2, p. 630; p. 633)**

22.8   A 67-year-old woman is receiving chemotherapy for non-small-cell adenocarcinoma of the lung. She currently complains of low mood, hopelessness, poor appetite, and chemotherapy-induced nausea. Which of the following antidepressants
may be helpful for its antiemetic and appetite-stimulating effects?

A. Mirtazapine.
B. Sertraline.
C. Citalopram.
D. Paroxetine.

The correct response is option A: Mirtazapine.

Mirtazapine's antiemetic and appetite-stimulating effects may make it a good
choice for anorexic-cachectic depressed cancer patients or for those experiencing
nausea or vomiting from chemotherapy (option A is correct). For patients experiencing significant nausea, mirtazapine should be considered over a selective serotonin reuptake inhibitor (options B, C, and D are incorrect). **Chapter 22 (p. 651),
Chapter 36 (p. 1192)**

References

Abrahams HJG, Gielissen MFM, Schmits IC, et al: Risk factors, prevalence, and course of severe
fatigue after breast cancer treatment: a meta-analysis involving 12 327 breast cancer survivors.
Ann Oncol 27(6):965–974, 2016 26940687

Carney CP, Jones L, Woolson RF, et al: Relationship between depression and pancreatic cancer in
the general population. Psychosom Med 65(5):884–888, 2003 14508036

Fang F, Fall K, Mittleman MA, et al: Suicide and cardiovascular death after a cancer diagnosis. N Engl
J Med 366(14):1310–1318, 2012 22475594

Green AI, Austin CP: Psychopathology of pancreatic cancer. A psychobiologic probe (review). Psychosomatics 34(3):208–221, 1993 8493302

Haque R, Shi J, Schottinger JE, et al: Tamoxifen and antidepressant drug interaction in a cohort of
16,887 breast cancer survivors. J Natl Cancer Inst 108(3): 2016 26631176

Joffe RT, Rubinow DR, Denicoff KD, et al: Depression and carcinoma of the pancreas. Gen Hosp
Psychiatry 8(4):241–245, 1986 3744031

Leon-Ferre RA, Majithia N, Loprinzi CL: Management of hot flashes in women with breast cancer
receiving ovarian function suppression. Cancer Treat Rev 52:82–90, 2017 27960127

Pirl WF: Evidence report on the occurrence, assessment, and treatment of depression in cancer patients. J Natl Cancer Inst Monogr 32(32):32–39, 2004 15263039

Rodin G, Walsh A, Zimmermann C, et al: The contribution of attachment security and social support to depressive symptoms in patients with metastatic cancer. Psychooncology 16(12):1080–
1091, 2007 17464942

Strong V, Waters R, Hibberd C, et al: Emotional distress in cancer patients: the Edinburgh Cancer
Centre symptom study. Br J Cancer 96(6):868–874, 2007 17311020

CHAPTER 23

Hematology

23.1 Which of the following is most likely to be seen in patients with folate deficiency anemia?

A. Hashimoto's thyroiditis.
B. Vegetarian diet.
C. Depression.
D. Subacute combined degeneration of the spinal cord.

The correct response is option C: Depression.

Vitamin B_{12} deficiency and folate deficiency have similar consequences on the nervous system and lead to megaloblastic anemia. Symptoms of folate deficiency are similar to those of B_{12} deficiency; however, subacute combined degeneration of the spinal cord is specific to B_{12} deficiency (option D is incorrect), and depression is more common in folate deficiency (Reynolds 2006) (option C is correct). Supplementation of B_{12} and folate in patients has not been shown to reduce depressive symptoms (de Koning et al. 2016; Okereke et al. 2015; Sharpley et al. 2014). Folic acid is found in both animal products and leafy green vegetables (option B is incorrect). Pernicious anemia is the most common cause of B_{12} deficiency (Toh et al. 1997) and is associated with other autoimmune disorders, including thyroiditis, diabetes mellitus, Addison's disease, Graves' disease, vitiligo, myasthenia gravis, Lambert-Eaton myasthenic syndrome, and hypoparathyroidism (Carmel et al. 2003; Toh et al. 1997) (option A is incorrect). **Chapter 23 (pp. 661–664)**

23.2 Which of the following is a major neuropsychiatric manifestation of sickle cell disease (SCD)?

A. Depression and anxiety related to stigma, unpredictable pain crises, and high mortality rates.
B. Depression and anxiety secondary to substance abuse.
C. Central nervous system damage resulting from opiate drug overuse.
D. Poor cognitive performance from frequent school absences.

The correct response is option A: Depression and anxiety related to stigma, unpredictable pain crises, and high mortality rates.

The neuropsychiatric manifestations of SCD can be divided into three main categories: 1) depression and anxiety resulting from living with a chronic stigmatizing disease associated with unpredictable, painful crises and high morbidity and mortality (option A is correct); 2) problems related to living with chronic and acute pain (often undertreated), control of which involves long-term use of analgesics, potentially leading to opioid dependency, addiction, and pseudoaddiction (option B is incorrect); and 3) central nervous system damage resulting from cerebral vascular accidents, primarily during childhood (option C is incorrect). SCD patients have been found to have lower scores in language skills and auditory discrimination as early as kindergarten; thus, deficits cannot be attributed to school absences (Strouse et al. 2011) (option D is incorrect). **Chapter 23 (pp. 664–666)**

23.3   How does opioid treatment typically impact patients with sickle cell disease?

   A. Opioids help control pain but decrease functional capacity and can lead to tolerance and addiction.
   B. Opioids help control pain but increase hospitalizations and can lead to tolerance and addiction.
   C. Opioids help control pain but consistently lead to tolerance and addiction.
   D. Opioids help control pain, improve functional capacity, and decrease hospitalizations.

The correct response is option D: Opioids help control pain, improve functional capacity, and decrease hospitalizations.

Over the past 15 years, opioid treatment has gained mainstream acceptance for the treatment of SCD pain. Opioids help control pain, *improve* functional capacity, and *decrease* hospitalizations in patients with SCD (Ballas et al. 2012; Taylor et al. 2010) (option D is correct; options A and B are incorrect). Chronic opioid use may result in tolerance, physiological dependence as well as substance dependence, and abuse. The few studies that address addiction in SCD report a low prevalence of substance abuse (option C is incorrect). **Chapter 23 (pp. 665–666)**

23.4   Which best describes the risk of agranulocytosis with clozapine use?

   A. The highest risk is present during the first 3 weeks of treatment and then decreases significantly.
   B. A white blood cell (WBC) count lower than $1,000/mm^3$ or an absolute neutrophil count lower than $500/mm^3$ is an indication for immediate cessation of clozapine.
   C. The fatality rate of clozapine-induced agranulocytosis is 4.2%–16%.
   D. Stopping clozapine is not typically a sufficient intervention.

The correct response is option C: The fatality rate of clozapine-induced agranulocytosis is 4.2%–16%.

The highest risk of clozapine-induced agranulocytosis is present during the first 6 months of treatment and then decreases significantly (option A is incorrect). A WBC count lower than $2,000/mm^3$ or an absolute neutrophil count lower than $1,000/mm^3$ is an indication for immediate cessation of clozapine (option B is incorrect). The case fatality rate of clozapine-induced agranulocytosis is estimated at 4.2%–16%, depending on whether a granulocyte colony stimulating factor (G-CSF) is used (Schulte 2006) (option C is correct). Stopping clozapine usually leads to WBC recovery within 3 weeks (Opgen-Rhein and Dettling 2008) (option D is incorrect). **Chapter 23 (pp. 670–671)**

23.5   Which of the following is an indication for cessation of treatment with a selective serotonin reuptake inhibitor (SSRI)?

A. SSRIs should be discontinued before any major surgery.
B. The SSRI in use is sertraline or citalopram, and the patient needs warfarin.
C. The patient is at high risk of gastrointestinal hemorrhage.
D. The patient has other sources of bleeding risk that outweigh the benefits of antidepressant treatment.

The correct response is option D: The patient has other sources of bleeding risk that outweigh the benefits of antidepressant treatment.

SSRIs inhibit platelet function and have been associated with bruising and bleeding, especially if used concomitantly with aspirin or nonsteroidal anti-inflammatory drugs (NSAIDs) (Jiang et al. 2015; Kuo et al. 2014). SSRIs increase central nervous system 5-hydroxytryptamine (5-HT; serotonin) and reduce 5-HT in platelets (leading to reduced platelet aggregation). Platelets normally release serotonin at the site of a vascular tear, leading to further platelet aggregation and vasodilatation and permitting the sealing of the tear without thrombosis of the vessel (Mahdanian et al. 2014). Especially in the elderly, bleeding from the upper gastrointestinal tract may occur at a frequency ranging from 1 in 100 to 1 in 1,000 patient-years of exposure to drugs, such as the SSRIs, that have high affinity to 5-HT (de Abajo et al. 2006). Caution is advised in patients at high risk of gastrointestinal bleeding, for whom clinicians may consider prescribing an antidepressant with low serotonin reuptake inhibition. Patients who are at risk for gastrointestinal hemorrhage and who are taking antidepressants with high serotonin reuptake inhibition should generally use smaller doses or avoid aspirin and NSAIDs (Loke et al. 2008; Weinrieb et al. 2005) (option C is incorrect). As a result of their antiplatelet effects, SSRIs and serotonin-norepinephrine reuptake inhibitors (SNRIs) may also increase the risk of perioperative bleeding. A review of 19 studies reporting information on bleeding complications during surgery among patients taking antidepressants found inconsistent risks from SSRIs (Roose and Rutherford 2016). On the basis of this finding, clinicians are advised to weigh with patients the risk of bleeding complications versus the risks of discontinuation syndrome and of symptom recurrence before advising discontinuation of SSRIs or SNRIs preoperatively (option A is incorrect). Although some reviews have concluded that there is no increased risk from combining SSRIs with warfarin (Kurdyak et al. 2005), there have been case reports of bleeding with concomitant use. Among the SSRIs, fluoxetine is the most commonly reported offending agent (Skop and Brown 1996). The interactions between warfarin and antidepressants can have potentially serious consequences, resulting from either platelet inhibition or inhibition of the cytochrome P450 (CYP) system. Of the antidepressants, fluoxetine, fluvoxamine, and paroxetine appear to have the highest potential for interactions (Duncan et al. 1998; Halperin and Reber 2007), while citalopram and sertraline may be relatively less likely to interact with warfarin (Duncan et al. 1998) (option B is incorrect). In summary, practitioners should proceed cautiously when prescribing SSRIs and SNRIs for patients who have other sources of bleeding risk, including patients who use antiplatelet agents, such as those prescribed in post–myocardial infarction or post–cardiac catheterization patients, and patients with bleeding dyscrasias from liver failure or hematological disease (option D is correct). **Chapter 23 (pp. 671–673)**

23.6   Why is carbamazepine contraindicated in patients with a history of bone marrow depression?

A. Carbamazepine is directly toxic to bone marrow and can cause potentially fatal agranulocytosis and aplastic anemia.
B. Carbamazepine causes a transient reduction in platelet count in approximately 10% of patients during the first 4 months of treatment.
C. Carbamazepine stimulates WBC production, predominantly neutrophils.
D. Potentially fatal hematopoietic complications such as neutropenia, thrombocytopenia, and macrocytic anemia have been associated with carbamazepine.

The correct response is option A: Carbamazepine is directly toxic to bone marrow and can cause potentially fatal agranulocytosis and aplastic anemia.

Carbamazepine should be avoided in individuals with a history of bone marrow depression. Carbamazepine produces a transient reduction in WBC count in approximately 10% of patients during the first 4 months of treatment (Rall and Schleifer 1980), but this is not the greatest danger from its use (option B is incorrect). In very rare cases, carbamazepine can cause potentially fatal agranulocytosis and aplastic anemia. Agranulocytosis results from direct toxicity to the bone marrow (Sedky and Lippmann 2006) (option A is correct). Lithium stimulates WBC production, predominantly neutrophils (option C is incorrect). Potentially fatal hematopoietic complications such as neutropenia, thrombocytopenia, and macrocytic anemia have been associated with valproate (Nasreddine and Beydoun 2008) (option D is incorrect). **Chapter 23 (p. 673)**

References

Ballas SK, Gupta K, Adams-Graves P: Sickle cell pain: a critical reappraisal. Blood 120(18):3647–3656, 2012 22923496

Carmel R, Green R, Rosenblatt DS, Watkins D: Update on cobalamin, folate, and homocysteine. Hematology (Am Soc Hematol Educ Program) 62–81, 2003 14633777

de Abajo FJ, Montero D, Rodríguez LA, Madurga M: Antidepressants and risk of upper gastrointestinal bleeding. Basic Clin Pharmacol Toxicol 98(3):304–310, 2006 16611206

de Koning EJ, van der Zwaluw NL, van Wijngaarden JP, et al: Effects of two-year vitamin B12 and folic acid supplementation on depressive symptoms and quality of life in older adults with elevated homocysteine concentrations: additional results from the B-PROOF study, an RCT. Nutrients 8(11):E748, 2016 27886078

Duncan D, Sayal K, McConnell H, Taylor D: Antidepressant interactions with warfarin. Int Clin Psychopharmacol 13(2):87–94, 1998 9669190

Halperin D, Reber G: Influence of antidepressants on hemostasis. Dialogues Clin Neurosci 9(1):47–59, 2007 17506225

Jiang HY, Chen HZ, Hu XJ, et al: Use of selective serotonin reuptake inhibitors and risk of upper gastrointestinal bleeding: a systematic review and meta-analysis. Clin Gastroenterol Hepatol 13(1):42–50.e3, 2015 24993365

Kuo CY, Liao YT, Chen VC: Risk of upper gastrointestinal bleeding when taking SSRIs with NSAIDs or aspirin. Am J Psychiatry 171(5):582, 2014 24788285

Kurdyak PA, Juurlink DN, Kopp A, et al: Antidepressants, warfarin, and the risk of hemorrhage. J Clin Psychopharmacol 25(6):561–564, 2005 16282838

Loke YK, Trivedi AN, Singh S: Meta-analysis: gastrointestinal bleeding due to interaction between selective serotonin uptake inhibitors and non-steroidal anti-inflammatory drugs. Aliment Pharmacol Ther 27(1):31–40, 2008 17919277

Mahdanian AA, Rej S, Bacon SL, et al: Serotonergic antidepressants and perioperative bleeding risk: a systematic review. Expert Opin Drug Saf 13(6):695–704, 2014 24717049

Nasreddine W, Beydoun A: Valproate-induced thrombocytopenia: a prospective monotherapy study. Epilepsia 49(3):438–445, 2008 18031547

Okereke OI, Cook NR, Albert CM, et al: Effect of long-term supplementation with folic acid and B vitamins on risk of depression in older women. Br J Psychiatry 206(4):324–331, 2015 25573400

Opgen-Rhein C, Dettling M: Clozapine-induced agranulocytosis and its genetic determinants. Pharmacogenomics 9(8):1101–1111, 2008 18681784

Rall TW, Schleifer LS: Drugs effective in the therapy of the epilepsies, in The Pharmacological Basis of Therapeutics, 6th Edition. Edited by Gilman AG, Goldman LG, Gilman A. New York, Macmillan, 1980, pp 448–474

Reynolds E: Vitamin B12, folic acid, and the nervous system. Lancet Neurol 5(11):949–960, 2006 17052662

Roose SP, Rutherford BR: Selective serotonin reuptake inhibitors and operative bleeding risk: a review of the literature. J Clin Psychopharmacol 36(6):704–709, 2016 27684291

Schulte P: Risk of clozapine-associated agranulocytosis and mandatory white blood cell monitoring. Ann Pharmacother 40(4):683–688, 2006 16595571

Sedky K, Lippmann S: Psychotropic medications and leukopenia. Curr Drug Targets 7(9):1191–1194, 2006 17017894

Sharpley AL, Hockney R, McPeake L, et al: Folic acid supplementation for prevention of mood disorders in young people at familial risk: a randomised, double blind, placebo controlled trial. J Affect Disord 167:306–311, 2014 25010374

Skop BP, Brown TM: Potential vascular and bleeding complications of treatment with selective serotonin reuptake inhibitors. Psychosomatics 37(1):12–16, 1996 8600488

Strouse JJ, Lanzkron S, Urrutia V: The epidemiology, evaluation and treatment of stroke in adults with sickle cell disease. Expert Rev Hematol 4(6):597–606, 2011 22077524

Taylor LE, Stotts NA, Humphreys J, et al: A review of the literature on the multiple dimensions of chronic pain in adults with sickle cell disease. J Pain Symptom Manage 40(3):416–435, 2010 20656451

Toh BH, van Driel IR, Gleeson PA: Pernicious anemia. N Engl J Med 337(20):1441–1448, 1997 9358143

Weinrieb RM, Auriacombe M, Lynch KG, Lewis JD: Selective serotonin re-uptake inhibitors and the risk of bleeding. Expert Opin Drug Saf 4(2):337–344, 2005 15794724

CHAPTER 24

Rheumatology

24.1 What class of pharmacological management of rheumatoid arthritis (RA) is associated with a lower prevalence of depressive and anxiety disorders?

A. Nonsteroidal anti-inflammatory drugs (NSAIDs).
B. Methotrexate and antimalarials.
C. Corticosteroids.
D. Biological response modifiers.

The correct response is option D: Biological response modifiers.

The use of medications that block peripheral proinflammatory cytokine activity (e.g., tumor necrosis factor antagonists) is associated with a lower prevalence of major depressive disorder and anxiety disorders independent of clinical status (Raison and Miller 2013; Uguz et al. 2009).

Biological treatments that target inflammation have been found to reduce disease activity and improve symptoms of fatigue in RA (Genty et al. 2017), consistent with the ability of etanercept to reduce depressive symptoms in patients with psoriasis (Tyring et al. 2006) (option D is correct). NSAIDs control symptoms and signs of local inflammation, although they do not appear to alter the eventual course of the disease; at high doses, NSAIDs may have psychiatric side effects including depression, anxiety, paranoia, hallucinations, reduced concentration, hostility, confusion, and delirium (option A is incorrect). Methotrexate and antimalarials alter the course of the disease by reducing inflammation; psychiatric side effects of antimalarials such as hydroxychloroquine include confusion, psychosis, mania, depression, nightmares, anxiety, aggression, and delirium (option B is incorrect). Corticosteroids can be used to reduce signs of inflammation by systemic administration (oral or parenteral) or by local injection and have been shown to cause a variety of psychiatric syndromes, including depression and anxiety (option C is incorrect). **Chapter 24 (pp. 684, 686, 695, 700; Table 24–3, p. 701)**

24.2 What is the *strongest* proximal risk factor for depression in RA?

A. Burden of chronic physical symptoms.
B. Personal losses resulting from RA.

301

C. Major life stressors, including interpersonal stress and social rejection.

D. Disability.

The correct response is option C: Major life stressors, including interpersonal stress and social rejection.

Major life stressors, especially those involving interpersonal stress and social rejection, are among the strongest proximal risk factors for depression in RA (Slavich and Irwin 2014) (option C is correct). Chronic psychosocial and interpersonal stressors not only contribute to depression but also increase cellular and molecular markers of inflammation, which can lead to worsening of RA disease activity and further exacerbation and perpetuation of disease-related stress and depressive symptoms (Margaretten et al. 2009; Slavich and Irwin 2014). The burden of chronic physical symptoms, disability, and personal losses resulting from RA contribute to an increased risk of depression (options A, B, and D are incorrect). **Chapter 24 (p. 685)**

24.3   Which cluster symptom in RA is associated with greater pain?

A. Sleep difficulties.

B. Depressed mood.

C. Fatigue.

D. Functional disability.

The correct response is option B: Depressed mood.

Depression is associated with greater pain, whereas sleep difficulties are associated with fatigue, depression, and pain (Drewes et al. 1998; Nicassio et al. 2002) (option B is correct; options A and C are incorrect). Sleep disturbance is thought to contribute to pain, fatigue, and depressed mood in patients with RA, and several studies have shown that subjective sleep complaints correlate with fatigue, functional disability (option D is incorrect), greater joint pain, and more depressive symptoms in these patients (Moldofsky 2001). **Chapter 24 (p. 689)**

24.4   What is the single strongest marker of central nervous system (CNS) risk in systemic lupus erythematosus (SLE) patients?

A. Articular manifestation or discoid rash.

B. Antinuclear antibody (ANA)–negative.

C. Antiphospholipid antibodies.

D. Drug-induced SLE.

The correct response is option C: Antiphospholipid antibodies.

Antiphospholipid antibodies may be the single strongest marker of CNS risk because they are associated with stroke, cognitive dysfunction, and epilepsy (Coín et al. 2015) (option C is correct). Patients with mainly articular manifestations or discoid rash (option A is incorrect) have a much lower risk of neuropsychiatric lupus, as do those few who are ANA-negative (option B is incorrect) and those with drug-induced SLE (option D is incorrect). **Chapter 24 (p. 692)**

24.5 To define neuropsychiatric lupus according to the American College of Rheumatology Ad Hoc Committee on Neuropsychiatric Lupus Nomenclature (1999), which disorder is the *most* common?

A. Cognitive dysfunction.
B. Anxiety.
C. Depression.
D. Mania.

The correct response is option A: Cognitive dysfunction.

Cognitive dysfunction is the most common neuropsychiatric disorder in patients with SLE, with a prevalence estimated at 80% in one systematic review (Meszaros et al. 2012) (option A is correct). Anxiety is quite common in SLE patients, often as a reaction to the illness (option B). Depression is the second most common neuropsychiatric disorder in SLE (option C is incorrect). In patients with SLE, the most common cause of mania is corticosteroid therapy (option D is incorrect). **Chapter 24 (p. 694)**

24.6 Which of the following is more likely due to a CNS lupus flare-up than a corticosteroid-induced psychiatric reaction?

A. Increases in indices of inflammation.
B. Mania or mixed states.
C. Exacerbation of symptoms in response to corticosteroids.
D. SLE symptoms preceding the onset of psychiatric symptoms.

The correct response is option A: Increases in indices of inflammation.

Increases in indices of inflammation in laboratory tests are associated with CNS lupus flare-up (option A is correct). Mania or mixed states, exacerbation of symptoms in response to corticosteroids, and the presence of SLE symptoms that precede onset of psychiatric symptoms are associated with corticosteroid-induced psychiatric reaction (options B, C, and D are incorrect). **Chapter 24 (Table 24–2, p. 697)**

24.7 As a wide variety of diseases can mimic neuropsychiatric SLE, which of the following may be mistaken for CNS lupus but is characterized by a negative ANA?

A. Mixed or undifferentiated connective tissue disease.
B. Hepatitis C.
C. Wegener's granulomatosis.
D. Multiple sclerosis.

The correct response is option C: Wegener's granulomatosis.

A third group of diseases, characterized by a negative ANA, also may be mistaken for CNS lupus. This group includes polyarteritis nodosa, microscopic angiitis, Wegener's granulomatosis (option C is correct), chronic fatigue syndrome, fibromyalgia, temporal arteritis, and Behçet's syndrome. A group of diseases, associated with a medium to high ANA titer (>1:160), includes Sjögren's syndrome and mixed or undifferentiated connective tissue disease (option A is incorrect). Finally, a group of diseases associated with a low ANA titer (<1:160) includes multiple sclerosis (option D is incorrect) and, less commonly, ANA-positive RA, sarcoidosis, and hepatitis C (option B is incorrect). **Chapter 24 (p. 696)**

24.8   CNS involvement is rare in which of the following rheumatological conditions?

A. Sjögren's syndrome.
B. Temporal arteritis.
C. Granulomatosis with polyangiitis.
D. RA.

The correct response is option D: RA.

Despite RA's multisystem manifestations, neurological complications are not common. The most common neurological manifestation is peripheral neuropathy. Direct CNS involvement is rare (option D is correct). Sjögren's syndrome may be difficult to distinguish from CNS SLE (and the two syndromes may overlap); involvement has been reported in 9%–44% of cases of primary Sjögren's syndrome (Bougea et al. 2015) (option A is incorrect). Neuropsychiatric manifestations of temporal arteritis arise because of involvement of arteries supplying blood to the CNS (option B is incorrect). The insults to the CNS in temporal arteritis can be ischemic or hemorrhagic. In granulomatosis with polyangiitis, CNS involvement has included chronic meningitis, hemorrhage, and mass lesions (Huang et al. 2015) (option C is incorrect). **Chapter 24 (pp. 685, 696, 698, 700)**

24.9   Which rheumatological disorder is *not* likely to respond to corticosteroid treatment?

A. Systemic sclerosis (scleroderma).
B. Temporal arteritis.
C. RA.
D. SLE.

The correct response is option A: Systemic sclerosis (scleroderma).

No known treatment is available to prevent progression of scleroderma (although some medications alleviate symptoms), and the prognosis can be poor because of renal failure and pulmonary hypertension (option A is correct). In temporal arteritis, treatment with high-dose corticosteroids should commence as soon as the diagnosis has been made on clinical grounds, before results of arterial biopsy are available, to prevent disease progression (Buttgereit et al. 2016) (option B is incorrect). The spectrum of treatment options for SLE is similar to that for RA, namely, NSAIDs, antimalarials (e.g., hydroxychloroquine), corticosteroids, and other immunosuppressants (e.g., azathioprine, mycophenolate mofetil, methotrexate, cyclophosphamide) (options C and D are incorrect)). **Chapter 24 (pp. 690, 698, 699)**

24.10 Which medication is likely to cause confusion, psychosis, mania, nightmares, and aggression?

A. Infliximab.
B. Tocilizumab.
C. Hydroxychloroquine.
D. Mycophenolate mofetil.

The correct response is option C. Hydroxychloroquine.

Hydroxychloroquine is known to have the following psychiatric side effects: confusion, psychosis, mania, depression, nightmares, anxiety, aggression, and delirium (option C is correct). There is no reported psychiatric side effect associated with infliximab or tocilizumab (options A and B are incorrect). Anxiety, depression, and sedation may rarely manifest with mycophenolate mofetil (option D is incorrect). **Chapter 24 (p. 701, Table 24–3)**

References

American College of Rheumatology Ad Hoc Committee on Neuropsychiatric Lupus Nomenclature: The American College of Rheumatology nomenclature and case definitions for neuropsychiatric lupus syndromes. Arthritis Rheum 42(4):599–608, 1999 10211873

Bougea A, Anagnostou E, Konstantinos G, et al: A systematic review of peripheral and central nervous system involvement of rheumatoid arthritis, systemic lupus erythematosus, primary Sjögren's syndrome, and associated immunological profiles. Int J Chronic Dis 2015:910352, 2015 26688829

Buttgereit F, Dejaco C, Matteson EL, Dasgupta B: Polymyalgia rheumatica and giant cell arteritis: a systematic review. JAMA 315(22):2442–2458, 2016 27299619

Coín MA, Vilar-López R, Peralta-Ramírez I, et al: The role of antiphospholipid autoantibodies in the cognitive deficits of patients with systemic lupus erythematosus. Lupus 24(8):875–879, 2015 25697771

Drewes AM, Svendsen L, Taagholt SJ, et al: Sleep in rheumatoid arthritis: a comparison with healthy subjects and studies of sleep/wake interactions. Br J Rheumatol 37(1):71–81, 1998 9487254

Genty M, Combe B, Kostine M, et al: Improvement of fatigue in patients with rheumatoid arthritis treated with biologics: relationship with sleep disorders, depression and clinical efficacy. A prospective, multicentre study. Clin Exp Rheumatol 35(1):85–92, 2017 27749229

Huang YH, Ro LS, Lyu RK, et al: Wegener's granulomatosis with nervous system involvement: a hospital-based study. Eur Neurol 73(3-4):197–204, 2015 25791920

Margaretten M, Yelin E, Imboden J, et al: Predictors of depression in a multiethnic cohort of patients with rheumatoid arthritis. Arthritis Rheum 61(11):1586–1591, 2009 19877099

Meszaros ZS, Perl A, Faraone SV: Psychiatric symptoms in systemic lupus erythematosus: a systematic review. J Clin Psychiatry 73(7):993–1001, 2012 22687742

Moldofsky H: Sleep and pain. Sleep Med Rev 5(5):385–396, 2001 12531004

Nicassio PM, Moxham EG, Schuman CE, Gevirtz RN: The contribution of pain, reported sleep quality, and depressive symptoms to fatigue in fibromyalgia. Pain 100(3):271–279, 2002 12467998

Raison CL, Miller AH: Role of inflammation in depression: implications for phenomenology, pathophysiology and treatment. Mod Trends Pharmacopsychiatry 28:33–48, 2013 25224889

Slavich GM, Irwin MR: From stress to inflammation and major depressive disorder: a social signal transduction theory of depression. Psychol Bull 140(3):774–815, 2014 24417575

Tyring S, Gottlieb A, Papp K, et al: Etanercept and clinical outcomes, fatigue, and depression in psoriasis: double-blind placebo-controlled randomised phase III trial. Lancet 367(9504):29–35, 2006 16399150

Uguz F, Akman C, Kucuksarac S, Tufekci O: Anti-tumor necrosis factor-alpha therapy is associated with less frequent mood and anxiety disorders in patients with rheumatoid arthritis. Psychiatry Clin Neurosci 63(1):50–55, 2009 19154212

CHAPTER 25

Chronic Fatigue and Fibromyalgia Syndromes

25.1   Which of the following statements most accurately describes chronic fatigue syndrome (CFS) and fibromyalgia syndrome (FMS)?

A. CFS and FMS are as firmly based in disease pathology as any other medical condition.
B. CFS and FMS are symptom-defined somatic syndromes in which biological, psychological, and social factors play a role.
C. CFS and FMS are social constructions based on psychological amplification of somatic sensation.
D. CFS and FMS are syndromes in which psychological conflicts are expressed in physical symptoms.

The correct response is option B: CFS and FMS are symptom-defined somatic syndromes in which biological, psychological, and social factors play a role.

The history of CFS and FMS has been notorious for disputes about whether these disorders are "organic" or "psychogenic" (Asbring and Närvänen 2003). The extreme organic position argues that they will eventually become as firmly based in disease pathology as any other medical condition, whereas the extreme psychogenic view is that they are pseudo-diseases, rooted not in biology but rather in social constructions based on the psychological amplification of somatic sensations (Shorter 1992). Neither of these extreme positions is satisfactorily sustained by the evidence or, indeed, helpful in managing patients (options A, C, and D are incorrect). The extreme organic view encourages the doctor to endlessly seek pathology while the patient is left without treatment. The extreme psychological view may encourage the doctor to dismiss the patient's symptoms as "all in the mind." As with most illnesses, an etiologically neutral and integrated perspective that simultaneously recognizes the reality of the symptoms and acknowledges the contribution of biological, psychological, and social factors is the best basis for clinical practice (Engel 1977) (option B is correct). **Chapter 25 (p. 710)**

25.2 A patient presents with 7 months of fatigue and malaise after exercising and reports that sleep is not restorative. What is an additional physical symptom that would support the diagnosis of CFS?

A. Chest pain.
B. Gastrointestinal problems.
C. Sore throat.
D. Chronic pelvic pain.

The correct response is option C: Sore throat.

The core symptom of CFS is persistent physical and mental fatigue that is exacerbated by exertion. Disrupted and unrefreshing sleep is almost universally described, and widespread pain is common (Prins et al. 2006). Diagnostic criteria for CFS based on an international consensus case definition requires clinically evaluated, medically unexplained fatigue of at least 6 months' duration that is of new onset (not lifelong), not the result of ongoing exertion, and not substantially alleviated by rest and is associated with a substantial reduction in previous level of activities. In addition to fatigue, four or more of the following symptoms must be present to diagnose CFS: subjective memory impairment, sore throat (option C is correct), tender lymph nodes, muscle pain, joint pain, headache, unrefreshing sleep, and postexertional malaise lasting more than 24 hours. Other functional syndromes include noncardiac chest pain, hyperventilation, irritable bowel and functional upper gastrointestinal disorders, idiopathic pruritus, migraine, chronic pelvic pain and vulvodynia, and several other pain syndromes (options A, B, and D are incorrect). **Chapter 25 (p. 711; Table 25–1, p. 712)**

25.3 Which of the following is an accurate statement about the revised 2010 American College of Rheumatology (ACR) criteria for FMS?

A. Patient must have a minimum number of tender point sites on palpation.
B. Patient must have widespread pain of at least 6 months' duration.
C. Patient must report fatigue, waking unrefreshed, cognitive symptoms, or somatic symptoms.
D. A distinguishing diagnostic feature is the presence of distressing bodily symptoms.

The correct response is option C: Patient must report fatigue, waking unrefreshed, cognitive symptoms, or somatic symptoms.

In 1990, the ACR adopted the term *fibromyalgia* and developed criteria for its classification (Wolfe et al. 1990); the criteria were updated in 2010 (Wolfe et al. 2010). The core feature of fibromyalgia is chronic widespread pain. Although the 1990 criteria require tenderness at 11 or more of 18 specific sites on the body, the 2010 update does *not* require the presence of tender points (option A is incorrect). The ACR criteria specify widespread pain of at least 3 months' duration (option B is incorrect). Fatigue, sleep disturbance, musculoskeletal tenderness, and subjective cognitive impairment (memory and concentration) are common; ACR criteria for fibromyalgia require widespread pain index (WPI) ≥7 and symptom severity (SS) scale score ≥5 or WPI 3–6 and SS scale score ≥9. The SS scale score rates fatigue, waking unrefreshed, cognitive symptoms, and somatic symptoms in general (option C is correct). Distressing bodily symptoms is a criterion for somatoform disorder that distinguishes it from illness anxiety disorder (option D is incorrect). **Chapter 11 (p. 307), Chapter 25 (pp. 711–712; Table 25–2, p. 713)**

25.4   Which of the following statements most accurately describes the association between CFS and FMS with psychiatric disorders?

A. Incidence of major depressive disorder (MDD) in patients with CFS and FMS is similar.
B. CFS, but not FMS, is associated with increased prevalence of posttraumatic stress disorder.
C. After adjusting for hierarchical rules that subsume generalized anxiety disorder (GAD) under MDD, the prevalence of GAD in patients with CFS and FMS is similar to that in the general population.
D. Most patients with CFS and FMS would meet criteria for somatic symptom disorder.

The correct response is option A: Incidence of major depressive disorder (MDD) in patients with CFS and FMS is similar.

Many patients who have received a diagnosis of CFS or FMS also meet criteria for a psychiatric diagnosis; some symptoms of CFS or FMS (e.g., fatigue, sleep disturbance, poor concentration) overlap with the symptoms of depression and anxiety. A study of patients with CFS reported that more than 25% had a current *Diagnostic and Statistical Manual of Mental Disorders* (DSM) MDD diagnosis and 50%–75% had a lifetime diagnosis (Afari and Buchwald 2003). In one study (Epstein et al. 1999) of FMS patients in a specialist clinic, 32% had a depressive disorder (22% had MDD) (option A is correct). The prevalence of posttraumatic stress disorder has been reported to be higher in patients with CFS (Dansie et al. 2012) and much higher in patients with FMS (Coppens et al. 2017) than in the general population (option B is incorrect). One study reported finding GAD in as many as half of clinic patients with CFS or FMS when the hierarchical rules that subsumed GAD under MDD were suspended (Fischler et al. 1997) (option C is incorrect). In DSM-5 (American Psychiatric Association 2013), the diagnosis somatic symptom disorder replaced the DSM-IV (American Psychiatric Association 1994) diagnosis of somatoform disorder. The DSM-5 disorder emphasizes the presence of excessive concern about somatic symptoms rather than the absence of identified physical disease (Dimsdale et al. 2013). Although it could be argued that most patients with FMS or CFS would meet criteria for DSM-IV somatoform disorder, the percentage who would meet criteria for DSM-5 somatic symptom disorder is uncertain but may be considerably smaller (Häuser et al. 2015) (option D is incorrect). **Chapter 25 (pp. 714–715)**

25.5 Which of the following is a predictor of poor outcome in CFS?

A. Short duration of illness.
B. Younger age.
C. Minimal symptom severity.
D. Belief that the illness has a physical cause.

The correct response is option D: Belief that the illness has a physical cause.

The prognosis for patients with CFS or FMS is variable; these illnesses typically have a chronic but fluctuating course. Prospective studies of CFS and FMS in the general population have reported that in about half of cases, the syndrome is in partial or complete remission by 2–3 years after diagnosis (Granges et al. 1994; Nisenbaum et al. 2003). Poor outcome in CFS and FMS is predicted by longer illness duration, more severe symptoms, older age (options A, B, and C are incorrect), depression, and lack of social support (van der Werf et al. 2002), and in CFS by a strong belief in a physical cause (Cairns and Hotopf 2005) (option D is correct). Both CFS and FMS are more common in women (Jones et al. 2015; Reyes et al. 2003). CFS and FMS are both associated with substantial loss of function and work disability; unemployment in patients with CFS and FMS accessing specialist services in the United States is as high as 50% (Bombardier and Buchwald 1996). **Chapter 25 (pp. 716–717)**

25.6 Which of the following statements regarding predisposing and precipitating factors for CFS is most supported by currently available evidence?

A. There is a strong heritable component to CFS and FMS, including likely candidate genes.
B. Certain personality types are predictive of developing CFS and FMS.
C. Patients with CFS and FMS often had highly active lives prior to onset of illness.
D. Chronic back pain is known to precipitate the onset of FMS and may of CFS also.

The correct response is option C: Patients with CFS and FMS often had highly active lives prior to onset of illness.

The etiologies of CFS and FMS remain unknown. The available evidence suggests that a combination of environmental factors and individual vulnerability initiates a series of biological, psychological, and social processes that lead to the development of CFS or FMS; however, most research in this area is based on small case–control studies with insufficient power to control for confounding, thereby limiting the ability to draw strong causal inferences about any of the findings reported below. Modest evidence from family and twin studies suggests that genetic factors play a part in predisposing individuals to CFS or to FMS; claims for the role of specific genes in the etiology of these conditions remain so far unproven (option A is incorrect). Although obsessional or perfectionistic personality type has been proposed as a risk factor for CFS and for chronic pain, there is limited evidence for this (option B is incorrect). The clinical observation that CFS and FMS patients lead abnormally active lives or have high levels of exercise before becoming ill has some empirical support (Harvey et al. 2008) (option C is correct). The role of physical injury in the etiology of CFS and FMS has been controversial; limited evidence indicates that both conditions may be precipitated by injury, particularly to the neck (option D is incorrect). **Chapter 25 (pp. 717–718; Table 25–3, p. 718)**

25.7   A 35-year-old man presents with symptoms suggestive of CFS, which he reports began a few months ago when he was offered a lucrative and exciting job promotion that would require frequent travel, but he felt pressured by family to decline when they learned he was the best human leukocyte antigen match for his critically ill brother who was awaiting renal transplantation. What type of stress does this patient demonstrate that may be relevant to the etiology of CFS?

A. Denial.
B. Fear.
C. Dilemma.
D. Altruism.

The correct response is option C: Dilemma.

Clinical experience indicates that patients often report that CFS or FMS has an onset during a stressful period in their lives. The evidence for life stress or life events as precipitants for FMS and CFS is, however, both limited and retrospective (Anderberg et al. 2000; Theorell et al. 1999). One of the best studies so far examined 64 patients and a similar number of matched control subjects. An excess of severe life events and difficulties was found in the CFS patients for the year prior to onset. More specifically, a certain type of life event called a *dilemma*—defined as an event in which the person must choose between two equally undesirable outcomes to circumstances—was reported by one-third of the patients with CFS and none of the control subjects (Hatcher and House 2003) (option C is correct). The patient in this scenario had to choose between a job promotion that would benefit himself or consider becoming a living kidney donor for the benefit of his brother and family. *Denial* is the conscious or unconscious repudiation of all or part of the total available meanings of an event to allay fear, anxiety, or other unpleasant affects; denial can be adaptive or maladaptive, based on how it influences a person's response to the realities of a stressful situation (option A is incorrect). Anger, fear, grief, and shame are common emotional responses to medical illness or other life stressors (option B is incorrect). Altruism is a mature defense mechanism, and altruistic behavior is an example of an adaptive response to stress or illness; through helping others, for example, some people feel a sense of purpose and gratification that can help improve their mood (option D is incorrect). **Chapter 3 (Table 3–2, p. 65; pp. 66, 69, 72), Chapter 25 (p. 718)**

25.8   In a patient with severe fatigue, which of the findings below would be most sup-
        portive of a diagnosis of CFS or FMS?

   A. Elevated interleukin-6 (IL-6).
   B. Low cortisol.
   C. Myoglobinuria.
   D. Positive Epstein-Barr virus test.

The correct response is option B: Low cortisol.

Changes in the level and response of neuroendocrine stress hormones have been
found in both CFS and FMS (Tak et al. 2011). Low blood cortisol and poor cortisol
response to stress have been reported (Parker et al. 2001) (option B is correct). These
observations differ from findings in depression (in which blood levels of cortisol
are typically elevated) but are similar to findings in other stress and anxiety states.
There is evidence that these low cortisol levels rise in response to successful cognitive-behavioral therapy (Roberts et al. 2009). Immunological factors, especially
cytokines, have been investigated in CFS and FMS, not only because of the possible
triggering effect of infection but also because immune-activating agents, such as interferons, are recognized to cause fatigue and myalgia. Systemic reviews, however,
have found only suggestive evidence of any consistent abnormality in CFS (Blundell et al. 2015; Nijs et al. 2014) (option A is incorrect). In patients with CFS or FMS,
there are no proven pathological or biochemical abnormalities of muscle or muscle
metabolism other than those expected with deconditioning (option C is incorrect).
There has been much interest in the potential role of ongoing infection and associated immunological factors, especially in CFS. It was previously thought that
chronic Epstein-Barr virus was a cause of CFS, but that hypothesis has been rejected (option D is incorrect). **Chapter 25 (p. 719)**

25.9   What measures should a therapist recommend that might improve the recovery
        of a patient with CFS/FMS?

   A. Graded exercise therapy.
   B. Avoiding activities that might lead to an increase in symptoms.
   C. Keeping a daily symptom record.
   D. Active involvement in a CFS/FMS patient support group.

The correct response is option A: Graded exercise therapy.

Graded exercise therapy has been found in systematic reviews to be of benefit for
both CFS and FMS (Bidonde et al. 2017; Larun et al. 2017) (option A is correct). A
fear-avoidance phenomenon—in which fear of exacerbating symptoms leads to
avoidance of activity—has been well described in both CFS and FMS (Nijs et al.
2013). Objective assessment has confirmed that patients with CFS and FMS have
reduced overall activity, with a quarter being pervasively inactive. This reduced
activity produces deconditioning, and hence inactivity is a target for treatment

(option B is incorrect). Another potentially important coping behavior is symptom vigilance, defined as the focusing of attention on symptoms (Roelofs et al. 2003). This behavior is associated with catastrophizing beliefs and greater perceived symptom intensity and therefore offers another target for treatment (Hughes et al. 2017) (option C is incorrect). A striking social aspect of CFS and FMS is the vocal patient support and advocacy organizations, often supported by social media. These organizations often campaign against rehabilitation and against psychological and psychiatric involvement in patient care, both of which are seen as threats to the "medical status" of their illness (Murphy et al. 2016). Studies have suggested that patients who are members of patient support and advocacy groups have poorer outcomes and poorer response to rehabilitation (Bentall et al. 2002) (option D is incorrect). **Chapter 25 (pp. 720–721, 729)**

25.10 What is the most appropriate initial approach to evaluate CFS or FMS for a new patient presenting with 3 weeks of fatigue and generalized pain?

A. Follow-up visit at 1 month.
B. Viral and immunological studies for CFS.
C. Discontinuing statin medication.
D. Sleep study.

The correct response is option A: Follow-up visit at 1 month.

The medical differential diagnosis for CFS and FMS is lengthy because so many diseases can present with pain and/or fatigue (Sharpe and Wilks 2002; Yunus 2002). Both physical and mental status examinations must be performed in every case to assess for alternative medical and physical diagnoses. The duration of symptoms is important because 75% of patients presenting to primary care with symptoms such as fatigue and pain improve within 2–4 weeks (Kroenke 2003) (option A is correct). For persistent symptoms, most of the common medical disorders can be diagnosed from standard history, physical examination, and basic laboratory studies. Initial investigation focuses on the clinical signs, symptoms, and time course. When symptom duration exceeds 4–6 weeks, an initial basic screening workup is appropriate. If there are no specific indications for special investigations, adequate screening tests include the following: thyrotropin, erythrocyte sedimentation rate, or similar measures of inflammation (sensitive for any condition with systemic inflammation), complete blood count, basic chemistries, and withdrawal of potential culprit medications (particularly statins, which typically require 4–6 weeks for symptom resolution after cessation) (option C is incorrect). Special investigations should be carried out only if clearly indicated by the history or examination. Immunological and virological tests are generally unhelpful (option B is incorrect). Sleep studies can be useful in excluding sleep apnea, narcolepsy, nocturnal myoclonus, and restless legs syndrome (option D is incorrect). **Chapter 25 (p. 723; Table 25–4, pp. 724–725)**

25.11   What would be the most effective medication to prescribe to a 30-year-old otherwise healthy depressed patient with FMS and widespread pain?

A. Nonsteroidal anti-inflammatory drugs (NSAIDs).
B. Nortriptyline.
C. Fluoxetine.
D. Citalopram.

The correct response is option B: Nortriptyline.

Antidepressant drug treatment is indicated when patients have depressive and
anxiety syndromes. Also, these agents can provide relief from pain and improve
sleep, even in the absence of depression. Overall, there is evidence for the short-
term efficacy of antidepressants in FMS (Häuser et al. 2009), but there is less evidence in CFS. The tricyclic antidepressants are more effective (option B is correct)
than the selective serotonin reuptake inhibitors for relieving pain and for induc-
ing sleep (options C and D are incorrect). Patients with CFS or FMS frequently
take NSAIDs to relieve pain. However, no evidence from clinical trials indicates
that NSAIDs are effective (Derry et al. 2017) (option A is incorrect). In summary,
the available evidence suggests that drug therapy currently has a limited role in
the management of these conditions, and nonpharmacological therapies are preferred. **Chapter 25 (pp. 727–728)**

References

Afari N, Buchwald D: Chronic fatigue syndrome: a review. Am J Psychiatry 160(2):221–236, 2003
    12562565
American Psychiatric Association: Diagnostic and Statistical Manual of Mental Disorders, 4th Edi-
    tion. Washington, DC, American Psychiatric Association, 1994
American Psychiatric Association: Diagnostic and Statistical Manual of Mental Disorders, 5th Edi-
    tion. Arlington, VA, American Psychiatric Association, 2013
Anderberg UM, Marteinsdottir I, Theorell T, von Knorring L: The impact of life events in female
    patients with fibromyalgia and in female healthy controls. Eur Psychiatry 15(5):295–301, 2000
    10954873
Asbring P, Närvänen AL: Ideal versus reality: physicians perspectives on patients with chronic fa-
    tigue syndrome (CFS) and fibromyalgia. Soc Sci Med 57(4):711–720, 2003 12821018
Bentall RP, Powell P, Nye FJ, Edwards RH: Predictors of response to treatment for chronic fatigue
    syndrome. Br J Psychiatry 181:248–252, 2002 12204931
Bidonde J, Busch AJ, Schachter CL, et al: Aerobic exercise training for adults with fibromyalgia.
    Cochrane Database Syst Rev 6(6):CD012700, 2017 28636204
Blundell S, Ray KK, Buckland M, White PD: Chronic fatigue syndrome and circulating cytokines:
    a systematic review. Brain Behav Immun 50:186–195, 2015 26148446
Bombardier CH, Buchwald D: Chronic fatigue, chronic fatigue syndrome, and fibromyalgia. Dis-
    ability and health-care use. Med Care 34(9):924–930, 1996 8792781
Cairns R, Hotopf M: A systematic review describing the prognosis of chronic fatigue syndrome.
    Occup Med (Lond) 55(1):20–31, 2005 15699087
Coppens E, Van Wambeke P, Morlion B, et al: Prevalence and impact of childhood adversities and
    post-traumatic stress disorder in women with fibromyalgia and chronic widespread pain. Eur
    J Pain 21(9):1582–1590, 2017 28543929

Dansie EJ, Heppner P, Furberg H, et al: The comorbidity of self-reported chronic fatigue syndrome, post-traumatic stress disorder, and traumatic symptoms. Psychosomatics 53(3):250–257, 2012 22296866

Derry S, Wiffen PJ, Häuser W, et al: Oral nonsteroidal anti-inflammatory drugs for fibromyalgia in adults. Cochrane Database Syst Rev 3(3):CD012332, 2017 28349517

Dimsdale JE, Creed F, Escobar J, et al: Somatic symptom disorder: an important change in DSM. J Psychosom Res 75(3):223–228, 2013 23972410

Engel GL: The need for a new medical model: a challenge for biomedicine. Science 196(4286):129–136, 1977 847460

Epstein SA, Kay G, Clauw D, et al: Psychiatric disorders in patients with fibromyalgia. A multicenter investigation. Psychosomatics 40(1):57–63, 1999 9989122

Fischler B, Cluydts R, De Gucht Y, et al: Generalized anxiety disorder in chronic fatigue syndrome. Acta Psychiatr Scand 95(5):405–413, 1997 9197905

Granges G, Zilko P, Littlejohn GO: Fibromyalgia syndrome: assessment of the severity of the condition 2 years after diagnosis. J Rheumatol 21(3):523–529, 1994 8006897

Harvey SB, Wadsworth M, Wessely S, Hotopf M: Etiology of chronic fatigue syndrome: testing popular hypotheses using a national birth cohort study. Psychosom Med 70(4):488–495, 2008 18378866

Hatcher S, House A: Life events, difficulties and dilemmas in the onset of chronic fatigue syndrome: a case-control study. Psychol Med 33(7):1185–1192, 2003 14580073

Häuser W, Bernardy K, Uçeyler N, Sommer C: Treatment of fibromyalgia syndrome with antidepressants: a meta-analysis. JAMA 301(2):198–209, 2009 19141768

Häuser W, Bialas P, Welsch K, Wolfe F: Construct validity and clinical utility of current research criteria of DSM-5 somatic symptom disorder diagnosis in patients with fibromyalgia syndrome. J Psychosom Res 78(6):546–552, 2015 25864805

Hughes AM, Chalder T, Hirsch CR, Moss-Morris R: An attention and interpretation bias for illness-specific information in chronic fatigue syndrome. Psychol Med 47(5):853–865, 2017 27894380

Jones GT, Atzeni F, Beasley M, et al: The prevalence of fibromyalgia in the general population: a comparison of the American College of Rheumatology 1990, 2010, and modified 2010 classification criteria. Arthritis Rheumatol 67(2):568–575, 2015 25323744

Kroenke K: Patients presenting with somatic complaints: epidemiology, psychiatric comorbidity and management. Int J Methods Psychiatr Res 12(1):34–43, 2003 12830308

Larun L, Brurberg KG, Odgaard-Jensen J, Price JR: Exercise therapy for chronic fatigue syndrome. Cochrane Database Syst Rev 4(4):CD003200, 2017 28444695

Murphy M, Kontos N, Freudenreich O: Electronic support groups: an open line of communication in contested illness. Psychosomatics 57(6):547–555, 2016 27421707

Nijs J, Roussel N, Van Oosterwijck J, et al: Fear of movement and avoidance behaviour toward physical activity in chronic-fatigue syndrome and fibromyalgia: state of the art and implications for clinical practice. Clin Rheumatol 32(8):1121–1129, 2013 23639990

Nijs J, Nees A, Paul L, et al: Altered immune response to exercise in patients with chronic fatigue syndrome/myalgic encephalomyelitis: a systematic literature review. Exerc Immunol Rev 20:94–116, 2014 24974723

Nisenbaum R, Jones JF, Unger ER, et al: A population-based study of the clinical course of chronic fatigue syndrome. Health Qual Life Outcomes 1:49, 2003 14613572

Parker AJ, Wessely S, Cleare AJ: The neuroendocrinology of chronic fatigue syndrome and fibromyalgia. Psychol Med 31(8):1331–1345, 2001 11722149

Prins JB, van der Meer JW, Bleijenberg G: Chronic fatigue syndrome. Lancet 367(9507):346–355, 2006 16443043

Reyes M, Nisenbaum R, Hoaglin DC, et al: Prevalence and incidence of chronic fatigue syndrome in Wichita, Kansas. Arch Intern Med 163(13):1530–1536, 2003 12860574

Roberts AD, Papadopoulos AS, Wessely S, et al: Salivary cortisol output before and after cognitive behavioural therapy for chronic fatigue syndrome. J Affect Disord 115(1-2):280–286, 2009 18937978

Roelofs J, Peters ML, McCracken L, Vlaeyen JW: The pain vigilance and awareness questionnaire (PVAQ): further psychometric evaluation in fibromyalgia and other chronic pain syndromes. Pain 101(3):299–306, 2003 12583873

Sharpe M, Wilks D: Fatigue. BMJ 325(7362):480–483, 2002 12202331

Shorter E: From Paralysis to Fatigue: A History of Psychosomatic Illness in the Modern Era. New York, Free Press, 1992

Tak LM, Cleare AJ, Ormel J, et al: Meta-analysis and meta-regression of hypothalamic-pituitary-adrenal axis activity in functional somatic disorders. Biol Psychol 87(2):183–194, 2011 21315796

Theorell T, Blomkvist V, Lindh G, Evengård B: Critical life events, infections, and symptoms during the year preceding chronic fatigue syndrome (CFS): an examination of CFS patients and subjects with a nonspecific life crisis. Psychosom Med 61(3):304–310, 1999 10367610

van der Werf SP, de Vree B, Alberts M, et al; Netherlands Fatigue Research Group Nijmegen: Natural course and predicting self-reported improvement in patients with chronic fatigue syndrome with a relatively short illness duration. J Psychosom Res 53(3):749–753, 2002 12217448

Wolfe F, Smythe HA, Yunus MB, et al: The American College of Rheumatology 1990 criteria for the classification of fibromyalgia: report of the Multicenter Criteria Committee. Arthritis Rheum 33(2):160–172, 1990 2306288

Wolfe F, Clauw DJ, Fitzcharles MA, et al: The American College of Rheumatology preliminary diagnostic criteria for fibromyalgia and measurement of symptom severity. Arthritis Care Res (Hoboken) 62(5):600–610, 2010 20461783

Yunus MB: A comprehensive medical evaluation of patients with fibromyalgia syndrome. Rheum Dis Clin North Am 28(2):201–217, v–vi, 2002

CHAPTER 26

Infectious Diseases

26.1 After returning from a summer trip to North Carolina where he was bitten by a tick, an otherwise healthy young man developed fever and a rash with erythematous macules that eventually progressed to maculopapular lesions with central petechiae. What organism is most likely responsible for this clinical presentation?

A. *Borrelia burgdorferi.*
B. *Treponema pallidum.*
C. *Tropheryma whipplei.*
D. *Rickettsia rickettsii.*

The correct response is option D: *Rickettsia rickettsii.*

The etiological agent for Rocky Mountain spotted fever (RMSF) is *Rickettsia rickettsii*. RMSF is a tick-borne disease with a seasonal distribution paralleling human contact with ticks, peaking May through September. Its name is misleading because half of U.S. cases are in the South Atlantic region, and rickettsial spotted fevers occur worldwide. RMSF typically (although not invariably) includes fever and a rash characterized by erythematous macules that later progress to maculopapular lesions with central petechiae (option D is correct). Central nervous system (CNS) involvement occurs in 25% of cases and manifests as lethargy, confusion, and occasionally fulminant delirium. Subtle changes such as irritability, personality changes, and apathy may occur before the rash, particularly in children.

Syphilis is a chronic systemic disease caused by the spirochetal bacterium *Treponema pallidum* (option B is incorrect).

Lyme disease is caused by the spirochete *Borrelia burgdorferi,* which is transmitted by deer ticks. Disease onset is marked by erythema migrans, a characteristic (more than 90% of cases) spreading rash with central clearing (option A is incorrect). Acute disseminated disease includes fatigue, arthralgia, headache, fever, and stiff neck. If untreated, Lyme disease may disseminate to other organs and produce subacute or chronic disease.

Whipple's disease is a rare infection caused by the bacterium *Tropheryma whipplei* (option C is incorrect). Most patients experience arthralgia, diarrhea, and weight loss. Neurological involvement has been reported in 6%–63% of patients, may occur without intestinal involvement (Mohamed et al. 2011), and can mimic almost any neurological syndrome. Psychiatric symptoms (e.g., depression, personality change) are present in about half of patients with neurological involvement. Cognitive deficits are even more common and may extend to dementia. **Chapter 26 (pp. 740–741, 742, 744, 748)**

26.2 Which microorganism classically causes muscle stiffness signs, such as "lockjaw" and *risus sardonicus*?

A. *Salmonella typhi.*
B. *Clostridium tetani.*
C. Group A beta-hemolytic streptococci.
D. *Leptospira interrogans.*

The correct response is option B: *Clostridium tetani.*

Pediatric acute-onset neuropsychiatric syndrome (PANS) refers to a syndrome in children with obsessive-compulsive and tic disorders (Chang et al. 2015; Murphy et al. 2015). Most cases of PANS are suspected to be postinfectious in origin. PANDAS is the term for a subgroup of PANS in which the symptoms appear to have been triggered by an infection with group A beta-hemolytic streptococci (option C is incorrect).

Typhoid fever is an enteric fever caused by salmonellae. Abdominal pain, headache, and fever are the classic presentation. However, when typhoid fever is endemic or is not treated promptly, psychiatric symptoms may appear. *Salmonella typhi* enters a bacteremic phase, and the typhoid bacilli can localize in the CNS (option A is incorrect).

Clostridium tetani produces a potent neurotoxin called *tetanospasmin*, which is the cause of tetanus. The classic symptom is muscle stiffness, particularly in the muscles of mastication—hence the descriptive term "lockjaw." If muscle stiffness extends across the entire face, *risus sardonicus* occurs, an expression of continuous grimace (option B is correct).

Leptospirosis is another protean spirochetal disease that occurs globally. The organism is spread through the urine of many species of mammals. Most infections resemble influenza and are relatively benign. The more severe form of leptospirosis is a multiorgan disease affecting liver, kidneys, lung, and brain (e.g., meningoencephalitis, aseptic meningitis). Confusion and delirium are common, and initial presentation with mania and psychosis have also been reported (Semiz et al. 2005) (option D is incorrect). **Chapter 26 (pp. 739, 741–742, 746)**

26.3 Which of the following serological tests can be used to confirm a diagnosis of syphilis after a positive screening test?

A. Microhemagglutination assay of *T. pallidum* (MHA-TP).
B. Rapid plasma reagin test.
C. Venereal Disease Research Laboratory test.
D. Monospot test.

The correct response is option A: Microhemagglutination assay of *T. pallidum* (MHA-TP).

Serological testing is based on both nontreponemal and anti-treponemal antibodies. The Venereal Disease Research Laboratory and the rapid plasma reagin tests are the most commonly used tests for detecting nontreponemal (nonspecific) antibodies (options B and C are incorrect). A treponemal test is the microhemagglutination assay of *T. pallidum* (MHA-TP). This assay is used as a confirmatory test, typically after a positive rapid plasma reagin test result (option A is correct).

Ebstein-Barr virus, one of the herpesviruses, commonly causes infectious mononucleosis ("mono") in children and adults. Diagnosis is based on the combination of typical clinical symptoms and a positive heterophil antibody test (Monospot) (option D is incorrect). **Chapter 26 (p. 743; Table 26–2, p. 744; p. 756)**

26.4   Which stage of syphilis infection is characterized by tabes dorsalis?

A. Primary syphilis.
B. Secondary syphilis.
C. Tertiary syphilis.
D. Acute syphilitic infection.

The correct response is option C: Tertiary syphilis.

In adults, syphilis passes through several stages. If the chancre of *primary syphilis* is untreated, it will disappear, followed 6–24 weeks later by *secondary syphilis* (option A is incorrect). During this stage, many different organ systems, including the CNS, may become involved. Most symptoms are constitutional (malaise, fatigue, anorexia, and weight loss). Most syphilitic meningitis occurs within the first year of infection. Symptoms of headache, stiff neck, nausea, and vomiting prevail, and focal neurological findings may be present. Often, signs and symptoms of secondary syphilis disappear, and the infection becomes latent (option B is incorrect). *Tertiary syphilis* refers to infection years to decades after initial infection, and neurosyphilis is the predominant form of tertiary syphilis (Gliatto and Caroff 2001). Neurosyphilis is divided into asymptomatic, meningeal, meningovascular, and parenchymatous forms. Meningeal syphilis may occur early in the course of the disease (as previously noted) or late. Meningovascular syphilis typically occurs 4–7 years after infection, with symptoms including changes in memory and personality, dizziness, and other symptoms mimicking atherosclerotic disease (e.g., transient ischemic attack, multi-infarct dementia). Parenchymatous neurosyphilis syndromes are tabes dorsalis and general paresis (option C is correct). Tabes dorsalis occurs 20–25 years after infection (option D is incorrect) and results from demyelination of the posterior columns and dorsal roots. **Chapter 26 (pp. 742–743)**

26.5   What AIDS-associated opportunistic infection characteristically causes nerve de-myelination and manifests with multiple focal neurological deficits?

A. Progressive multifocal leukoencephalopathy.
B. Cryptococcal meningitis.
C. Central nervous system (CNS) lymphoma.
D. Toxoplasmosis.

The correct response is option A: Progressive multifocal leukoencephalopathy.

Infection with *Toxoplasma gondii* generally occurs in 30% of patients with fewer than 100 CD4 cells/mm^3 (Kaplan et al. 2009). In patients with AIDS, toxoplasmosis, affecting between 2% and 4% of the AIDS population, is the most common cause of intracranial masses. Head computed tomography usually shows multiple bilateral, ring-enhancing lesions in the basal ganglia or at the gray-white matter junction. Symptoms of CNS infection are fever, reduced alertness, headache, confusion, focal neurological signs (approximately 80% of cases), and partial or generalized seizures (approximately 30% of cases) (option D is incorrect).

Although meningitis caused by *Cryptococcus neoformans* is rare in immunocompetent persons, it is a devastating illness occurring in approximately 8%–10% of AIDS patients in the Unites States and in up to 30% of AIDS patients in other parts of the world (Powderly 2000). Patients generally present with fever and delirium. Meningeal signs are not universally seen. Seizures and focal neurological deficits occur in about 10% of cases, and intracranial pressure is elevated in about 50% (option B is incorrect).

Progressive multifocal leukoencephalopathy is a demyelinating disease caused by the reactivation of the John Cunningham virus in immunocompromised patients. The clinical syndrome consists of multiple focal neurological deficits, such as monoparetic or hemiparetic limb weakness, dysarthria, gait disturbances, sensory deficits, and progressive dementia with eventual coma and death (option A is correct).

Lymphoma is the most common neoplasm seen in AIDS patients, affecting between 0.6% and 3% of patients. AIDS is the most common condition associated with primary CNS lymphoma. The patient is generally afebrile; may develop a single lesion with focal neurological signs or small, multifocal lesions; and most commonly presents with mental status change. Seizures occur in about 15% of cases. CNS lymphoma manifests late in the course of HIV infection and has a very poor prognosis (option C is incorrect). **Chapter 26 (pp. 749–750)**

26.6   Which of the following is a risk factor for HIV-associated neurocognitive disorder (HAND)?

A. Younger age.
B. Absence of cerebrovascular disease.
C. Higher CD4 nadir.
D. Co-infection with hepatitis C.

The correct response is option D: Co-infection with hepatitis C.

HAND is the term for the spectrum of cognitive dysfunction due to primary HIV CNS infection, which ranges from asymptomatic changes demonstrable only in neurocognitive testing to HIV-associated dementia (Antinori et al. 2007). Mild neurocognitive disorder, characterized by mild to moderate difficulties in daily functioning, affects 2%–8% of this population (Antinori et al. 2007). Risks factors for HAND include older age, lower CD4 nadir, co-infection with hepatitis C, alcohol and/or substance use, cerebrovascular disease, and psychiatric disorders. Several of these factors are independent risk factors for cognitive impairment as well (option D is correct; options A, B, and C are incorrect). **Chapter 26 (p. 751)**

26.7   Which of the following is true regarding HIV infection and depression?

   A. Depression has no effect on adherence to HIV treatment.
   B. Major depressive disorder is not a risk factor for HIV infection.
   C. HAND and other HIV-related CNS conditions can produce a flat, apathetic state that is often misdiagnosed as depression.
   D. Fatigue has been found to be more associated with HIV disease progression than with depression.

The correct response is option C: HAND and other HIV-related CNS conditions can produce a flat, apathetic state that is often misdiagnosed as depression.

Depression is a significant problem among persons with HIV and AIDS. The estimated prevalence of major depressive disorder (MDD) in HIV-infected patients has been reported as 19%–43% (Cysique et al. 2007; Gibbie et al. 2007). Depression has well-documented negative effects on adherence to treatment (Tao et al. 2018), quality of life (Lenz and Demal 2000; Meltzer-Brody and Davidson 2000), and treatment outcomes (option A is incorrect). MDD is a risk factor for HIV infection (McDermott et al. 1994) via intensification of substance use, exacerbation of self-destructive behaviors, and promotion of poor sexual partner choice (option B is incorrect). HIV increases the risk of developing MDD through a variety of mechanisms, including direct injury to the subcortex, chronic stress, worsening social isolation, and intense demoralization. HAND and other HIV-related CNS conditions can produce a flat, apathetic state that is often misdiagnosed as depression (option C is correct). Fatigue has been found to be more associated with depression than with HIV disease progression (option D is incorrect). **Chapter 26 (pp. 752–753)**

26.8   Which of the following best describes the relationship between bipolar disorder and HIV infection?

   A. Patients with bipolar disorder are less likely to engage in behaviors that place them at risk for HIV infection.
   B. Irritable mood is a prominent feature of "AIDS mania."

C. The prevalence of mania is about the same in patients with AIDS as in the general population.

D. Mania remains a common manifestation of AIDS.

The correct response is option B: Irritable mood is a prominent feature of "AIDS mania."

Patients with bipolar disorder may be more likely to engage in behaviors that place them at risk for HIV infection, including unprotected sex, sex with partners with unknown HIV status, and drug use (option A is incorrect). The prevalence of mania is higher in patients with AIDS compared with the general population (Atkinson et al. 2009) (option C is incorrect). Before the availability of effective antiretroviral therapy, patients with low CD4 cell counts often presented with a constellation of symptoms described as "AIDS mania." Irritable mood was often a prominent feature (option B is correct), but elevated mood was observed as well. AIDS mania was usually quite severe in its manifestation and malignant in its course (Lyketsos et al. 1993, 1997). It is rarely seen in the era of antiretroviral therapy (option D is incorrect). **Chapter 26 (pp. 754–755)**

26.9 What potential drug-drug interaction can occur when erythromycin is coadministered with the following medications?

A. Antipsychotics and tricyclic antidepressants—prolongation of QT interval.

B. Alprazolam—decrease in alprazolam levels.

C. Buspirone—decrease in buspirone levels.

D. Carbamazepine—decrease in carbamazepine levels.

The correct response is option A: Antipsychotics and tricyclic antidepressants—prolongation of QT interval.

Erythromycin (and similar antibiotics, such as clarithromycin) and ketoconazole (and similar antifungals) may cause QT interval prolongation and ventricular arrhythmias when given to a patient taking other QT-prolonging drugs, including tricyclic antidepressants and many antipsychotics (option A is correct). Erythromycin inhibits cytochrome P450 (CYP) 3A4 and therefore may increase the levels of drugs metabolized by this isoenzyme, including alprazolam, buspirone, and carbamazepine (Westphal 2000) (options B, C, and D are incorrect). **Chapter 26 (p. 767; Table 26–5, p. 770) and Westphal (2000)**

26.10 Which of the following antiretroviral drugs is known to cause vivid dreams and nightmares?

A. Maraviroc.

B. Atazanavir.

C. Zidovudine.

D. Efavirenz.

The correct response is option D: Efavirenz.

Maraviroc is a CCR5 receptor antagonist that may cause dizziness and insomnia (option A is incorrect). Atazanavir is a protease inhibitor, and depression and insomnia are potential side effects (option B is incorrect). Zidovudine is a nucleoside reverse transcriptase inhibitor and can cause anxiety, agitation, restlessness, insomnia, mild confusion, mania, and psychosis (option C is incorrect). Efavirenz is a nonnucleoside reverse transcriptase inhibitor that is known to cause high rates of neuropsychiatric side effects, including vivid dreams, nightmares, insomnia, and mood changes—these side effects commonly peak in the first 2 weeks of treatment (Kenedi and Goforth 2011) (option D is correct). **Chapter 26 (Table 26–4, p. 769)** and **Kenedi and Goforth (2011)**

References

Antinori A, Arendt G, Becker JT, et al: Updated research nosology for HIV-associated neurocognitive disorders. Neurology 69(18):1789–1799, 2007 17914061

Atkinson JH, Higgins JA, Vigil O, et al: Psychiatric context of acute/early HIV infection. The NIMH Multisite Acute HIV Infection Study: IV. AIDS Behav 13(6):1061–1067, 2009 19517225

Chang K, Frankovich J, Cooperstock M, et al; PANS Collaborative Consortium: Clinical evaluation of youth with pediatric acute-onset neuropsychiatric syndrome (PANS): recommendations from the 2013 PANS Consensus Conference. J Child Adolesc Psychopharmacol 25(1):3–13, 2015 25325534

Cysique LA, Deutsch R, Atkinson JH, et al; HNRC GrouP: Incident major depression does not affect neuropsychological functioning in HIV-infected men. J Int Neuropsychol Soc 13(1):1–11, 2007 17166298

Gibbie T, Hay M, Hutchison CW, Mijch A: Depression, social support and adherence to highly active antiretroviral therapy in people living with HIV/AIDS. Sex Health 4(4):227–232, 2007 18082064

Gliatto MF, Caroff SN: Neurosyphilis: a history and clinical review. Psychiatr Ann 31(3):153–161, 2001

Kaplan JE, Benson C, Holmes KK, et al; Centers for Disease Control and Prevention (CDC); National Institutes of Health; HIV Medicine Association of the Infectious Diseases Society of America: Guidelines for prevention and treatment of opportunistic infections in HIV-infected adults and adolescents: recommendations from CDC, the National Institutes of Health, and the HIV Medicine Association of the Infectious Diseases Society of America. MMWR Recomm Rep 58(RR-4):1–207, quiz CE1–CE4, 2009

Kenedi CA, Goforth HW: A systematic review of the psychiatric side-effects of efavirenz. AIDS Behav 15(8):1803–1818, 2011 21484283

Lenz G, Demal U: Quality of life in depression and anxiety disorders: an exploratory follow-up study after intensive inpatient cognitive behaviour therapy. Psychopathology 33(6):297–302, 2000 11060512

Lyketsos CG, Hanson AL, Fishman M, et al: Manic syndrome early and late in the course of HIV. Am J Psychiatry 150(2):326–327, 1993 8422087

Lyketsos CG, Schwartz J, Fishman M, Treisman G: AIDS mania. J Neuropsychiatry Clin Neurosci 9(2):277–279, 1997 9144109

McDermott BE, Sautter FJ Jr, Winstead DK, Quirk T: Diagnosis, health beliefs, and risk of HIV infection in psychiatric patients. Hosp Community Psychiatry 45(6):580–585, 1994 8088739

Meltzer-Brody S, Davidson JR: Completeness of response and quality of life in mood and anxiety disorders. Depress Anxiety 12 (Suppl 1):95–101, 2000 11098422

Mohamed W, Neil E, Kupsky WJ, et al: Isolated intracranial Whipple's disease--report of a rare case and review of the literature. J Neurol Sci 308(1-2):1–8, 2011 21696776

Murphy TK, Patel PD, McGuire JF, et al: Characterization of the pediatric acute-onset neuropsychiatric syndrome phenotype. J Child Adolesc Psychopharmacol 25(1):14–25, 2015 25314221

Powderly WG: Cryptococcal meningitis in HIV-infected patients. Curr Infect Dis Rep 2(4):352–357, 2000 11095877

Semiz UB, Turhan V, Basoglu C, et al: Leptospirosis presenting with mania and psychosis: four consecutive cases seen in a military hospital in Turkey. Int J Psychiatry Med 35(3):299–305, 2005 16480244

Tao J, Vermund SH, Qian HZ: Association between depression and antiretroviral therapy use among people living with HIV: a meta-analysis. AIDS Behav 22(5):1542–1550, 2018 28439754

Westphal JF: Macrolide - induced clinically relevant drug interactions with cytochrome P-450A (CYP) 3A4: an update focused on clarithromycin, azithromycin and dirithromycin. Br J Clin Pharmacol 50(4):285–295, 2000 11012550

CHAPTER 27

Dermatology

27.1 Studies of patients with psychogenic purpura suggest which of the following to be a likely etiologic process?

A. Autoimmune.
B. Factitious.
C. Psychotic.
D. Infectious.

The correct response is option A: Autoimmune.

Severe emotional stress, conversion (including religious stigmata) and dissociation symptoms (Gupta et al. 2017b), and other psychological factors (Ivanov et al. 2009; Ratnoff 1980, 1989) have been observed in the majority of cases of psychogenic purpura. However, there is a marked heterogeneity of psychological findings, and the exact role of psychological factors in psychogenic purpura remains unclear. An underlying autoimmune process has been suggested (option A is correct). Psychogenic purpura should be differentiated from factitious purpura, which is a type of self-induced factitious dermatitis (option B is incorrect). Delusional infestation is most commonly a psychotic disorder. Chronic stress may suppress cutaneous immunity, reactivating latent viral infections such as herpes viruses (Dhabhar 2013). Psychogenic purpura is not thought to be due to a psychotic or infectious etiology (options C and D are incorrect). **Chapter 27 (pp. 782, 793)**

27.2 Which of the following findings is most consistent with somatoform pruritus?

A. The lesions on the skin are in areas where it is difficult for patients to reach with their hands.
B. The pruritus wakes patients from sleep.
C. The pruritus is associated with a starvation state.
D. The pruritus first started after a traumatic experience.

The correct response is option D: The pruritus first started after a traumatic experience.

Starvation in eating disorders has been associated with pruritus (Gupta et al. 1992b), and rapid refeeding can lead to a flare-up of acne, most likely because of rising androgen levels (Gupta and Gupta 2001). It has been suggested that an-orexia nervosa should be considered in all patients with low body weight and pru-ritus (Morgan and Lacey 1999) (option C is incorrect). *Dermatitis artifacta* refers to cutaneous lesions that are wholly self-inflicted; however, the patient typically de-nies responsibility. The lesions in dermatitis artifacta vary widely; thus, they can mimic a variety of cutaneous disorders. The lesions typically occur in regions that are accessible by hand (option A is incorrect). *Somatoform pruritus* is defined as pruritus in which psychological factors play a critical role in the onset, intensity, exacerbation, or persistence of the symptoms (Weisshaar et al. 2012) (option D is correct). Patients' perceptions of pruritus, irrespective of its etiology, can be mod-ulated by psychological factors. Persons with mental distress were found to be twice as likely to experience itching as those without (Dalgard et al. 2007). Soma-toform pruritus rarely disturbs sleep (Weisshaar et al. 2012); however, pruritus due to PTSD is often associated with nocturnal awakenings from traumatic night-mares (Gupta 2006) (option B is incorrect). **Chapter 27 (pp. 790, 792)**

27.3   In which dermatological disorder do a predominance of those affected experience onset of symptoms during childhood, onset frequently occurring after a stressful event, higher rates of attention-deficit/hyperactivity disorder (ADHD) and de-pression and suicidality, and blunted cortisol responsiveness to a stressor?

A. Psoriasis.
B. Atopic dermatitis.
C. Acne.
D. Chronic urticaria.

The correct response is option B: Atopic dermatitis.

Atopic dermatitis (AD) can occur at any age; however, in up to 90% of cases, onset is before the age of 5 years. The onset or exacerbation of AD often follows stressful life events, such as parental divorce (Suárez et al. 2012). AD patients have been shown to exhibit an overactive sympathetic response to histamine-induced itch and scratching compared with non-AD control subjects (Tran et al. 2010). There is at-tenuated hypothalamic-pituitary-adrenal (HPA)–axis responsiveness, as evidenced by a blunted cortisol response to a stressor in AD (Buske-Kirschbaum et al. 2006). Studies have demonstrated higher than average rates of suicidal ideation and be-havior in adolescent and adult populations (Gupta and Gupta 1998; Kimata 2006; Lee and Shin 2017) and elevated rates of ADHD (Schmitt et al. 2009) (option B is correct). Psoriasis can occur at any age; in approximately 75% of patients, onset is before age 40 years. Evidence suggests the possibility of higher underlying sym-pathetic tone in psoriasis. It has been proposed that stress-reactive psoriasis is as-sociated with a hyporesponsive HPA-axis cortisol response and possibly more severe psoriasis (Arnetz et al. 1985; Evers et al. 2010; Richards et al. 2005). The rate of suicidality in psoriasis may be higher than for any other dermatological condi-tion (option A is incorrect). Acne vulgaris has a peak incidence during adoles-cence. Psychosocial stress can exacerbate acne in more than 60% of cases. Acne often coexists with depressive disorders, eating disorders, and body dysmorphic disorder and may be more likely to be associated with ADHD. In one study, relative to adolescents who reported "no/little acne," those who reported "very much" acne reported suicidal ideation about twice as often among the girls and three times as often among the boys (Halvorsen et al. 2011) (option C is incorrect). Urticaria can occur at any age (Grattan and Black 2008). Psychogenic factors are reported to be important in around 50% of cases (Gupta 2009). Some patients with chronic urticaria have been shown to have lower serum levels of dehydroepiandrosterone sulfate (DHEAS) during the active period of the disease (Kasperska-Zajac et al. 2008). Urticaria may commonly co-occur with depressive and anxiety disorders and obsessive-compulsive disorder (Ozkan et al. 2007; Staubach et al. 2006; Uguz et al. 2008) (option D is incorrect). **Chapter 27 (pp. 793–798, 800–802)**

27.4 Patients with body dysmorphic disorder (BDD) are overrepresented in dermatological treatment settings, with dermatological concerns being the most common reason for seeking nonpsychiatric treatment. Which of the following patterns of treatment-seeking behavior is most likely among patients with BDD?

A. The interventions most commonly requested by patients with BDD in dermatological practice are systemic acne treatments.
B. Patients with BDD are likely to report satisfaction with their treatment outcome.
C. Patients with BDD are more likely to agree to a trial of isotretinoin than the general acne population.
D. Patients seeking dermatological care for more severe acne have higher rates of having a diagnosis of BDD.

The correct response is option C: Patients with BDD are more likely to agree to a trial of isotretinoin than the general acne population.

Acne is a major concern among patients with BDD, and dermatological treatments are the most frequently sought after and received nonpsychiatric treatments in BDD, the most common being topical acne agents (Crerand et al. 2005) (option A is incorrect). Most studies of BDD patients who underwent surgery for cosmetic procedures found that patients either experienced no change in BDD severity or experienced emergence of new BDD-related ideation, and most patients reported dissatisfaction with treatment outcome (Crerand et al. 2010) (option B is incorrect). Patients requiring systemic isotretinoin therapy were twice as likely to have BDD as those who had never used it (Bowe et al. 2007) (option C is correct). In a study of acne patients ages 16–35 years, 36.7% of patients with clinically "minimal to nonexistent acne" and 32.9% with clinically mild acne met criteria for BDD (Bowe et al. 2007) (option D is incorrect). **Chapter 27 (pp. 789, 801)**

27.5 Which of the following psychotropic medications is approved by the U.S. Food and Drug Administration (FDA) for management of a condition with both dermatological and psychiatric manifestations?

A. Pimozide (for delusional infestation).
B. Doxepin topical cream (for atopic dermatitis [AD]).

C. Lamotrigine (for skin-picking disorder).

D. Venlafaxine (for the mucocutaneous dysesthesias).

The correct response is option B: Doxepin topical cream (for atopic dermatitis [AD]).

Currently, no orally administered psychotropic agents are approved by the FDA for the treatment of a primary dermatological disorder; 5% topical doxepin cream is FDA approved for short-term (up to 8 days) management of moderate pruritus in adults with conditions such as AD (option B is correct). There are many reports of the use of pimozide for delusional infestation, but no evidence demonstrates the superiority of pimozide over other antipsychotics (Mothi and Sampson 2013) (option A is incorrect). Lamotrigine has been associated with a reduction in skin-picking disorder severity but was not superior to placebo (Grant et al. 2010) (option C is incorrect). The mucocutaneous dysesthesias are usually treated with the same agents used for the treatment of neuropathic pain, such as tricyclic antidepressants, serotonin-norepinephrine reuptake inhibitors, or anticonvulsants such as gabapentin (Thornsberry and English 2013), but controlled clinical trials are lacking (option D is incorrect). **Chapter 27 (pp. 784, 786, 788, 792)**

27.6 Which of the following disorders that manifest in the skin and in psychological ways is best categorized as a somatic symptom disorder?

A. Excoriation (skin-picking) disorder.

B. Body dysmorphic disorder.

C. Dermatitis artefacta.

D. Morgellon's disease.

The correct response is option C: Dermatitis artefacta.

In DSM-5 (American Psychiatric Association 2013), the *body-focused repetitive behaviors*—excoriation (skin-picking) disorder and trichotillomania (hair-pulling disorder)—and *body dysmorphic disorder* are grouped in the newly created category of *obsessive-compulsive and related disorders* (options A and B are incorrect). Dermatitis artefacta refers to cutaneous lesions that are wholly self-inflicted; however, the patient typically denies responsibility. Dermatitis artefacta is a factitious disorder, with no underlying motive to provide false information or behave deceptively, and therefore does not represent malingering (Gieler et al. 2013) (option C is correct). Delusional infestation (previously delusional parasitosis) is classified as a *delusional disorder, somatic type* (American Psychiatric Association 2013) and is characterized by a fixed false belief that one is infested by parasites or other living or inanimate (e.g., fibers, wax, crystals, needles, particles) pathogens (delusional infestation with inanimate pathogens is also known as Morgellon's disease) (Foster et al. 2012; Lepping et al. 2015) (option D is incorrect). **Chapter 27 (pp. 785–786, 790)**

27.7   Which of the following is a known dermatological manifestation of binge-eating disorder?

A. Acne.
B. Russell's sign.
C. Pruritus.
D. Subconjunctival hemorrhage.

The correct response is option A: Acne.

Patients with *anorexia nervosa* or *bulimia nervosa* can initially present with dermatological symptoms (Gupta et al. 1987; Strumia 2013) resulting from malnutrition (e.g., lanugo-like body hair, carotenodermia) or abnormal peripheral vascular response (leading to perniosis or *erythema ab igne* [Dessinioti et al. 2016]) or from bingeing and purging (e.g., knuckle calluses or Russell's sign, periorbital petechiae/ subconjunctival hemorrhage, gingivitis, perimylolysis, flare-ups of acne) (options B and D are incorrect). Acne and eating disorders often coexist (Strumia 2013), and binge eating can be associated with acne flare-ups, while starvation, which can result in lower androgen levels, may improve acne (Gupta et al. 1992a) (option A is correct). Starvation in eating disorders has been associated with pruritus (Gupta et al. 1992b), and rapid refeeding can lead to a flare-up of acne, most likely because of rising androgen levels (option C is incorrect). **Chapter 27 (pp. 790, 801)**

27.8   In which scenario should the clinician be most concerned for Stevens-Johnson syndrome/toxic epidermal necrolysis (SJS/TEN) for a patient taking carbamazepine for bipolar disorder?

A. New addition of lithium.
B. Use of carbamazepine for more than 1 year.
C. Recent ketoconazole treatment of a fungal infection.
D. A patient of Caucasian ancestry.

The correct response is option C: Recent ketoconazole treatment of a fungal infection.

The greatest risk for development of SJS/TEN is within the first 8 weeks of therapy (option B is incorrect). Use of multiple anticonvulsants and higher dosages increases the risk. It is well recognized that lithium can precipitate or exacerbate psoriasis, sometimes within the first few months but usually within the first few years of treatment. The absolute increased risk is quite small (Brauchli et al. 2009) (option A is incorrect). Ketoconazole inhibits cytochrome P450 (CYP) 3A4 isoenzymes, increasing carbamazepine levels (option C is correct). The risk of developing SJS/TEN with anticonvulsants (most often carbamazepine) is significantly increased in individuals with particular variants of the human leukocyte antigen (HLA) alleles, specifically HLA-B*1502 and HLA-A*3101 (U.S. Food and Drug Administration 2007). The B*1502 allele variant is more common in Asian populations. The FDA has recommended that individuals of Asian (including South

Asian Indians) ancestry be screened for the B*1502 variant prior to commencing treatment with carbamazepine (U.S. Food and Drug Administration 2007). The A*3101 variant is found in numerous populations, including Caucasians, and is associated with a number of diverse cutaneous drug reactions, including SJS/TEN and drug hypersensitivity syndrome. At present, the FDA does not explicitly advocate genotyping for the A*3101 variant prior to commencing carbamazepine (option D is incorrect). **Chapter 27 (pp. 804, 805; Table 27–4, p. 807)**

27.9 A dermatologist consults a psychiatrist for help with a patient who has diffuse pruritus and repetitive scratching that is causing lesions, leading to more scratching. What recommendation might the psychiatrist suggest as part of the evaluation and management?

A. Initiation of olanzapine.
B. Review of the patient's sleep patterns.
C. Discontinuation of the patient's benzodiazepines.
D. Referral for meaning-centered psychotherapy.

The correct response is option B: Review of the patient's sleep patterns.

A range of psychiatric medications may be used to manage symptoms, based on the factors underlying the pruritus. Antipsychotics would not be first-line in absence of psychotic symptoms (option A is incorrect). Sleep-wake disorders such as insomnia disorder, obstructive sleep apnea (Gupta et al. 2017a), and circadian rhythm sleep-wake disorders can exacerbate pruritus and immune-mediated dermatological disorders such as psoriasis and AD (Gupta and Gupta 2013) and should be ruled out (option B is correct). Benzodiazepine withdrawal may further exacerbate pruritus (option C is incorrect). Psychological therapies (Daunton et al. 2016; Evers et al. 2016; Schut et al. 2016), including CBT, relaxation training for arousal reduction, and habit-reversal therapy, may be helpful in interrupting the itch-scratch cycle, and there are reports of the benefits of hypnosis. Meaning-centered psychotherapy is a treatment used primarily in palliative care/end-of-life situations (option D is incorrect). **Chapter 27 (pp. 784, 793, 795), Chapter 39 (p. 1323)**

References

American Psychiatric Association: Diagnostic and Statistical Manual of Mental Disorders, 5th Edition. Arlington, VA, American Psychiatric Association, 2013

Arnetz BB, Fjellner B, Eneroth P, Kallner A: Stress and psoriasis: psychoendocrine and metabolic reactions in psoriatic patients during standardized stressor exposure. Psychosom Med 47(6):528–541, 1985 4070523

Bowe WP, Leyden JJ, Crerand CE, et al: Body dysmorphic disorder symptoms among patients with acne vulgaris. J Am Acad Dermatol 57(2):222–230, 2007 17498840

Brauchli YB, Jick SS, Curtin F, Meier CR: Lithium, antipsychotics, and risk of psoriasis. J Clin Psychopharmacol 29(2):134–140, 2009 19512974

Buske-Kirschbaum A, Ebrecht M, Kern S, Hellhammer DH: Endocrine stress responses in TH1-mediated chronic inflammatory skin disease (psoriasis vulgaris)–do they parallel stress-induced endocrine changes in TH2-mediated inflammatory dermatoses (atopic dermatitis)? Psychoneuroendocrinology 31(4):439–446, 2006 16359823

Crerand CE, Phillips KA, Menard W, Fay C: Nonpsychiatric medical treatment of body dysmorphic disorder. Psychosomatics 46(6):549–555, 2005 16288134

Crerand CE, Menard W, Phillips KA: Surgical and minimally invasive cosmetic procedures among persons with body dysmorphic disorder. Ann Plast Surg 65(1):11–16, 2010 20467296

Dalgard F, Lien L, Dalen I: Itch in the community: associations with psychosocial factors among adults. J Eur Acad Dermatol Venereol 21(9):1215–1219, 2007 17894708

Daunton A, Bridgett C, Goulding JM: Habit reversal for refractory atopic dermatitis: a review. Br J Dermatol 174(3):657–659, 2016 26384717

Dessinioti C, Katsambas A, Tzavela E, et al: Erythema ab igne in three girls with anorexia nervosa. Pediatr Dermatol 33(2):e149–e150, 2016 26822102

Dhabhar FS: Psychological stress and immunoprotection versus immunopathology in the skin. Clin Dermatol 31(1):18–30, 2013 23245970

Evers AW, Verhoeven EW, Kraaimaat FW, et al: How stress gets under the skin: cortisol and stress reactivity in psoriasis. Br J Dermatol 163(5):986–991, 2010 20716227

Evers AW, Schut C, Gieler U, et al: Itch management: psychotherapeutic approach. Curr Probl Dermatol 50:64–70, 2016 27578073

Foster AA, Hylwa SA, Bury JE, et al: Delusional infestation: clinical presentation in 147 patients seen at Mayo Clinic. J Am Acad Dermatol 67(4):673.e1–673.e10, 2012 22264448

Gieler U, Consoli SG, Tomás-Aragones L, et al: Self-inflicted lesions in dermatology: terminology and classification--a position paper from the European Society for Dermatology and Psychiatry (ESDaP). Acta Derm Venereol 93(1):4–12, 2013 23303467

Grant JE, Odlaug BL, Chamberlain SR, Kim SW: A double-blind, placebo-controlled trial of lamotrigine for pathological skin picking: treatment efficacy and neurocognitive predictors of response. J Clin Psychopharmacol 30(4):396–403, 2010 20531220

Grattan CEH, Black AK: Urticaria and angioedema, in Dermatology, 2nd Edition, Vol 1. Edited by Bolognia JL, Jorizzo JL, Rapini RP. London, Mosby Elsevier, 2008, pp 261–276

Gupta MA: Somatization disorders in dermatology. Int Rev Psychiatry 18(1):41–47, 2006 16451879

Gupta MA: Stress and urticaria, in Neuroimmunology of the Skin: Basic Science to Clinical Practice. Edited by Granstein RD, Luger TA. Berlin, Heidelberg, Germany, Springer-Verlag, 2009, pp 209–217

Gupta MA, Gupta AK: Depression and suicidal ideation in dermatology patients with acne, alopecia areata, atopic dermatitis and psoriasis. Br J Dermatol 139(5):846–850, 1998 9892952

Gupta MA, Gupta AK: The psychological comorbidity in acne. Clin Dermatol 19(3):360–363, 2001 11479049

Gupta MA, Gupta AK: Sleep-wake disorders and dermatology. Clin Dermatol 31(1):118–126, 2013 23245983

Gupta MA, Gupta AK, Haberman HF: Dermatologic signs in anorexia nervosa and bulimia nervosa. Arch Dermatol 123(10):1386–1390, 1987 3310913

Gupta MA, Gupta AK, Ellis CN, Voorhees JJ: Bulimia nervosa and acne may be related: a case report. Can J Psychiatry 37(1):58–61, 1992a 1532340

Gupta MA, Gupta AK, Voorhees JJ: Starvation-associated pruritus: a clinical feature of eating disorders. J Am Acad Dermatol 27(1):118–120, 1992b 1619062

Gupta MA, Simpson FC, Vujcic B, Gupta AK: Obstructive sleep apnea and dermatologic disorders. Clin Dermatol 35(3):319–327, 2017a 28511831

Gupta MA, Vujcic B, Gupta AK: Dissociation and conversion symptoms in dermatology. Clin Dermatol 35(3):267–272, 2017b 28511823

Halvorsen JA, Stern RS, Dalgard F, et al: Suicidal ideation, mental health problems, and social impairment are increased in adolescents with acne: a population-based study. J Invest Dermatol 131(2):363–370, 2011 20844551

Ivanov OL, Lvov AN, Michenko AV, et al: Autoerythrocyte sensitization syndrome (Gardner-Diamond syndrome): review of the literature. J Eur Acad Dermatol Venereol 23(5):499–504, 2009 19192020

Kasperska-Zajac A, Brzoza Z, Rogala B: Lower serum dehydroepiandrosterone sulphate concentration in chronic idiopathic urticaria: a secondary transient phenomenon? Br J Dermatol 159(3):743–744, 2008 18616787

Kimata H: Prevalence of suicidal ideation in patients with atopic dermatitis. Suicide Life Threat Behav 36(1):120–124, 2006 16676633

Lee S, Shin A: Association of atopic dermatitis with depressive symptoms and suicidal behaviors among adolescents in Korea: the 2013 Korean Youth Risk Behavior Survey. BMC Psychiatry 17(1):3, 2017 28049449

Lepping P, Huber M, Freudenmann RW: How to approach delusional infestation. BMJ 350:h1328, 2015 25832416

Morgan JF, Lacey JH: Scratching and fasting: a study of pruritus and anorexia nervosa. Br J Dermatol 140(3):453–456, 1999 10233265

Mothi M, Sampson S: Pimozide for schizophrenia or related psychoses. Cochrane Database Syst Rev (11):CD001949, 2013 24194433

Ozkan M, Oflaz SB, Kocaman N, et al: Psychiatric morbidity and quality of life in patients with chronic idiopathic urticaria. Ann Allergy Asthma Immunol 99(1):29–33, 2007 17650826

Ratnoff OD: The psychogenic purpuras: a review of autoerythrocyte sensitization, autosensitization to DNA, "hysterical" and factitial bleeding, and the religious stigmata. Semin Hematol 17(3):192–213, 1980 7006087

Ratnoff OD: Psychogenic purpura (autoerythrocyte sensitization): an unsolved dilemma. Am J Med 87(3N):16N–21N, 1989 2486528

Richards HL, Ray DW, Kirby B, et al: Response of the hypothalamic-pituitary-adrenal axis to psychological stress in patients with psoriasis. Br J Dermatol 153(6):1114–1120, 2005 16307645

Schmitt J, Romanos M, Schmitt NM, et al: Atopic eczema and attention-deficit/hyperactivity disorder in a population-based sample of children and adolescents. JAMA 301(7):724–726, 2009 19224748

Schut C, Mollanazar NK, Kupfer J, et al: Psychological interventions in the treatment of chronic itch. Acta Derm Venereol 96(2):157–161, 2016 26073701

Staubach P, Eckhardt-Henn A, Dechene M, et al: Quality of life in patients with chronic urticaria is differentially impaired and determined by psychiatric comorbidity. Br J Dermatol 154(2):294–298, 2006 16433799

Strumia R: Eating disorders and the skin. Clin Dermatol 31(1):80–85, 2013 23245978

Suárez AL, Feramisco JD, Koo J, Steinhoff M: Psychoneuroimmunology of psychological stress and atopic dermatitis: pathophysiologic and therapeutic updates. Acta Derm Venereol 92(1):7–15, 2012 22101513

Thornsberry LA, English JC 3rd: Scalp dysesthesia related to cervical spine disease. JAMA Dermatol 149(2):200–203, 2013 23565509

Tran BW, Papoiu AD, Russoniello CV, et al: Effect of itch, scratching and mental stress on autonomic nervous system function in atopic dermatitis. Acta Derm Venereol 90(4):354–361, 2010 20574599

Uguz F, Engin B, Yilmaz E: Axis I and Axis II diagnoses in patients with chronic idiopathic urticaria. J Psychosom Res 64(2):225–229, 2008 18222137

U.S. Food and Drug Administration: Information for healthcare professionals: dangerous or even fatal skin reactions—carbamazepine (marketed as Carbatrol, Equetro, Tegretol, and generics). December 2007. Available at: https://www.fda.gov/drugs/postmarket-drug-safety-information-patients-and-providers/information-carbamazepine-marketed-carbatrol-equetro-tegretol-and-generics. Accessed May 2, 2019.

Weisshaar E, Szepietowski JC, Darsow U, et al: European guideline on chronic pruritus. Acta Derm Venereol 92(5):563–581, 2012 22790094

CHAPTER 28

Surgery

28.1   In patients with which psychiatric illness is postoperative pain most likely to be underrecognized?

A. Depression.
B. Schizophrenia.
C. Body dysmorphic disorder (BDD).
D. Bipolar disorder.

The correct response is option B: Schizophrenia.

Depression has been associated with worse outcomes after a variety of operations. Depression has also been associated with worse outcomes after other procedures, including increased mortality after kidney transplant (Novak et al. 2010), increased cardiovascular events following vascular surgery for peripheral artery disease (Cherr et al. 2007), and complicated recovery after colorectal surgery (Balentine et al. 2011) (option A is incorrect). In comparison with healthy control subjects, patients with schizophrenia have been shown to have lower pain sensitivity, which can result in delayed diagnosis and treatment of conditions requiring surgical intervention and can complicate interpretation of postoperative pain (Engels et al. 2014) (option B is correct). In some individuals with BDD who seek cosmetic treatments, an area of concern is the risk of suicidality and violent behavior. Rates of suicidality—including suicidal ideation and suicide attempts—in individuals with BDD are quite high. In some cases, individuals with BDD can become depressed following cosmetic treatments because they are upset about the lack of improvement in their symptoms or what they perceive to be a procedure that made their appearance look worse (option C is incorrect). The psychological and physiological stress associated with surgery may result in destabilization of bipolar disorder with relapse of depressive, mixed, or manic symptoms. Mania in the perioperative period can significantly disrupt the surgical team's ability to provide care, increasing the risk of life-threatening complications (option D is incorrect). **Chapter 28 (pp. 822–824, 846)**

28.2 What is the most common theme in preoperative fears of anesthesia across multiple studies?

A. Fear of postoperative pain.
B. Fear of not waking up after surgery.
C. Fear of being nauseous or vomiting.
D. Fear of intraoperative awareness.

The correct response is option A: Fear of postoperative pain.

Preoperative fears of anesthesia are common. The reasons for these fears have been explored in a number of studies, with no clear consensus, although fear of postoperative pain seems to be a common theme (option A is correct). In a survey of 400 surgical patients during the preoperative anesthesiology visit, 81% reported experiencing preoperative anxiety (Mavridou et al. 2013). The main sources of anxiety were fear of postoperative pain (84%), fear of not waking up after surgery (64.8%), fear of being nauseous or vomiting (60.2%), and fear of drains and needles (59.5%). Another study found that 88% of the presurgical sample (N=400) experienced preoperative fear (Ruhaiyem et al. 2016). The top three sources of patient fears were fear of postoperative pain (77.3%), fear of intraoperative awareness (73.7%), and fear of delayed recovery of consciousness after anesthesia (69.5%) (options B, C, and D are incorrect). **Chapter 28 (p. 825)**

28.3 Which sedative used in postoperative intensive care unit (ICU) patients is associated with the lowest incidence of delirium?

A. Midazolam.
B. Dexmedetomidine.
C. Lorazepam.
D. Propofol.

The correct response is option B: Dexmedetomidine.

In ICUs, dexmedetomidine may be a suitable alternative to antipsychotic medications to reduce the incidence and/or duration of postoperative delirium, especially for patients considered to be at high risk. In a study of patients undergoing elective cardiac surgery, patients randomly assigned to receive dexmedetomidine after surgery had a 3% incidence of delirium, which was significantly lower than the delirium incidence with midazolam (50%) or propofol (50%) (Maldonado et al. 2009) (option B is correct; options A and D are incorrect). A meta-analysis of 16 randomized controlled trials (N=1,994 patients) comparing dexmedetomidine with other sedative agents (i.e., lorazepam, midazolam, or propofol) in ICU patients found significant reductions in ICU length of stay, mechanical ventilation duration, and delirium incidence in patients receiving dexmedetomidine (Constantin et al. 2016) (option C is incorrect). **Chapter 28 (p. 830)**

28.4 Which common type of bariatric surgery is most effective at promoting weight loss?

A. Sleeve gastrectomy.
B. Biliopancreatic bypass with duodenal switch.
C. Laparoscopic adjustable gastric banding.
D. Laparoscopic Roux-en-Y gastric bypass.

The correct response is option D: Laparoscopic Roux-en-Y gastric bypass.

There are three main bariatric surgery procedures currently offered in North America: laparoscopic adjustable gastric banding, sleeve gastrectomy, and laparoscopic Roux-en-Y gastric bypass (LRYGB) (Figures 28–1 through 28–3). LRYGB involves creation of a small gastric pouch with a small outlet; the malabsorptive element involves bypass of the distal stomach, the entire duodenum, and about 20–40 cm of the proximal jejunum. Bariatric surgery promotes weight loss through two primary mechanisms, namely, restriction and malabsorption. LRYGB uses both restriction and malabsorption and has been shown to result in greater sustained weight loss and more durable resolution of metabolic comorbidities compared with the other two common bariatric surgical procedures (option D is correct; options A and C are incorrect).

A fourth procedure, the biliopancreatic bypass with duodenal switch, removes a large portion of the stomach (to restrict meal sizes), reroutes food away from much of the small intestine (to prevent absorption), and reroutes bile (which impairs digestion). There are no clear indications for this procedure, but it is usually considered only for morbidly obese patients, given its superior weight-loss results but higher complication rates compared with LRYGB (SAGES Guidelines Committee 2008) (option B is incorrect). **Chapter 28 (pp. 837–840)**

28.5 BDD is *most* common in patients seeking which type of surgery?

A. Cosmetic.
B. Bariatric.
C. Healthy limb amputation.
D. Strabismus correction.

The correct response is option A: Cosmetic.

Research suggests that many patients who seek consultation for a cosmetic procedure meet criteria for a psychiatric disorder such as BDD, narcissistic personality disorder, or histrionic personality disorder (Ishigooka et al. 1998). BDD is one of the most common psychiatric diagnoses in patients seeking cosmetic and dermatological surgery (see also Chapter 27, "Dermatology"). In a systematic review of 33 studies examining the prevalence of BDD in plastic surgery and dermatology patients, BDD was found in 15% (range, 2.21%–56.67%) of plastic surgery patients (mean age, 35 years; 74% women) and 13% (range, 4.52%–35.16%) of dermatology patients (mean age, 28 years; 76% women) (Ribeiro 2017).

Most individuals with BDD continue to be dissatisfied with their appearance following cosmetic treatment. In a sample of 200 patients with BDD who received cosmetic surgery, the most common outcome was no change in the severity of BDD symptoms (Phillips et al. 2001). Another 5-year follow-up study showed that cosmetic surgery had no significant effects on BDD diagnosis, disability, or psychiatric comorbidity (Tignol et al. 2007). In a sample of individuals with BDD who received surgical and minimally invasive procedures for their appearance concerns, 25% showed a longer-term improvement in their preoccupation with the treated body part, but only 2.3% of surgical and minimally invasive procedures led to longer-term improvement in overall BDD symptoms (Crerand et al. 2010) (option A is correct).

Presurgical eating disorders are common in bariatric surgery candidates. In a review of 25 studies (Dawes et al. 2016), the lifetime prevalence of binge-eating disorder in patients seeking bariatric surgery was 17%, which is higher than the lifetime prevalence in the general population (option B is incorrect).

Rarely, patients may request that a healthy limb be amputated, usually in the context of body integrity identity disorder (BIID; First 2005) (option C is incorrect).

In a study in which patients with childhood-onset strabismus were evaluated prior to corrective surgery at ages 15–25 years (Menon et al. 2002), more than 75% of the patients reported experiencing social problems because of their continuous squint, being ridiculed at school and work, and having fewer employment opportunities. After corrective surgery, more than 90% reported improved self-confidence and self-esteem (option D is incorrect). **Chapter 28 (pp. 840, 842–843, 844, 845)**

28.6   Which type of drug forms the pharmacological basis of burn pain management?

A. Nonsteroidal anti-inflammatory agents.
B. Benzodiazepines.
C. Acetaminophen.
D. Opioids.

The correct response is option D: Opioids.

Potent opioids form the basis of pharmacological pain control in patients with extensive burns (option D is correct). However, nonsteroidal anti-inflammatory agents and acetaminophen are still of value when combined with opioids, as the analgesia they provide lessens the dosage requirements for opioids (options A and C are incorrect). Because burn pain has well-defined components (i.e., background, procedural, breakthrough, and postoperative pain), pharmacological choices for analgesia should target each pain pattern individually. Analgesic regimens should be continuously evaluated and reassessed to avoid undermedication or overmedication. If there are sleep and anxiety concerns, then benzodiazepines may provide benefit (option B is incorrect). **Chapter 28 (pp. 835–836)**

28.7 Concerns about bodily noises occur commonly after what type of surgery?

A. Bariatric.
B. Limb amputation.
C. Ostomies.
D. Prostatectomy.

The correct response is option C: Ostomies.

Ostomy-related issues, including sexual problems, depressive symptoms, gas and/or constipation, dissatisfaction with appearance, clothing adaptations, travel difficulties, fatigue, and worry about noises from the ostomy, were summarized in a recent review by Vonk-Klaassen et al. (2016) (option C is correct).

Common eating problems after bariatric surgery include grazing behavior (eating small quantities of food continuously over a long period of time), compulsive eating, and emotional eating. Clinically, it is important to mention that certain behaviors or concerns commonly reported after gastric bypass surgery—such as vomiting in response to early adjustment to decreased intake capacity or the sensation that food is "stuck" in the pouch—should not be confused with disordered eating (option A is incorrect).

Many amputees experience phantom limb sensations, which range from pleasant warmth to discomfort such as pain, paresthesias, and itching, and chronic phantom limb pain (Brodie et al. 2007) (option B is incorrect).

Although most patients report problems in sexual/urinary function, global quality of life does not appear to be compromised after prostatectomy (Zelefsky and Eid 1998). Some men may occasionally lose a little urine when lifting objects or coughing (i.e., stress incontinence). Other men are left with very little control over urine flow (option D is incorrect). **Chapter 28 (pp. 836–837, 841, 843)**

28.8 Which of the following is a risk factor for intraoperative awareness during surgery?

A. Male gender.
B. Inpatient surgery.
C. Cardiac surgery.
D. Absence of serious systemic illness.

The correct response is option C: Cardiac surgery.

Risk factors for intraoperative awareness, according to findings from epidemiological studies, have been classified by Nunes et al. (2012) into three main groups: 1) *patient-related* (females are more susceptible, as are children, the elderly, patients with a history of substance use, patients with an American Society of Anesthesiologists classification of III ["patient with severe systemic disease"] or IV ["patient with severe systemic disease that is a constant threat to life"], and patients with difficult-to-intubate airways) (options A and D are incorrect); 2) *procedure-related* (obstetric, cardiac, and trauma surgeries convey a higher incidence) (option C is correct); and 3) *anesthetic technique–related*. Even though it is not possible to prevent all cases of intraoperative awareness (and it may be even more difficult as outpatient surgery becomes more common), preoperative preparation of the patient for the unlikely possibility of accidental awareness during anesthesia may be helpful (option B is incorrect). **Chapter 28 (p. 827)**

28.9   Which sensation associated with limb amputation may patients with body integrity identity disorder (BIID) experience?

A. Phantom limb.
B. Stump pain.
C. Overcompleteness.
D. Residual pain.

The correct response is option C: Overcompleteness.

The term *phantom limb* refers to the experience of feeling as if an amputated part is still present. Phantom limb pain was first described by Ambrose Paré (1649). Many amputees experience phantom limb sensations, which range from pleasant warmth to discomfort such as pain, paresthesias, and itching. Chronic phantom limb pain occurs in up to 85% of amputees and is a cause of significant disability and impaired quality of life (see Brodie et al. 2007 for summary).

Many previous studies of phantom limb pain were complicated by a failure to distinguish between stump pain and various types of phantom limb phenomena (Richardson et al. 2006). *Stump pain* is defined as pain located in the residual portion of the stump (option B is incorrect), whereas *phantom limb pain* stems from painful sensations in the part of the limb that no longer exists (option A is incorrect). Risk factors for phantom limb pain include female sex, upper-extremity amputation, presence of preamputation pain, and experience of residual pain in the remaining limb (option D is incorrect).

Rarely, patients may request that a healthy limb be amputated, usually in the context of BIID. BIID is an extreme form of body image disturbance in which patients experience a sense of alienation and "overcompleteness" in regard to a specific limb (First 2005). Individuals with BIID do not suffer from delusions or psychosis and have insight into the bizarre nature of their wish. As a result, patients with BIID often seek surgical consultation for amputation or in extreme cases resort to self-amputation when they have not found a surgeon to perform the procedure (option C is correct). **Chapter 28 (pp. 842–843)**

28.10   Which is most likely to be the best predictor of postoperative posttraumatic stress disorder (PTSD)?

A. Quality of prior emotional adjustment.
B. Severity of condition requiring surgery.
C. Alcohol use.
D. Presence of acute stress disorder during acute ICU hospitalization.

The correct response is option D: Presence of acute stress disorder during acute ICU hospitalization.

Among patients receiving follow-up medical and surgical care after experiencing physical trauma, approximately 25% develop PTSD (Alarcon et al. 2012; Warren et al. 2014). Several studies have tried to identify factors that predict the emergence of PTSD. As expected, better prior emotional adjustment and social support are relatively protective (option A is incorrect). Neither severity of the physical injury nor severity of the illness requiring surgery is clearly correlated with emergence of PTSD (option B is incorrect). The evidence for alcohol use as a predictive factor for PTSD after surgery is mixed (option C is incorrect). A systematic review of 44 studies examining predictors of PTSD after motor vehicle accidents identified the following risk factors: rumination about the trauma, perceived threat to life, lower social support, higher acute stress disorder symptom severity, persistent physical health issues, previous emotional problems, history of an anxiety disorder, and involvement of litigation/compensation (Heron-Delaney et al. 2013). Perhaps the best predictor of PTSD at 1 year is the presence of acute stress disorder symptoms during the acute ICU hospitalization (Davydow et al. 2013) (option D is correct). **Chapter 28 (p. 830)**

References

Alarcon LH, Germain A, Clontz AS, et al: Predictors of acute posttraumatic stress disorder symptoms following civilian trauma: highest incidence and severity of symptoms after assault. J Trauma Acute Care Surg 72(3):629–635, discussion 635–637, 2012

Balentine CJ, Hermosillo-Rodriguez J, Robinson CN, et al: Depression is associated with prolonged and complicated recovery following colorectal surgery. J Gastrointest Surg 15(10):1712–1717, 2011 21786060

Brodie EE, Whyte A, Niven CA: Analgesia through the looking-glass? A randomized controlled trial investigating the effect of viewing a 'virtual' limb upon phantom limb pain, sensation and movement. Eur J Pain 11(4):428–436, 2007 16857400

Cherr GS, Wang J, Zimmerman PM, Dosluoglu HH: Depression is associated with worse patency and recurrent leg symptoms after lower extremity revascularization. J Vasc Surg 45(4):744–750, 2007 17303367

Constantin JM, Momon A, Mantz J, et al: Efficacy and safety of sedation with dexmedetomidine in critical care patients: a meta-analysis of randomized controlled trials. Anaesth Crit Care Pain Med 35(1):7–15, 2016 26700947

Crerand CE, Menard W, Phillips KA: Surgical and minimally invasive cosmetic procedures among persons with body dysmorphic disorder. Ann Plast Surg 65(1):11–16, 2010 20467296

Davydow DS, Zatzick D, Hough CL, Katon WJ: A longitudinal investigation of posttraumatic stress and depressive symptoms over the course of the year following medical-surgical intensive care unit admission. Gen Hosp Psychiatry 35(3):226–232, 2013 23369507

Dawes AJ, Maggard-Gibbons M, Maher AR, et al: Mental health conditions among patients seeking and undergoing bariatric surgery: a meta-analysis. JAMA 315(2):150–163, 2016 26757464

Engels G, Francke AL, van Meijel B, et al: Clinical pain in schizophrenia: a systematic review. J Pain 15(5):457–467, 2014 24365324

First MB: Desire for amputation of a limb: paraphilia, psychosis, or a new type of identity disorder. Psychol Med 35(6):919–928, 2005 15997612

Heron-Delaney M, Kenardy J, Charlton E, Matsuoka Y: A systematic review of predictors of post-traumatic stress disorder (PTSD) for adult road traffic crash survivors. Injury 44(11):1413–1422, 2013 23916902

Ishigooka J, Iwao M, Suzuki M, et al: Demographic features of patients seeking cosmetic surgery. Psychiatry Clin Neurosci 52(3):283–287, 1998 9681579

Maldonado JR, Wysong A, van der Starre PJ, et al: Dexmedetomidine and the reduction of post-operative delirium after cardiac surgery. Psychosomatics 50(3):206–217, 2009 19567759

Mavridou P, Dimitriou V, Manataki A, et al: Patient's anxiety and fear of anesthesia: effect of gender, age, education, and previous experience of anesthesia. A survey of 400 patients. J Anesth 27(1):104–108, 2013 22864564

Menon V, Saha J, Tandon R, et al: Study of the psychosocial aspects of strabismus. J Pediatr Ophthalmol Strabismus 39(4):203–208, 2002 12148552

Novak M, Molnar MZ, Szeifert L, et al: Depressive symptoms and mortality in patients after kidney transplantation: a prospective prevalent cohort study. Psychosom Med 72(6):527–534, 2010 20410250

Nunes RR, Porto VC, Miranda VT, et al: Risk factor for intraoperative awareness. Rev Bras Anestesiol 62(3):365–374, 2012 22656682

Paré A: The Works of That Famous Chirurgion, Ambrose Parey. Translated from the Latin and compared with the French by T. Johnson. London, Cotes, 1649

Phillips KA, Grant J, Siniscalchi J, Albertini RS: Surgical and nonpsychiatric medical treatment of patients with body dysmorphic disorder. Psychosomatics 42(6):504–510, 2001 11815686

Ribeiro RVE: Prevalence of body dysmorphic disorder in plastic surgery and dermatology patients: a systematic review with meta-analysis. Aesthetic Plast Surg 41(4):964–970, 2017 28411353

Richardson C, Glenn S, Nurmikko T, Horgan M: Incidence of phantom phenomena including phantom limb pain 6 months after major lower limb amputation in patients with peripheral vascular disease. Clin J Pain 22(4):353–358, 2006 16691088

Ruhaiyem ME, Alshehri AA, Saade M, et al: Fear of going under general anesthesia: A cross-sectional study. Saudi J Anaesth 10(3):317–321, 2016 27375388

SAGES Guidelines Committee: SAGES guideline for clinical application of laparoscopic bariatric surgery. Surg Endosc 22(10):2281–2300, 2008 18791862

Tignol J, Biraben-Gotzamanis L, Martin-Guehl C, et al: Body dysmorphic disorder and cosmetic surgery: evolution of 24 subjects with a minimal defect in appearance 5 years after their request for cosmetic surgery. Eur Psychiatry 22(8):520–524, 2007 17900876

Vonk-Klaassen SM, de Vocht HM, den Ouden MEM, et al: Ostomy-related problems and their impact on quality of life of colorectal cancer ostomates: a systematic review. Qual Life Res 25(1):125–133, 2016 26123983

Warren AM, Foreman ML, Bennett MM, et al: Posttraumatic stress disorder following traumatic injury at 6 months: associations with alcohol use and depression. J Trauma Acute Care Surg 76(2):517–522, 2014 24458060

Zelefsky MJ, Eid JF: Elucidating the etiology of erectile dysfunction after definitive therapy for prostatic cancer. Int J Radiat Oncol Biol Phys 40(1):129–133, 1998 9422568

CHAPTER 29

Organ Transplantation

29.1   For which organ is the U.S. transplant wait list the largest?

A. Heart.
B. Lung.
C. Liver.
D. Kidney.

The correct response is option D: Kidney.

The number of wait-listed individuals has increased far beyond the availability of donated organs. Currently, nearly 130,000 persons are active on the U.S. waiting list. Patients awaiting kidney transplant (the most common transplant performed) account for 80% of wait-listed patients (option D is correct). By contrast, slightly less than 15,000 patients are waiting for a liver, 4,000 for a heart, and nearly 1,500 for a lung (Organ Procurement and Transplantation Network 2017) (options A, B, and C are incorrect). **Chapter 29 (p. 859)**

29.2   Which group of patients has the best 10-year survival rate?

A. Living-donor liver transplant.
B. Deceased-donor liver transplant.
C. Deceased-donor kidney transplant.
D. Heart transplant.

The correct response is option A: Living-donor liver transplant.

Following transplantation, living-donor kidney and living-donor liver recipients experience the highest long-term survival rates (78% and 73%, respectively, alive at 10 years posttransplantation; Figure 29–1; U.S. Department of Health and Human Services 2012) (option A is correct). Recipients of deceased-donor kidneys, livers, and hearts have somewhat lower 10-year survival (63%, 61%, and 58%, respectively) (Organ Procurement and Transplantation Network 2017) (options B, C, and D are incorrect). **Chapter 29 (p. 860; Figure 29–1, p. 861)**

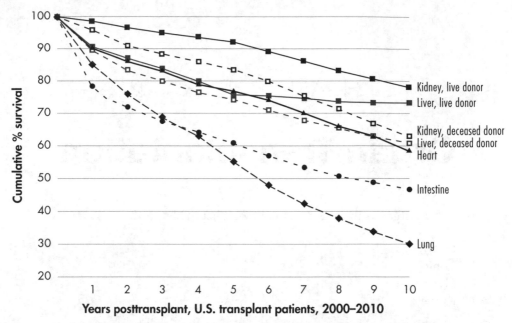

FIGURE 29–1.   Survival rates of transplant recipients, by organ type.

Source.   U.S. Department of Health and Human Services, Health Resources and Services Administration, Scientific Registry of Transplant Recipients: Organ Procurement and Transplantation Network (OPTN) and Scientific Registry of Transplant Recipients (SRTR) 2011 Annual Data Report. Rockville, MD, U.S. Department of Health and Human Services, Health Resources and Services Administration, Healthcare Systems Bureau, Division of Transplantation, 2012. Available at: https://srtr.transplant.hrsa.gov/annual_reports/2011/Default.aspx. Accessed September 26, 2017.

29.3   Which pretransplant psychiatric condition has consistently been shown to be associated with early graft loss and patient death?

A. Schizophrenia.
B. Bipolar.
C. Depression.
D. Anxiety.

The correct response is option C: Depression.

In meta-analysis, depression, either pretransplant or posttransplant, predicted poorer survival (Dew et al. 2015) (option C is correct). Anxiety was not associated with poorer outcomes (option D is incorrect). A review of a national renal transplant database found <1% of kidney recipients had bipolar disorder or schizophrenia, with no significant difference between these recipients and the general transplant group on length of transplant hospitalization, frequency of acute rejection episodes, graft function, or patient or graft survival (Butler et al. 2017) (options A and B are incorrect). These complex psychiatric patients may receive optimal management to ensure normal survival rates. **Chapter 29 (pp. 866, 871, 881)**

29.4   Which is the correct list of organs according to psychosocial stringency of clearance?

   A. Heart, liver, kidney.
   B. Heart, kidney, liver.
   C. Liver, kidney, heart.
   D. Lung, kidney, liver.

The correct response is option A: Heart, liver, kidney.

Cardiac transplant programs are more likely than liver transplant programs to consider psychosocial issues as contraindications, and liver transplant programs in turn are more stringent than kidney transplant programs (Butt et al. 2014) (option A is correct; options B, C, and D are incorrect). **Chapter 29 (p. 870)**

29.5   Which strategy has demonstrated its ability to improve adherence to medical regimes posttransplantation?

   A. Excluding patients with severe personality disorders from transplant.
   B. Allowing occasional missed doses to improve alliance with the patient.
   C. Implementing mobile phone apps.
   D. Reviewing standard deviation of tacrolimus blood levels.

The correct response is option C: Implementing mobile phone apps.

Mobile phone apps have been demonstrated to improve adherence (DeVito Dabbs et al. 2009; Dobbels et al. 2017; McGillicuddy et al. 2013; Reese et al. 2017) (option C is correct). Even occasional missing of a dose can have deleterious consequences, with some studies suggesting that less than 95% adherence is sufficient to produce poorer outcomes (Fine et al. 2009; Nevins et al. 2017) (option B is incorrect). A high standard deviation of tacrolimus blood levels can predict rejection episodes but has not been studied as an intervention tool (Stuber et al. 2008) (option D is incorrect). Patients with severe personality disorders have been shown to successfully maintain adequate adherence to medication regimens (Carlson et al. 2000) (option A is incorrect). **Chapter 29 (pp. 870–873)**

29.6   Nicotine replacement, despite dose adjustment, is relatively contraindicated in which of these potential organ transplant patients?

   A. Kidney.
   B. Liver.
   C. Heart.
   D. Lung.

The correct response is option C: Heart.

Nicotine replacement is relatively contraindicated in patients with serious heart disease because of the potential for worsening angina, increasing heart rate, and possibly exacerbating arrhythmias (option C is correct). Nicotine replacement strategies have been safely used in patients with advanced liver and lung disease, but severe renal disease may affect nicotine clearance (options A, B, and D are incorrect). When nicotine replacement therapy has been combined with bupropion, cases of severe hypertension have been reported, so careful monitoring of blood pressure is indicated. **Chapter 29 (p. 877)**

29.7 Which is a standard treatment for hepatic or portosystemic encephalopathy?

A. Benztropine.
B. Shunting to relieve portal hypertension.
C. Osmotic laxatives.
D. High-protein diets.

The correct response is option C: Osmotic laxatives.

Treatment strategies for hepatic or portosystemic encephalopathy include administration of lactulose (an osmotic laxative to flush out ammonia) (option C is correct) and nonabsorbable antibiotics (to reduce levels of intestinal bacteria that convert protein to ammonia). Medications that potentially contribute to symptoms of encephalopathy—anticholinergic drugs, tranquilizers, and sedatives—should be avoided (option A is incorrect). Patients who undergo shunting procedures to relieve portal hypertension are at increased risk of ammonia buildup with subsequent hepatic encephalopathy (Riggio et al. 2008) (option B is incorrect). High-protein diets for cirrhosis have been controversial given the need to rebuild lost muscle, but this is considered still relatively contraindicated in some people with hepatic encephalopathy (Nguyen and Morgan 2014) (option D is incorrect). **Chapter 29 (p. 884)** and **Nguyen and Morgan (2014)**

29.8 Which of the following has become an increasing concern for solid organ donors in the United States?

A. Regret after poor recipient outcomes.
B. Financial hardship.
C. Coercion to donate.
D. Postdonation decrease in general well-being.

The correct response is option B: Financial hardship.

Liver and kidney donors report that out-of-pocket costs are burdensome, and they experience financial stress from lost work and wages for both themselves and their family caregivers (option B is correct). Living donors almost uniformly report that they do not regret having donated and feel a deep sense of gratification at being able to help another person (option A is incorrect). Potential donors who are being coerced to donate are routinely ruled out for living donation (option C is incorrect). Health-related quality of life assessments show that postdonation donors' well-being, on average, meets or exceeds that reported in the general population (option D is incorrect). **Chapter 29 (pp. 886, 888)**

29.9 A 55-year-old male with bipolar disorder, alcohol use disorder, in full sustained remission, and hepatic encephalopathy receives a liver transplant complicated by acute cellular rejection. He remains in the surgical intensive care unit and develops mania on postoperative day 7. Which medication is most likely contributing to the secondary mania?

A. Tacrolimus.
B. Mycophenolate mofetil.
C. Methylprednisolone.
D. Cyclosporine.

The correct response is option C: Methylprednisolone.

Many medications are associated with secondary mania. Acute cellular rejection occurs in 20%–70% of liver transplant recipients, typically within the first 3 weeks posttransplant, resulting in transient graft dysfunction. Sixty-five percent to 80% of cases are effectively treated with high-dose steroids, which are a cause of secondary mania (option C is correct). Cyclosporine is used as a primary immunosuppressive agent. Side effects are usually mild and include tremor, restlessness, and headache (Wijdicks et al. 1999). About 12% of patients on cyclosporine experience more serious neurotoxicity, characterized by acute confusional states, psychosis, seizures, speech apraxia, cortical blindness, and coma (de Groen et al. 1987; Wijdicks et al. 1995, 1996; Wilson et al. 1988) (option D is incorrect). Although tacrolimus is more potent and possibly less toxic than cyclosporine, the neuropsychiatric side effects of the two drugs appear to be similar (DiMartini et al. 1991; Freise et al. 1991). With tacrolimus, as with cyclosporine, neuropsychiatric side effects are more common with intravenous administration and diminish with oral administration and dosage reduction. Common symptoms include tremulousness, headache, restlessness, insomnia, vivid dreams, hyperesthesias, anxiety, and agitation (Fung et al. 1991) (option A is incorrect). Few neuropsychiatric symptoms have been reported with mycophenolate mofetil (option B is incorrect). **Chapter 9 (Table 9–4, p. 262), Chapter 29 (pp. 890–893)**

29.10 A 25-year-old female with borderline personality disorder receives a liver transplant after fulminant hepatic failure from an acetaminophen overdose. She is transferred to inpatient psychiatry on daily tacrolimus, prednisone, and oxycodone as needed. Which psychotropic should be used with the most caution given the risk of posterior reversible encephalopathy syndrome?

A. Venlafaxine.
B. Fluoxetine.
C. Paroxetine.
D. Sertraline.

The correct response is option B: Fluoxetine.

Specific cytochrome P450 (CYP) 3A4 inhibitors capable of interacting adversely with immunosuppressants, in decreasing order of inhibition, are as follows: fluvoxamine > nefazodone > fluoxetine > sertraline, TCAs, paroxetine > venlafaxine (option B is correct; options A, C, and D are incorrect). Oxycodone is another substrate for the 3A4 enzyme. Both cyclosporine and tacrolimus are associated with posterior reversible (leuko)encephalopathy syndrome, an uncommon neurotoxic syndrome involving demyelination (particularly in the parieto-occipital region and centrum semiovale) (Ahn et al. 2003; Bartynski and Boardman 2007; Small et al. 1996). **Chapter 29 (pp. 892, 894)**

References

Ahn KJ, Lee JW, Hahn ST, et al: Diffusion-weighted MRI and ADC mapping in FK506 neurotoxicity. Br J Radiol 76(912):916–919, 2003 14711782

Bartynski WS, Boardman JF: Distinct imaging patterns and lesion distribution in posterior reversible encephalopathy syndrome. AJNR Am J Neuroradiol 28(7):1320–1327, 2007 17698535

Butler MI, McCartan D, Cooney A, et al: Outcomes of renal transplantation in patients with bipolar affective disorder and schizophrenia: a national retrospective cohort study. Psychosomatics 58(1):69–76, 2017 27887740

Butt Z, Levenson J, Olbrisch ME: Psychosocial screening practices and criteria for kidney transplantation: a survey of U.S. transplant centers. Presentation at the annual meeting of the Society of Behavioral Medicine, April 26, 2014

Carlson J, Potter L, Pennington S, et al: Liver transplantation in a patient at psychosocial risk. Prog Transplant 10(4):209–214, 2000 11232551

de Groen PC, Aksamit AJ, Rakela J, et al: Central nervous system toxicity after liver transplantation. The role of cyclosporine and cholesterol. N Engl J Med 317(14):861–866, 1987 3306386

DeVito Dabbs A, Dew MA, Myers B, et al: Evaluation of a hand-held, computer-based intervention to promote early self-care behaviors after lung transplant. Clin Transplant 23(4):537–545, 2009 19473201

Dew MA, Rosenberger EM, Myaskovsky L, et al: Depression and anxiety as risk factors for morbidity and mortality after organ transplantation: a systematic review and meta-analysis. Transplantation 100(5):988–1003, 2015 26492128

DiMartini A, Pajer K, Trzepacz P, et al: Psychiatric morbidity in liver transplant patients. Transplant Proc 23(6):3179–3180, 1991 1721399

Dobbels F, De Bleser L, Berben L, et al: Efficacy of a medication adherence enhancing intervention in transplantation: The MAESTRO-Tx trial. J Heart Lung Transplant 36(5):499–508, 2017 28162931

Fine RN, Becker Y, De Geest S, et al: Nonadherence consensus conference summary report. Am J Transplant 9(1):35–41, 2009 19133930

Freise CE, Rowley H, Lake J, et al: Similar clinical presentation of neurotoxicity following FK 506 and cyclosporine in a liver transplant recipient. Transplant Proc 23(6):3173–3174, 1991 1721397

Fung JJ, Alessiani M, Abu-Elmagd K, et al: Adverse effects associated with the use of FK 506. Transplant Proc 23(6):3105–3108, 1991 1721372

McGillicuddy JW, Gregoski MJ, Weiland AK, et al: Mobile health medication adherence and blood pressure control in renal transplant recipients: a proof-of-concept randomized controlled trial. JMIR Res Protoc 2(2):e32, 2013 24004517

Nevins TE, Nickerson PW, Dew MA: Understanding medication nonadherence after kidney transplantation. J Am Soc Nephrol 28(8):2290–2301, 2017 28630231

Nguyen DL, Morgan T: Protein restriction in hepatic encephalopathy is appropriate for selected patients: a point of view. Hepatol Int 8(2):447–451, 2014 25525477

Organ Procurement and Transplantation Network: Data. 2017. Available at: https://optn .transplant.hrsa.gov/data/. Accessed September 26, 2017.

Reese PP, Bloom RD, Trofe-Clark J, et al: Automated reminders and physician notification to promote immunosuppression adherence among kidney transplant recipients: a randomized trial. Am J Kidney Dis 69(3):400–409, 2017 27940063

Riggio O, Angeloni S, Salvatori FM, et al: Incidence, natural history, and risk factors of hepatic encephalopathy after transjugular intrahepatic portosystemic shunt with polytetrafluoro-ethylene-covered stent grafts. Am J Gastroenterol 103(11):2738–2746, 2008 18775022

Small SL, Fukui MB, Bramblett GT, Eidelman BH: Immunosuppression-induced leukoencephalopathy from tacrolimus (FK506). Ann Neurol 40(4):575–580, 1996 8871576

Stuber ML, Shemesh E, Seacord D, et al: Evaluating non-adherence to immunosuppressant medications in pediatric liver transplant recipients. Pediatr Transplant 12(3):284–288, 2008 18331387

U.S. Department of Health and Human Services, Health Resources and Services Administration, Healthcare Systems Bureau, Division of Transplantation: Organ Procurement and Transplantation Network (OPTN) and Scientific Registry of Transplant Recipients (SRTR) 2011 Annual Data Report. Rockville, MD, U.S. Department of Health and Human Services, Health Resources and Services Administration, Healthcare Systems Bureau, Division of Transplantation, 2012. Available at: https://srtr.transplant.hrsa.gov/annual_reports/ 2011/Default.aspx. Accessed September 26, 2017.

Wijdicks EF, Wiesner RH, Krom RA: Neurotoxicity in liver transplant recipients with cyclosporine immunosuppression. Neurology 45(11):1962–1964, 1995 7501141

Wijdicks EF, Plevak DJ, Wiesner RH, Steers JL: Causes and outcome of seizures in liver transplant recipients. Neurology 47(6):1523–1525, 1996 8960738

Wijdicks EF, Dahlke LJ, Wiesner RH: Oral cyclosporine decreases severity of neurotoxicity in liver transplant recipients. Neurology 52(8):1708–1710, 1999 10331708

Wilson SE, de Groen PC, Aksamit AJ, et al: Cyclosporin A-induced reversible cortical blindness. J Clin Neuroophthalmol 8(4):215–220, 1988 2977135

CHAPTER 30

Neurology and Neurosurgery

30.1   Of the following common and observable poststroke changes in brain function, which should be specifically tested for because it is easily overlooked?

A. Dementia.
B. Delirium.
C. Vascular cognitive impairment.
D. Strategic infarction.

The correct response is option B: Delirium.

Delirium affects 30%–40% of patients during the first week after a stroke, especially after a hemorrhagic stroke (Gustafson et al. 1993; Langhorne et al. 2000; Rahkonen et al. 2000). If not specifically inquired about, delirium will often be missed (option B is correct). Dementia following stroke is common; dementia is found to be present in up to one-third of patients at 3 months poststroke (option A is incorrect). The common occurrence of relatively subtle cognitive decline, falling short of frank dementia, in the context of cerebrovascular disease has given rise to the broader concept of "vascular cognitive impairment" (option C is incorrect). The term "strategic infarction" refers to the occurrence of unexpectedly severe cognitive impairment following limited infarction, often in the absence of classic signs such as hemiplegia (option D is incorrect). **Chapter 30 (pp. 908–910)**

30.2   In which of the following poststroke behavioral changes does recognition of the deficit remain intact?

A. Affective dysprosody.
B. Anosognosia.
C. Somatoparaphrenia.
D. Wernicke's aphasia.

The correct response is option A: Affective dysprosody.

Affective dysprosody involves impairment in the production and comprehension of language components used to communicate inner emotional states in speech. Affective dysprosody is not associated with an actual deficit in the ability to *experience* emotions. A depressed patient with dysprosody will appear depressed and say that he or she is depressed, but the patient will not "sound" depressed (option A is correct). This is in contrast to anosognosia, a partial or complete unawareness of a deficit, which occurs frequently after right-sided cerebral lesions (including stroke) (Breier et al. 1995; Jehkonen et al. 2006). Anosognosia can occur with reference to any function, and it is commonly associated with visual and language dysfunction. A patient with anosognosia will both appear and sound depressed but may deny that he or she is depressed (option B is incorrect). Anosognosia for hemiplegia is perhaps the most often described form of the condition; for example, patients may attempt to walk normally despite the hemiplegia, yet paradoxically, accept a wheelchair, all while continuing to maintain that their functioning is intact. In extreme cases of anosognosia, ownership of the limb is denied—or, exceptionally, "extra" phantom limb sensations ("somatoparaphrenia") can occur (option C is incorrect). Wernicke's aphasia is characterized by a lack of insight, with the patient unable to comprehend that he or she cannot communicate (Lazar et al. 2000) (option D is incorrect). **Chapter 30 (pp. 910–911)**

30.3   Which of the following statements about poststroke depression is *most* supported by current research consensus?

A. Poststroke depression affects fewer than 5% of stroke patients.
B. Left frontal lesions are associated with an increased rate of depressive illness.
C. SSRIs (selective serotonin reuptake inhibitors) are ineffective in treating depression after stroke.
D. Silent infarcts are a risk factor for poststroke depression.

The correct response is option D: Silent infarcts are a risk factor for poststroke depression.

Recent research consensus has developed around subcortical small-vessel disease, large infarct volumes, and silent infarcts as risk factors for poststroke depression (Ferro et al. 2016) (option D is correct). A meta-analysis concluded that available scientific literature did not support the hypothesis that left frontal lesions are associated with an increased rate of depressive illness (Carson et al. 2000) (option B is incorrect). Poststroke depression is a common problem, affecting about one-quarter of stroke patients (Ferro et al. 2016) (option A is incorrect). There is clear evidence based on reviews of many randomized controlled trials that SSRIs are effective in treating depression after stroke (Ferro et al. 2016) (option C is incorrect). **Chapter 30 (p. 911)**

30.4   Which of the following is relatively rare poststroke?

A. Anxiety.
B. Hyposexuality.

C. Self-directed anger or frustration.

D. Impairment of executive function.

The correct response is option D: Impairment of executive function.

Executive function, including decision making, judgment, and social cognition, is regulated by complex systems that are relatively resistant to damage after stroke (Carota et al. 2002; Zinn et al. 2007) (option D is correct). Anxiety disorders are common after stroke and probably share the same risk factors as depression (Aström 1996). Estimates of prevalence have varied markedly, depending on whether the investigators subsumed anxiety symptoms within the construct of major depressive disorder. The reported prevalence of poststroke anxiety is around 20% (Ferro et al. 2016) (option A is incorrect). Hyposexuality is a common complaint after stroke in both men and women (see also Chapter 15, "Sexual Dysfunctions"). In some studies, close to 60% of stroke patients report sexual dysfunction; the most common dysfunctions are low desire, erectile dysfunction, premature or delayed ejaculation, and dyspareunia (option B is incorrect). Catastrophic reactions manifest as disruptive emotional behavior, typically self-directed anger or frustration, precipitated when a patient finds a task unsolvable (Goldstein 1939). This symptom is often associated with aphasia, and it has been suggested that damage to language areas is a critical part of the etiology (Carota et al. 2001) (option C is incorrect). **Chapter 15 (p. 417), Chapter 30 (pp. 912–914)**

30.5 What medication is *best* supported in the literature for the treatment of psychosis in the setting of Parkinson's disease (PD)?

A. Quetiapine.

B. Clozapine.

C. Pimavanserin.

D. Cholinesterase inhibitors.

The correct response is option B: Clozapine.

The atypical antipsychotic drug clozapine is the only antipsychotic that has been demonstrated in randomized controlled trials to reduce psychosis without worsening motor symptoms (Cummings 1999; Rabinstein and Shulman 2000) (option B is correct). Quetiapine is ineffective (Shotbolt et al. 2010), and high-potency typical antipsychotics and risperidone should be avoided (option A is incorrect). There has been recent interest in and promising results for the use of pimavanserin, a selective serotonin 2A (5-HT$_{2A}$) inverse agonist (Cummings et al. 2014), to treat PD psychosis. Pimavanserin produced substantial reductions in symptoms and showed a good side-effect profile in motor and nonmotor domains, but its cost may limit widespread use (Kianirad and Simuni 2017) (option C is incorrect). Secondary analyses of data from PD dementia trials suggest that cholinesterase inhibitors may have a role in the treatment of PD psychosis (Emre et al. 2004), as well as a good safety profile and an action that targets visual hallucinations that result from loss of central cholinergic function (option D is incorrect). **Chapter 30 (p. 916)**

30.6 Which of the following symptoms is *most* useful in diagnosing depression in patients with PD?

A. Preoccupation with health.
B. Sleep disturbance.
C. Anhedonia.
D. Attention deficit.

The correct response is option C: Anhedonia.

The diagnosis of depression in PD is difficult because many depressive symptoms overlap with the core features of PD—motor retardation, attention deficit, sleep disturbance, hypophonia, impotence, weight loss, fatigue, preoccupation with health, and reduced facial expression (options A, B, and D are incorrect). Therefore, anhedonia and sustained sadness are important diagnostic features, particularly if they are out of proportion to the severity of motor symptoms (Brooks and Doder 2001) (option C is correct). **Chapter 30 (p. 916)**

30.7 Which of the following statements about symptoms that commonly occur with multiple sclerosis (MS) is correct?

A. Fatigue is the most common single symptom in MS.
B. Cognitive impairment is uncommon with MS.
C. Mood symptoms comorbid with MS are a depressive psychological reaction to the illness.
D. There is no increased risk of psychosis with MS.

The correct response is option A: Fatigue is the most common single symptom in MS.

Fatigue affects up to 80% of individuals with the disease (option A is correct); it is important to differentiate fatigue from depression, sleepiness, adverse medication side effects, or pure physical exhaustion secondary to gait abnormalities. Cognitive impairment affects at least half of all patients with MS (Beatty et al. 1989; Heaton et al. 1985; Rao 1986; Rao et al. 1991) (option B is incorrect). Impairment, when present, is generally a "subcortical dementia," with impaired attention and speed of processing as the hallmark signs. Mood disorders are common in MS, with more than half of MS patients reporting depressive symptoms; mania and emotional lability are also common (Joffe et al. 1987; Sadovnick et al. 1996). A recent systematic review found a pooled prevalence rate of depression of 30.5% (Boeschoten et al. 2017). Depression may be a direct physiologically mediated consequence of the disease, a psychological reaction to the illness, a complication of pharmacotherapy, or coincidental (option C is incorrect). Well-conducted population studies have challenged the perceived orthodoxy that MS is not associated with an increased risk of psychosis, reporting that the population baseline rate of psychosis (1%) was increased in patients with MS to 2%–3%, with the highest prevalence (4%) in the 15- to 24-year-old population (Patten et al. 2005) (option D is incorrect). **Chapter 30 (pp. 919–922)**

30.8 Which of the following is *most* helpful in differentiating epileptic seizures from psychogenic nonepileptic seizures?

A. Frequent occurrence of seizures in public spaces.
B. Tremulous movements of varying frequency.
C. Resistance to attempted eye opening.
D. Acceptance that psychological factors contribute to the illness.

The correct response is option B: Tremulous movements of varying frequency.

At the core of psychogenic nonepileptic seizures (also called "dissociative seizures" and "pseudoseizures") is a distinct seizure semiology (with tremulous movements, often of varying frequency) that differs from the evolving jerky movements of epilepsy (option B is correct). Breathing is maintained during dissociative seizures. Some patients fall down and lie still without movement for prolonged periods. Clinical clues suggesting dissociative or psychogenic nonepileptic seizures include a preexisting somatoform disorder; atypical varieties of seizure, especially the occurrence of frequent and prolonged seizures in the face of normal intellectual function and normal interictal electroencephalogram; a preponderance of seizures in public places (option A is incorrect), especially in clinics and hospitals; and behavior during an apparent generalized seizure that suggests preservation of awareness (e.g., resistance to attempted eye opening) (option C is incorrect). Compared with patients who have epilepsy, those with recent-onset dissociative seizures are more likely to believe that psychological factors are less important than somatic ones and have a greater tendency to deny nonhealth life stresses (Stone et al. 2004) (option D is incorrect). **Chapter 30 (p. 934)**

30.9 Which of the following is *true* regarding the relationship between depression and epilepsy?

A. Depression is an independent risk factor for unprovoked seizures.
B. The prevalence of depression is similar in people with or without epilepsy.
C. Antidepressant medication should be avoided in people with epilepsy.
D. Anticonvulsant medication has no association with increased risk for suicide.

The correct response is option A: Depression is an independent risk factor for unprovoked seizures.

Depression is an independent risk factor for unprovoked seizures (Hesdorffer et al. 2000); the contribution of depression to risk appears to be particularly marked for partial seizures (option A is correct). The relationship between depression and epilepsy is bidirectional (i.e., each is a risk factor for the other). A meta-analysis that examined depression in people with epilepsy reported an overall prevalence 2.77 times the rate in people without epilepsy (Fiest et al. 2013) (option B is incorrect). Certain psychiatric drugs can lower the seizure threshold, thereby increasing the risk of seizures (see Chapter 36, "Psychopharmacology," for a review). The role of depression in exacerbating seizure risk is important, because many psychiatrists worry that antidepressant use will worsen epilepsy, when in fact it is the persistence of untreated depression that carries the greater threat (option C is incorrect). A 2008 U.S. Food and Drug Administration investigation of antiepileptic drugs concluded that all classes of antiepileptic drugs were associated with an increased risk of suicide (U.S. Department of Health and Human Services et al. 2008); suicidal behaviors were found in 0.43% of patients taking antiepileptic drugs, compared with 0.24% of control subjects taking a placebo. However, to date, there is no consensus across studies regarding which anticonvulsants carry the most risk, and the mechanism of this relationship is poorly understood; the elevated rates of psychiatric comorbidity in epilepsy likely account for at least some of this increased risk (Grimaldi-Bensouda et al. 2017) (option D is incorrect). **Chapter 30 (pp. 937–938)**

30.10 Which of the following signs or symptoms occurs with equal frequency in both functional neurological symptom disorders and organic neurological disorders?

A. Fixed dystonia.
B. *La belle indifférence.*
C. Depersonalization or derealization at the time of onset.
D. Tremor with variable frequency and entrainment.

The correct response is option B: *La belle indifférence.*

The presence of *la belle indifférence* was classically considered to be highly suggestive of conversion or functional neurological symptom disorder; however, this attitude is seen in only a minority of patients with conversion; it is seen with equal frequency in patients with organic neurological disorders (Stone et al. 2006) (option B is correct). Diagnosis of conversion disorder requires the presence of positive physical signs of internal inconsistency or marked incongruity with recognized neurological disorders. Helpful indicators suggestive of conversion disorder include the following: fixed dystonia, conversion weakness, and conversion tremor. Fixed dystonia describes the sustained posture of a limb, usually a clenched hand or an inverted or plantar-flexed foot (Hallett et al. 2005; Schrag et al. 2004) (option A is incorrect). Patients with conversion weakness will often describe symptoms suggestive of depersonalization or derealization at the time of onset, and symptom onset is most commonly associated with a physical trauma that is often minor (Pareés et al. 2014) (option C is incorrect). A conversion tremor typically demonstrates variable frequency and marked attenuation with distraction and entrainment (in which the frequency entrains to a contralateral limb voluntarily, making a 3- to 4-Hz movement) (option D is incorrect). **Chapter 30 (p. 943)**

30.11 Which of the following psychotropic medications appears to be *most* effective in treating fatigue associated with MS?

A. Amantadine.
B. Psychostimulants.
C. Modafinil.
D. Bupropion.

The correct response is option A: Amantadine.

A number of agents have been advocated for the treatment of MS fatigue, including amantadine, aminopyridines, psychostimulants, modafinil, and bupropion (options B, C, and D are incorrect). A recent meta-analysis concluded that only amantadine had relatively sufficient evidence of effectiveness (Yang et al. 2017); however, our experience with the drug has not been encouraging (option A is correct). **Chapter 30 (pp. 921–922)**

30.12 Which of the following cognitive impairments is typical of MS?

A. Procedural and implicit memory functions are impaired.
B. Aphasia and apraxia are common.
C. Cognitive impairment in MS is rare.
D. Impairment is usually a subcortical dementia.

The correct response is option D: Impairment is usually a subcortical dementia.

Cognitive impairment affects at least half of all patients with MS (Beatty et al. 1989; Heaton et al. 1985; Rao 1986; Rao et al. 1991) (option C is incorrect). Impairment, when present, is generally a "subcortical dementia," with impaired attention and speed of processing as the hallmark signs (option D is correct). Executive function deficits are common. Deficits in working, semantic, and episodic memory are reported, but procedural and implicit memory functions are generally preserved (option A is incorrect). Cortical syndromes such as aphasia, apraxia, and agnosia are relatively rare (option B is incorrect). **Chapter 30 (pp. 919)**

30.13 Which of the following psychiatric conditions is rarely associated with Wilson's disease?

A. Depression.
B. Dementia.
C. Schizophreniform psychosis.
D. Personality change.

The correct response is option C: Schizophreniform psychosis.

Wilson's disease is a rare progressive degenerative brain disease caused by a disorder of copper metabolism, which produces personality change, cognitive decline, extrapyramidal signs, and cirrhosis of the liver. The onset of Wilson's disease is most commonly in childhood or adolescence but can be as late as the fifth decade. Patients may present to psychiatrists with personality change, behavioral disturbance, depression, irritability, or dementia, or they may present to neurologists with a variety of extrapyramidal signs, including tremor, dysarthria and drooling, rigidity, bradykinesia, and dystonia (options A, B, and D are incorrect). Although commonly featured in psychiatry textbooks, schizophreniform psychosis is in fact rare (Shanmugiah et al. 2008) (option C is correct). **Chapter 30 (pp. 925–926)**

30.14 Which of the following findings of cognitive function is *most* likely to be observed in a patient with Wernicke-Korsakoff syndrome?

A. Severely impaired executive function.
B. Retrograde amnesia with relative sparing of anterograde memory.
C. Flattened affect with normal levels of motivation and interest.
D. Minimal difficulty on standard tasks of attention and working memory.

The correct response is option D: Minimal difficulty on standard tasks of attention and working memory.

Wernicke-Korsakoff syndrome results from thiamine depletion, and any cause of such depletion—including hyperemesis gravidarum, and gastric bypass surgery—can lead to the syndrome. However, the overwhelming majority of cases are associated with chronic alcohol abuse, which results in both decreased intake and decreased absorption of thiamine. Patients may present acutely with Wernicke's encephalopathy, which is characterized by confusion, ataxia, nystagmus, and ophthalmoplegia. Peripheral neuropathy may also be present. The chronic state of Korsakoff's syndrome, in the majority of cases, occurs following Wernicke's encephalopathy. On clinical examination, patients with Korsakoff's syndrome may perform well on standard tasks of attention and working memory (e.g., serial sevens, reverse digit span) (Kopelman 1985) (option D is correct), but they may struggle on more complex tasks involving shifting and dividing attention. Executive functions are commonly mildly affected, but this impairment may be secondary to chronic alcoholism rather than representing a specific deficit (option A is incorrect). A severe memory impairment involving both anterograde and retrograde deficits is present (Kopelman et al. 1999) (option B is incorrect). Defective encoding of new information is the core component of this memory disorder (Meudell and Mayes 1982). Disorientation and apathy, often with lack of curiosity about the past, are common, yet such disengaged patients frequently demonstrate labile irritability (option C is incorrect). **Chapter 30 (pp. 922–923)**

30.15 Which of the following is the *most* likely initial presentation of an autoimmune encephalitis?

A. Episodic impairment of working memory without focal neurologic deficits.
B. Acute onset of autonomic dysfunction, preceding psychiatric symptoms.

C. Numerous metastatic tumors on magnetic resonance imaging.

D. Subacute onset of psychiatric symptoms, with no identifiable tumor.

The correct response is option D: Subacute onset of psychiatric symptoms, with no identifiable tumor.

Limbic encephalitis (LE) is an autoimmune-mediated inflammation that may occur as a paraneoplastic phenomenon, or (more often) as a primary autoimmune disease. Primary autoimmune LE normally presents subacutely, over a couple of weeks but occasionally over a period as long as 3 months, with mood changes and sometimes psychosis evolving into confusion with seizures. Progressive impairment of working memory is thought to be a hallmark symptom, and focal central nervous system findings on examination are common (option A is incorrect). Particularly common is anti–N-methyl-D-aspartate receptor encephalitis, occurring in association with an occult ovarian teratoma in young women in about one-third of cases; this presents with rapid onset, with psychiatric disturbance and cognitive disturbance. Because of the initial psychiatric prodrome, patients may first present to psychiatrists, but the encephalopathic features quickly become apparent (option B is incorrect). Patients may have pressured speech or verbal reduction/mutism, movement disorder or dyskinesias or rigidity/abnormal posture, decreased level of consciousness, autonomic dysfunction, or central hypoventilation. Paraneoplastic LE is most commonly caused by small-cell lung cancer, but breast, ovarian, renal, and testicular carcinoma and lymphoma can also be responsible. The tumor may be quite small and sometimes is initially undetectable by imaging (option C is incorrect). Thus, with either paraneoplastic or primary autoimmune LE, patients may present subacutely over weeks to months, with mood changes and sometimes psychosis evolving into confusion with seizures; the tumor associated with the autoimmune inflammation may often be occult or initially undetectable by imaging (option D is correct). **Chapter 30 (pp. 927–928)**

References

Aström M: Generalized anxiety disorder in stroke patients. A 3-year longitudinal study. Stroke 27(2):270–275, 1996 8571422

Beatty WW, Goodkin DE, Beatty PA, Monson N: Frontal lobe dysfunction and memory impairment in patients with chronic progressive multiple sclerosis. Brain Cogn 11(1):73–86, 1989 2789818

Boeschoten RE, Braamse AMJ, Beekman ATF, et al: Prevalence of depression and anxiety in Multiple Sclerosis: A systematic review and meta-analysis. J Neurol Sci 372:331–341, 2017 28017241

Breier JI, Adair JC, Gold M, et al: Dissociation of anosognosia for hemiplegia and aphasia during left-hemisphere anesthesia. Neurology 45(1):65–67, 1995 7824138

Brooks DJ, Doder M: Depression in Parkinson's disease. Curr Opin Neurol 14(4):465–470, 2001 11470962

Carota A, Rossetti AO, Karapanayiotides T, Bogousslavsky J: Catastrophic reaction in acute stroke: a reflex behavior in aphasic patients. Neurology 57(10):1902–1905, 2001 11723287

Carota A, Staub F, Bogousslavsky J: Emotions, behaviours and mood changes in stroke. Curr Opin Neurol 15(1):57–69, 2002 11796952

Carson AJ, MacHale S, Allen K, et al: Depression after stroke and lesion location: a systematic review. Lancet 356(9224):122–126, 2000 10963248

Cummings JL: Managing psychosis in patients with Parkinson's disease. N Engl J Med 340(10):801–803, 1999 10072418

Cummings J, Isaacson S, Mills R, et al: Pimavanserin for patients with Parkinson's disease psychosis: a randomised, placebo-controlled phase 3 trial. Lancet 383(9916):533–540, 2014 24183563

Emre M, Aarsland D, Albanese A, et al: Rivastigmine for dementia associated with Parkinson's disease. N Engl J Med 351(24):2509–2518, 2004 15590953

Ferro JM, Caeiro L, Figueira ML: Neuropsychiatric sequelae of stroke. Nat Rev Neurol 12(5):269–280, 2016 27063107

Fiest KM, Dykeman J, Patten SB, et al: Depression in epilepsy: a systematic review and meta-analysis. Neurology 80(6):590–599, 2013 23175727

Goldstein K: The Organism: A Holistic Approach to Biology Derived From Pathological Data in Man. New York, American Books, 1939

Grimaldi-Bensouda L, Nordon C, Rossignol M, et al; PROTECT-WP6 study group: Antiepileptic drugs and risk of suicide attempts: a case-control study exploring the impact of underlying medical conditions. Pharmacoepidemiol Drug Saf 26(3):239–247, 2017 28052554

Gustafson Y, Olsson T, Asplund K, Hagg E: Acute confusional state (delirium) soon after stroke is associated with hypercortisolism. Cerebrovasc Dis 3:33–38, 1993

Hallett M, Lang AE, Fahn S, et al: Psychogenic Movement Disorders. Philadelphia, PA, American Neurological Association and Lippincott Williams & Wilkins, 2005

Heaton RK, Nelson LM, Thompson DS, et al: Neuropsychological findings in relapsing-remitting and chronic-progressive multiple sclerosis. J Consult Clin Psychol 53(1):103–110, 1985 3980815

Hesdorffer DC, Hauser WA, Annegers JF, Cascino G: Major depression is a risk factor for seizures in older adults. Ann Neurol 47(2):246–249, 2000 10665498

Jehkonen M, Laihosalo M, Kettunen J: Anosognosia after stroke: assessment, occurrence, subtypes and impact on functional outcome reviewed. Acta Neurol Scand 114(5):293–306, 2006 17022776

Joffe RT, Lippert GP, Gray TA, et al: Mood disorder and multiple sclerosis. Arch Neurol 44(4):376–378, 1987 3827692

Kianirad Y, Simuni T: Pimavanserin, a novel antipsychotic for management of Parkinson's disease psychosis. Expert Rev Clin Pharmacol 10(11):1161–1168, 2017 28817967

Kopelman MD: Rates of forgetting in Alzheimer-type dementia and Korsakoff's syndrome. Neuropsychologia 23(5):623–638, 1985 4058708

Kopelman MD, Stanhope N, Kingsley D: Retrograde amnesia in patients with diencephalic, temporal lobe or frontal lesions. Neuropsychologia 37(8):939–958, 1999 10426519

Langhorne P, Stott DJ, Robertson L, et al: Medical complications after stroke: a multicenter study. Stroke 31(6):1223–1229, 2000 10835436

Lazar RM, Marshall RS, Prell GD, Pile-Spellman J: The experience of Wernicke's aphasia. Neurology 55(8):1222–1224, 2000 11071506

Meudell P, Mayes AR: Normal and abnormal forgetting: some comments on the human amnesic syndrome, in Normality and Pathology in Cognitive Functions. Edited by Willis AW. London, Academic Press, 1982, pp 203–238

Pareés I, Kojovic M, Pires C, et al: Physical precipitating factors in functional movement disorders. J Neurol Sci 338(1-2):174–177, 2014 24439198

Patten SB, Svenson LW, Metz LM: Psychotic disorders in MS: population-based evidence of an association. Neurology 65(7):1123–1125, 2005 16217073

Rabinstein AA, Shulman LM: Management of behavioral and psychiatric problems in Parkinson's disease. Parkinsonism Relat Disord 7(1):41–50, 2000 11008195

Rahkonen T, Mäkelä H, Paanila S, et al: Delirium in elderly people without severe predisposing disorders: etiology and 1-year prognosis after discharge. Int Psychogeriatr 12(4):473–481, 2000 11263714

Rao SM: Neuropsychology of multiple sclerosis: a critical review. J Clin Exp Neuropsychol 8(5):503–542, 1986 3805250

Rao SM, Leo GJ, Bernardin L, Unverzagt F: Cognitive dysfunction in multiple sclerosis. I. Frequency, patterns, and prediction. Neurology 41(5):685–691, 1991 2027484

Sadovnick AD, Remick RA, Allen J, et al: Depression and multiple sclerosis. Neurology 46(3):628–632, 1996 8618657

Schrag A, Trimble M, Quinn N, Bhatia K: The syndrome of fixed dystonia: an evaluation of 103 patients. Brain 127(Pt 10):2360–2372, 2004 15342362

Shanmugiah A, Sinha S, Taly AB, et al: Psychiatric manifestations in Wilson's disease: a cross-sectional analysis. J Neuropsychiatry Clin Neurosci 20(1):81–85, 2008 18305288

Shotbolt P, Samuel M, David A: Quetiapine in the treatment of psychosis in Parkinson's disease. Ther Adv Neurol Disorder 3(6):339–350, 2010 21179595

Stone J, Binzer M, Sharpe M: Illness beliefs and locus of control: a comparison of patients with pseudoseizures and epilepsy. J Psychosom Res 57(6):541–547, 2004 15596160

Stone J, Smyth R, Carson A, et al: La belle indifférence in conversion symptoms and hysteria: systematic review. Br J Psychiatry 188:204–209, 2006 16507959

U.S. Department of Health and Human Services: Food and Drug Administration, Center for Evaluation and Research, et al: Statistical review and evaluation: antiepileptic drugs and suicidality. May 23, 2008. Available at: https://www.fda.gov/files/drugs/published/Statistical-Review-and-Evaluation--Antiepileptic-Drugs-and-Suicidality.pdf. Accessed May 2019.

Yang TT, Wang L, Deng XY, Yu G: Pharmacological treatments for fatigue in patients with multiple sclerosis: a systematic review and meta-analysis. J Neurol Sci 380:256–261, 2017 28870581

Zinn S, Bosworth HB, Hoenig HM, Swartzwelder HS: Executive function deficits in acute stroke. Arch Phys Med Rehabil 88(2):173–180, 2007 17270514

CHAPTER 31

Obstetrics and Gynecology

31.1 Which psychiatric disorder is *more* common among women with infertility?

A. Posttraumatic stress disorder.
B. Psychosis.
C. Major depressive disorder (MDD).
D. Anxiety disorder.

The correct response is option C: Major depressive disorder (MDD).

Although some studies show that women with infertility are distressed but do not meet criteria for a major psychiatric disorder, other studies reveal rates of MDD in infertile women that reach 40%, with anxiety disorders reaching 20% (Chen et al. 2004) (option C is correct; option D is incorrect). Both infertility and perinatal loss are associated with lower quality of life, marital discord, MDD, anxiety disorders, and posttraumatic stress disorder (Bhat and Byatt 2016) (option A is incorrect). Careful attention should be paid to the potential contribution of recent changes in drug regimens to recent-onset psychiatric symptoms such as depression, anxiety, mania, and psychosis. Clomiphene induces follicle-stimulating hormone (FSH) and has been associated with anxiety, insomnia, and psychosis (Burns 2007; Seeman 2015) (option B is incorrect). **Chapter 31 (pp. 967–968)**

31.2 Which psychiatric medication is most likely to be associated with infertility due to hyperprolactinemia?

A. Escitalopram.
B. Haloperidol.
C. Valproic acid.
D. Fluoxetine.

The correct response is option B: Haloperidol.

It is important to consider the impact of psychotropic medications on fertility. Selective serotonin reuptake inhibitors (SSRIs) have been shown to be associated with a small but increased risk of early miscarriage and postpartum hemorrhage

(Hanley et al. 2016) (options A and D are incorrect). Valproic acid is associated with polycystic ovarian syndrome (option C is incorrect), and many antipsychotic medications are associated with anovulation due to hyperprolactinemia (Joffe 2007) (option B is correct). **Chapter 31 (pp. 968–969)**

31.3   How does infertility most commonly impact a couple's mental health?

A. Duration of infertility does not affect the couple's mental health.
B. Fertility treatments themselves may have adverse effects on mental health.
C. Men show the same distress and guilt whether the infertility is attributed to male-factor etiology or female-factor etiology.
D. The rate of anxiety and depression is higher among men with infertility than women with infertility.

The correct response is option B: Fertility treatments themselves may have adverse effects on mental health.

Biological factors related to infertility that may affect mental health include the cause and duration of infertility (option A is incorrect), as well as the effects of fertility treatment. There is evidence that the difference in psychological profile between fertile and infertile couples increases with infertility duration (Baldur-Felskov et al. 2013)). Interestingly, men show greater distress and guilt when the infertility is attributable to male-factor etiology (Volgsten et al. 2010) (option C is incorrect). There are sex differences in the scope of psychiatric illness affecting couples with infertility, with men reporting more symptoms of anxiety and depression than men in the general population but far fewer than their female counterparts (Volgsten et al. 2008) (option D is incorrect). Fertility treatments themselves may have adverse effects on mental health (option B is correct). Interventions can be time-consuming, expensive, embarrassing, and invasive. The psychological effects, particularly mood alterations, of fertility-enhancing drugs are underappreciated. **Chapter 31 (pp. 967–968)**

31.4   Which of the following psychotropic medications reduces the efficacy of hormonal contraception?

A. Phenobarbital.
B. Valproate.
C. Lamotrigine.
D. Amitriptyline.

The correct response is option A: Phenobarbital.

The major pathway of metabolism for both the estrogen and progesterone components of hormonal contraception is through cytochrome P450 (CYP) 3A4 (Oesterheld et al. 2008). Psychotropic medications that induce CYP3A4, thus reducing the efficacy of hormonal contraception, include phenobarbital (option A is correct), oxcarbazepine, carbamazepine, topiramate (at dosages >200 mg/day), modafinil, and St. John's wort. Oral contraceptives can also inhibit the oxidation of various psychiatric medications via CYP1A2, 2B6, 2C19, and 3A4. This can result in increased levels of benzodiazepines and tricyclic antidepressants (option D is incorrect). Levels of valproate and lamotrigine can also be increased by oral contraceptives (options B and C are incorrect). **Chapter 31 (p. 971)**

31.5   Electroconvulsive therapy (ECT) is generally regarded as a safe and effective treatment for which one of the following conditions in pregnancy?

A. Hyperemesis.
B. All forms of MDD.
C. A patient with schizophrenia who is stable on medications.
D. Affective psychosis.

The correct response is option D: Affective psychosis.

Hyperemesis is no longer considered a psychiatric disorder. Mental health intervention can, however, help the patient and family cope until the condition resolves. Treatment is usually with standard antiemetics, but mirtazapine may be helpful in treatment-resistant cases (Guclu et al. 2005) (option A is incorrect). ECT is generally regarded as a safe and effective treatment for severe depression (option B is incorrect), affective psychosis (option D is correct), and catatonia during pregnancy and the puerperium. ECT is underused and should be considered in emergency situations in which the safety of the mother, fetus, or child is jeopardized; to avoid first-trimester exposure to teratogenic drugs; and in patients who have not responded to psychotropics (option C is incorrect) or who have previously had successful treatment with ECT (Stewart and Vigod 2016). **Chapter 31 (pp. 984–985, 992)**

31.6   Which of the following atypical antipsychotics is most likely to impair fertility?

A. Quetiapine.
B. Ziprasidone.
C. Risperidone.
D. Lurasidone.

The correct response is option C: Risperidone.

Atypical antipsychotics, other than risperidone (option C is correct), do not impair fertility as much as older antipsychotics and may result in unwanted pregnancies in women being treated for psychotic illnesses (options A, B, and D are incorrect). **Chapter 31 (p. 972)**

31.7 Which of the following is considered to be a risk factor for poor outcome after hysterectomy?

A. Preoperative pain.
B. Lack of psychiatric history.
C. Clear indications for hysterectomy.
D. Use of laparoscopic rather than robotic surgery.

The correct response is option A: Preoperative pain.

Risk factors for poor outcome appear to be related to preoperative pain, sexual dysfunction, and psychiatric morbidity (option A is correct; option B is incorrect). A study of 228 hysterectomy patients who underwent elective abdominal, laparoscopic, or robotic surgery found no difference in satisfaction, well-being, or dyspareunia scores among the three groups (Schiff et al. 2015) (option D is incorrect). Hartmann et al. (2004) reported that women with preoperative pain and depression had less improvement after hysterectomy than women without pain and depression preoperatively. Women with substantiated diagnoses and clear indications for hysterectomy have better physical and psychological outcomes than do women with less-defined symptoms and indicators such as chronic pelvic pain (option C is incorrect). **Chapter 31 (pp. 973–974)**

31.8 How does spontaneous abortion typically impact mental health?

A. Spontaneous abortion does not precipitate psychiatric consequences, as it is not associated with serious medical or obstetric complications.
B. Only women with repeated miscarriages are at risk of psychological sequelae.
C. Increased attention from health care providers exacerbates the emotional effect of spontaneous abortion.
D. The end of pregnancy through miscarriage or stillbirth is associated with an increase in anxiety and depression during a subsequent pregnancy.

The correct response is option D: The end of pregnancy through miscarriage or stillbirth is associated with an increase in anxiety and depression during a subsequent pregnancy.

Spontaneous abortion, like a stillbirth or neonatal death, may precipitate complicated grief, depression, or posttraumatic stress disorder (Engelhard et al. 2003; Kulathilaka et al. 2016) (option A is incorrect). Women with repeated miscarriages are at *greater* risk of psychological sequelae (option B is incorrect). Health care providers may have difficulty addressing the emotional effect of spontaneous abortion. They feel helpless to prevent it, and it is generally not associated with serious medical or obstetric complications. Psychiatrists can help them to understand and tolerate their patients' feelings and to appreciate the benefits of simply allowing patients to express them (option C is incorrect). The end of pregnancy through miscarriage or stillbirth is associated with an increase in anxiety and depression during a subsequent pregnancy (option D is correct). Data suggest that fears related to miscarriage may have a negative impact on pregnancy and intimate relationships (Haghparast et al. 2016). **Chapter 31 (pp. 974–975)**

31.9   Which one of the following pieces of a patient's history would indicate a risk for depression in pregnancy?

A. No prior psychiatric history.
B. Higher-powered, high-stress employment.
C. Intimate partner violence.
D. Fair social support.

The correct response is option C: Intimate partner violence.

Risk factors for depression during pregnancy include a history of depression (option A is incorrect), and major life stressors, especially intimate partner violence (option C is correct), as well as low socioeconomic status (option B is incorrect) and low levels of social support (option D is correct). **Chapter 31 (p. 981)**

31.10   Which of the following conditions is potentially increased, in either mother or fetus, with a selective serotonin reuptake inhibitor (SSRI) antidepressant use in pregnancy?

A. Cardiac malformation in fetus.
B. Persistent pulmonary hypertension of the newborn.
C. Risk of preeclampsia.
D. Renal hypoplasia in fetus.

The correct response is option B: Persistent pulmonary hypertension of the newborn.

Persistent pulmonary hypertension of the newborn is a rare but potentially fatal condition, with a background rate of about 1.2 per 1,000 births. One well-conducted study of 11,014 pregnancies exposed to an SSRI after the 20th gestational week found an adjusted odds ratio (aOR) of 2.1 (95% confidence interval [CI]: 1.5–3.0), representing an increase from 1.2 to 3 per 1,000 births; risk was similar across SSRI types (Kieler et al. 2012). A more recent study with 102,179 SSRI exposures and 26,771 non-SSRI antidepressant exposures found that whereas risks were increased from 2.1 per 1,000 births in unexposed pregnancies to 3.2 per 1,000 and 2.9 per 1,000 in SSRI and non-SSRI antidepressant–exposed pregnancies, respectively, the associations were not statistically significant after analyses were restricted to women with depression only and comprehensively adjusted for confounders (aOR: 1.10, 95% CI: 0.94–1.29 for SSRIs; aOR: 1.02, 95% CI: 0.77–1.35 for non-SSRIs) (Huybrechts et al. 2015) (option B is correct).
    Antidepressant use in pregnancy does not appear to be associated with increased risk for congenital malformations (option D is incorrect). Some studies

have suggested that it may be associated with a small absolute increased risk for specific cardiac defects (especially with paroxetine), but more rigorous studies do not support this interpretation. A U.S. study of more than 65,000 antidepressant exposures in pregnancy had sufficient sample size to explore specific antidepressants in a well-conducted propensity-matched analysis; this study found no association between antidepressant exposure in pregnancy and any type of cardiac malformation for paroxetine, sertraline, fluoxetine, tricyclic antidepressants, serotonin-norepinephrine reuptake inhibitors, bupropion, or other antidepressants (Huybrechts et al. 2014) (option A is incorrect). The highest-quality studies conducted to date suggest that SSRI exposure does not appear to increase the risk of hypertensive disorders of pregnancy. A U.S. study of 100,942 pregnant women with depression found no increased risk of preeclampsia from use of SSRIs during pregnancy (Palmsten et al. 2013) (option C is incorrect). **Chapter 31 (pp. 989–990)**

31.11 Which of the following is associated with untreated depression during pregnancy or the postpartum period?

A. No change in risk of morbidity in the mother and her offspring.
B. Increased risk of preterm birth.
C. No change in infant birth weight.
D. No change in risk related to substance use during pregnancy.

The correct response is option B: Increased risk of preterm birth.

Untreated depression during pregnancy or the postpartum period is associated with increased morbidity in the mother and her offspring (option A is incorrect). Potential complications in pregnancy and at delivery include increased risk of poor prenatal care, substance use during pregnancy, preterm birth, and low birth weight (Grigoriadis et al. 2013) (option B is correct; options C and D are incorrect). Women with depression in pregnancy are at high risk for postpartum depression and for impaired mother-infant interactions, which have been associated with poor developmental and emotional outcomes in the offspring (Stein et al. 2014). Unfortunately, depression is undertreated during pregnancy, with fewer than 20% of women seeking treatment (Byatt et al. 2016). **Chapter 31 (p. 988)**

31.12 Which one of the following medications is associated with the greatest risk of teratogenicity in the fetus?

A. Lorazepam.
B. Quetiapine.
C. Valproic acid.
D. Lithium.

The correct response is option C: Valproic acid.

A long-standing debate has existed regarding whether benzodiazepine use in pregnancy is associated with cleft lip or cleft palate; however, rigorously controlled studies do not support this assertion (Enato et al. 2011) (option A is incorrect). Data are emerging to suggest that most second-generation antipsychotics are reasonably low risk in pregnancy (option B is incorrect); high-potency antipsychotics, such as haloperidol, have been in use longer and are also considered to be reasonably low risk (Tosato et al. 2017). Early reports warned of congenital heart disease in infants exposed in utero to lithium carbonate, but subsequent analyses have shown these risks to be only slightly greater than those in the general population (Altshuler et al. 1996) (option D is incorrect). Other mood stabilizers, such as carbamazepine and valproic acid, are associated with greater teratogenicity than lithium (Stewart and Robinson 2001) (option C is correct). **Chapter 31 (p. 991)**

31.13 Which one of the following strategies should be implemented in the care of a pregnant woman being treated with lithium?

A. Divided dosing.
B. Keeping the daily dose of lithium the same throughout the pregnancy.
C. Checking lithium levels only at the beginning and at the end of the pregnancy.
D. Maintain the dose used during the pregnancy after delivery.

The correct response is option A: Divided dosing.

For women with unstable bipolar disorder, it is reasonable to continue lithium throughout pregnancy while carefully monitoring serum levels (option C is incorrect). Divided doses may be safer than once daily dosing (option A is correct). An ultrasound during the first trimester can identify possible congenital cardiac malformations. Dosage should be reduced after delivery to avoid lithium toxicity in the early postpartum period (option D is incorrect). An increase in the usual dosage of lithium carbonate may be required during the second and third trimesters to achieve therapeutic serum levels, with a decrease postpartum (option B is incorrect). **Chapter 31 (pp. 989, 991)**

31.14 The levels of which of the following psychotropic medications can be increased by oral contraceptives?

A. Modafinil.
B. Oxcarbazepine.
C. Lamotrigine.
D. Phenobarbital.

The correct response is option C: Lamotrigine.

Oral contraceptives can inhibit the oxidation of various psychiatric medications via CYP1A2, 2B6, 2C19, and 3A4. This can result in increased levels of benzodiazepines and tricyclic antidepressants. Levels of valproate and lamotrigine can also be increased by oral contraceptives (option C is correct). Psychotropic medications that induce CYP3A4, thus reducing the efficacy of hormonal contraception, include phenobarbital (option D is incorrect), oxcarbazepine (option B is incorrect), carbamazepine, topiramate (at dosages >200 mg/day), modafinil (option A is incorrect), and St. John's wort. **Chapter 31 (p. 971)**

References

Altshuler LL, Cohen L, Szuba MP, et al: Pharmacologic management of psychiatric illness during pregnancy: dilemmas and guidelines. Am J Psychiatry 153(5):592–606, 1996 8615404

Baldur-Felskov B, Kjaer SK, Albieri V, et al: Psychiatric disorders in women with fertility problems: results from a large Danish register-based cohort study. Hum Reprod 28(3):683–690, 2013 23223399

Bhat A, Byatt N: Infertility and perinatal loss: when the bough breaks. Curr Psychiatry Rep 18(3):31, 2016 26847216

Burns LH: Psychiatric aspects of infertility and infertility treatments. Psychiatr Clin North Am 30(4):689–716, 2007 17938041

Byatt N, Xiao RS, Dinh KH, Waring ME: Mental health care use in relation to depressive symptoms among pregnant women in the USA. Arch Women Ment Health 19(1):187–191, 2016 25846018

Chen TH, Chang SP, Tsai CF, Juang KD: Prevalence of depressive and anxiety disorders in an assisted reproductive technique clinic. Hum Reprod 19(10):2313–2318, 2004 15242992

Enato E, Moretti M, Koren G: The fetal safety of benzodiazepines: an updated meta-analysis. J Obstet Gynaecol Can 33(1):46–48, 2011 21272436

Engelhard IM, van den Hout MA, Kindt M, et al: Peritraumatic dissociation and posttraumatic stress after pregnancy loss: a prospective study. Behav Res Ther 41(1):67–78, 2003 12488120

Grigoriadis S, VonderPorten EH, Mamisashvili L, et al: The impact of maternal depression during pregnancy on perinatal outcomes: a systematic review and meta-analysis. J Clin Psychiatry 74(4):e321–e341, 2013 23656857

Guclu S, Gol M, Dogan E, Saygili U: Mirtazapine use in resistant hyperemesis gravidarum: report of three cases and review of the literature. Arch Gynecol Obstet 272(4):298–300, 2005 16007504

Haghparast E, Faramarzi M, Hassanzadeh R: Psychiatric symptoms and pregnancy distress in subsequent pregnancy after spontaneous abortion history. Pak J Med Sci 32(5):1097–1101, 2016 27882001

Hanley GE, Smolina K, Mintzes B, et al: Postpartum hemorrhage and use of serotonin reuptake inhibitor antidepressants in pregnancy. Obstet Gynecol 127(3):553–561, 2016 26855096

Hartmann KE, Ma C, Lamvu GM, et al: Quality of life and sexual function after hysterectomy in women with preoperative pain and depression. Obstet Gynecol 104(4):701–709, 2004 15458889

Huybrechts KF, Palmsten K, Avorn J, et al: Antidepressant use in pregnancy and the risk of cardiac defects. N Engl J Med 370(25):2397–2407, 2014 24941178

Huybrechts KF, Bateman BT, Palmsten K, et al: Antidepressant use late in pregnancy and risk of persistent pulmonary hypertension of the newborn. JAMA 313(21):2142–2151, 2015 26034955

Joffe H: Reproductive biology and psychotropic treatments in premenopausal women with bipolar disorder. J Clin Psychiatry 68(Suppl 9):10–15, 2007 17764379

Kieler H, Artama M, Engeland A, et al: Selective serotonin reuptake inhibitors during pregnancy and risk of persistent pulmonary hypertension in the newborn: population based cohort study from the five Nordic countries. BMJ 344:d8012, 2012 22240235

Kulathilaka S, Hanwella R, de Silva VA: Depressive disorder and grief following spontaneous abortion. BMC Psychiatry 16:100, 2016 27071969

Oesterheld JR, Cozza K, Sandson NB: Oral contraceptives. Psychosomatics 49(2):168–175, 2008 18354071

Palmsten K, Huybrechts KF, Michels KB, et al: Antidepressant use and risk for preeclampsia. Epidemiology 24(5):682–691, 2013 23873072

Schiff L, Wegienka G, Sangha R, Eisenstein D: Is cervix removal associated with patient-centered outcomes of pain, dyspareunia, well-being and satisfaction after laparoscopic hysterectomy? Arch Gynecol Obstet 291(2):371–376, 2015 25145555

Seeman MV: Transient psychosis in women on clomiphene, bromocriptine, domperidone and related endocrine drugs. Gynecol Endocrinol 31(10):751–754, 2015 26291819

Stein A, Pearson RM, Goodman SH, et al: Effects of perinatal mental disorders on the fetus and child. Lancet 384(9956):1800–1819, 2014 25455250

Stewart DE, Robinson G: Psychotropic drugs and electroconvulsive therapy during pregnancy and lactation, in Psychological Aspects of Women's Health Care: The Interface Between Psychiatry and Obstetrics and Gynecology, 2nd Edition. Edited by Stotland N, Stewart D. Washington, DC, American Psychiatric Press, 2001, pp 67–93

Stewart DE, Vigod S: Postpartum depression. N Engl J Med 375(22):2177–2186, 2016 27959754

Tosato S, Albert U, Tomassi S, et al: A systematized review of atypical antipsychotics in pregnant women: balancing between risks of untreated illness and risks of drug-related adverse effects. J Clin Psychiatry 78(5):e477–e489, 2017 28297592

Volgsten H, Skoog Svanberg A, Ekselius L, et al: Prevalence of psychiatric disorders in infertile women and men undergoing in vitro fertilization treatment. Hum Reprod 23(9):2056–2063, 2008 18583334

Volgsten H, Skoog Svanberg A, Ekselius L, et al: Risk factors for psychiatric disorders in infertile women and men undergoing in vitro fertilization treatment. Fertil Steril 93(4):1088–1096, 2010 19118826

CHAPTER 32

Pediatrics

32.1 A 9-year-old child has which of the following cognitive understandings of their body?

A. Ability to apply logic to his or her understanding of physical illness and is eager for factual information about the body.
B. Lack of capacity to create a narrative about his or her experience.
C. Ability to use abstract reasoning and can discuss body systems and not just individual organs.
D. Ability to understand basic concepts of cause and effect and is most aware of body parts he or she can directly sense, like the heart.

The correct response is option A: Ability to apply logic to his or her understanding of physical illness and is eager for factual information about the body.

Children's conceptions about their bodies vary widely and are influenced by their experiences. However, in general, children appear to follow a developmental path of understanding their bodies that roughly corresponds to Piaget's stages of cognitive development. *Sensorimotor children* (birth to approximately 2 years) are largely preverbal and do not have the capacity to create narratives to explain their experiences (option B is incorrect). Their perception of their body and of illness is therefore primarily built on sensory experiences and does not involve any formal reasoning. *Preoperational children* (approximately 2–7 years) also understand through perception, but they are able to use words and some very basic concepts of cause and effect. They tend to be most aware of parts of the body that they can directly sense, such as bones and heart (which they can feel) and blood (which they have seen come out of their bodies) (option D is incorrect). However, they do not have a clear sense of cause and effect and are therefore inclined to see events that are temporally related as causally related. They also have no real sense of organs but conceptualize blood and food as going into or coming out of their body as though the body were itself the container. This leads to many humorous but confusing assumptions and misunderstandings. *Concrete operational children* (approximately 7–11 years) are able to apply logic to their perceptions in a more integrative manner. However, the logic is quite literal or concrete and allows for only one cause for an effect. They tend to be eager to learn factual information about the body and illness but will have difficulty with any concepts that require abstract reasoning (option A is correct). *Formal operational children* (older than 11 years) are able to use a level of abstract reasoning that allows discussion of systems rather than simple organs and can incorporate multiple causations of illness (option C is incorrect). It should not be assumed, however, that all adolescents approach the understanding of illness and their body at this level of cognition. In fact, most adults function at this level of thought only in areas of their own expertise, if at all. **Chapter 32 (pp. 1011–1012)**

32.2   Which of the following statements is *true* about parents and their children in a medical system?

A. Parents may not be involved in significant aspects of their children's medical care.
B. Children do not let their parents' reactions to an illness determine how they should respond.
C. Parents (or legal guardian equivalents) are the legal decision makers for the child and thus are deeply involved in the child's care.
D. Heightened parental stress plays no role in how the child adjusts psychologically to illness.

The correct response is option C: Parents (or legal guardian equivalents) are the legal decision makers for the child and thus are deeply involved in the child's care.

No pediatric patient can be considered in isolation from his or her family (option A is incorrect). Parents are the legal decision makers for the child and thus are involved in all aspects of care (option C is correct). Children look to their parents to understand the world. It is partially from their reactions to the illness and treatment that the child determines how dangerous the illness is and how to respond (Cousino and Hazen 2013) (option B is incorrect). Given that heightened parental stress has been shown to predict poorer psychological adjustment in children with chronic illness (Cousino and Hazen 2013), addressing parental fear, helplessness, anger, or withdrawal is also helpful for their children (option D is incorrect). **Chapter 32 (p. 1012)**

32.3   Which of the following risk factors is *not* linked to illness- or treatment-related posttraumatic stress symptoms in children?

A. Premorbid psychopathology.
B. Female gender.
C. Maternal negative life events.
D. Older age.

The correct response is option D: Older age.

An area of increasing clinical focus is illness- or treatment-related (iatrogenic) posttraumatic stress symptoms in children who undergo medical procedures and/or have life-threatening conditions. Several risk factors have been identified as increasing vulnerability for iatrogenic medical trauma symptoms. Davydow et al. (2010) found that premorbid psychopathology (option A is incorrect), female gender (option B is incorrect), younger age (option D is correct), developmental problems, and maternal negative life events (option C is incorrect) increased the risk of psychiatric problems in pediatric survivors of critical illnesses. Other studies have highlighted the importance of peritraumatic factors as well. Having psychological or behavioral problems at the time of the trauma, a higher heart rate, and beliefs about the trauma being serious or life-threatening all increased the risk of initial symptom development (Brosbe et al. 2011). Once these preliminary symptoms developed, children's beliefs about their symptoms, use of thought suppression as a coping technique, and previous parental posttraumatic stress disorder (PTSD) further predisposed youth to developing acute stress disorder (Brosbe et al. 2011). While many of these cases focus on acute trauma reactions rather than full-fledged PTSD, these peritraumatic symptoms appear to predict decrements in functioning, quality of life, and psychological well-being well into adulthood (Agorastos et al. 2014). **Chapter 32 (p. 1013)**

32.4   Which of the following factors does *not* increase the risk of suicide in medically ill adolescents?

A. Suicidal intent and plan.
B. Recent improvement in depressive symptoms.
C. Family history of suicide.
D. Hypersomnia.

The correct response is option D: Hypersomnia.

Adolescents with suicidal intent and plan (option A is incorrect), family history of suicide (option C is incorrect), comorbid psychiatric disorder, intractable pain, persistent insomnia (option D is correct), lack of social support, inadequate coping skills, recent improvement in depressive symptoms (option B is incorrect), or impulsivity are at heightened risk of suicide (Glenn and Nock 2014; Horowitz et al. 2014). Although supportive and cognitive-behavioral interventions can lead to significant improvements in depressive symptoms (Gledhill and Hodes 2011; Hofmann et al. 2012), the combination of psychotherapy with a selective serotonin reuptake inhibitor (SSRI) may prove optimal. For some adolescents, thoughts about suicide provide an important source of control in the face of an unknown and uncontrollable illness course. Addressing the lack of perceived control, isolation, and distressing physical symptoms should be a top priority. Use of antidepressant medication in suicidal adolescents and young adults should be monitored closely, given the small chance of an increase in suicidal ideation. **Chapter 32 (p. 1015)**

32.5 Which of the following selective serotonin reuptake inhibitor (SSRI) medications is *not* considered first-line in the treatment of depression in medically ill youth?

A. Escitalopram.
B. Sertraline.
C. Citalopram.
D. Fluoxetine.

The correct response is option D: Fluoxetine.

In medically ill youth, citalopram, escitalopram, and sertraline should be considered as first-line in the treatment of depression (option D is correct; options A, B, and C are incorrect). These SSRIs are efficacious and tolerable for children with complex medical problems and are the least likely SSRIs to have drug interactions (Bursch and Forgey 2013). They may also be helpful in the treatment of anxiety and iatrogenic medical trauma symptoms (Bursch and Forgey 2013). Second-line, both risperidone and quetiapine have proven to be effective for more severe anxiety and trauma symptoms (Bursch and Forgey 2013). Low dosages of benzodiazepines are frequently prescribed by pediatricians for acute anxiety and agitation in the hospital because they can have a more immediate effect than SSRIs. However, benzodiazepines increase the risk of delirium, agitated (i.e., paradoxical) reactions, and/or posttraumatic stress symptoms and, therefore, should be avoided whenever possible (Bursch and Forgey 2013). **Chapter 32 (p. 1015)**

32.6 According to the chronic illness literature, which percentage is the most accurate estimate of nonadherence to prescribed treatment in pediatric patients?

A. 50%.
B. 10%.
C. 75%.
D. 90%.

The correct response is option A: 50%.

The term *adherence* is generally used to describe the extent to which a patient's health behavior is consistent with medical recommendations. Defined as such, adherence includes not only taking medications and attending clinic appointments but also engaging in recommended diet, exercise, and other lifestyle behaviors such as smoking abstinence and sunscreen use (Ahmed and Aslani 2014). Adherence is a difficult construct to study and measure, given that health behaviors vary across medical conditions and illness severity levels. Variables known to moderate adherence include self-efficacy, degree of concordance between patient and provider, and culturally mediated differences in the understanding of an illness's cause, course, and treatment (Ahmed and Aslani 2014). Overall, chronic illness literature estimates that at least 50% of pediatric patients are nonadherent to their prescribed treatment regimen (Duncan et al. 2014) (option A is correct; options B, C, and D are incorrect). Nonadherence is linked to increased health care spending, emergency room visits, hospitalizations, exacerbations in morbidity, and premature mortality (McGrady and Hommel 2013; Oliva et al. 2013; Simon et al. 2011). **Chapter 32 (p. 1016)**

32.7 Which of the following features is *not* considered more specific to pediatric delirium compared with delirium in adults?

A. Psychosis.
B. Inconsolability.
C. Autonomic dysregulation.
D. Purposeless actions.

The correct response is option A: Psychosis.

Pediatric delirium (see Chapter 4, "Delirium") has received little clinical and research attention compared with adult delirium (Schieveld and Janssen 2014; Smith et al. 2011, 2013). It is estimated that at least 30% of critically ill children experience delirium (Smith et al. 2013), although this may be an underestimation given that hypoactive delirium is commonly underdiagnosed (Smith et al. 2011). As in adults, critically ill children can develop delirium with hyperactive, hypoactive, mixed, or veiled presentations (Bursch and Forgey 2013; Smith et al. 2011). Across the life span, delirium may sometimes manifest with psychotic symptoms (Smith et al. 2013) (option A is correct). Several features, however, are considered unique or more common to pediatric populations, including labile affect, inconsolability, signs of autonomic dysregulation, and purposeless actions (Smith et al. 2013) (options B, C, and D are incorrect). Given the wide range of symptoms and presentations in pediatric delirium, reasons for psychiatric consultation requests can vary widely, from agitation and oppositionality to unexplained lethargy, depression, or confusion. **Chapter 32 (pp. 1018–1019)**

32.8 Which of the following is *not* a common psychiatric reason for consultation for patients with autism who have medical illness?

A. Difficulty coping with hospitalization/illness.
B. Nonadherence to treatment plan.
C. Substance abuse.
D. Homicidal ideation.

The correct response is option D: Homicidal ideation.

Common medical presentations of patients with autism include seizures, gastrointestinal symptoms (weight loss or gain, nausea, vomiting, constipation, diarrhea due to unusual eating habits, abnormal sensory signaling, or underlying gastrointestinal problems), injuries (due to self-injurious behavior, sensory signaling problems, physical altercations, lack of fear, inattentiveness, or clumsiness), pain or other sensory abnormalities, and substance use disorders (option C is incorrect). Additional reasons for psychiatric consultation might include requests for evaluation and recommendations regarding difficulty coping with hospitalization or illness (option A is incorrect), nonadherence to treatment plan (option B is incorrect), capacity to refuse treatment, or pretransplantation evaluations but not homicidal ideation (option D is correct). **Chapter 32 (p. 1025)**

32.9   Which statistic correctly represents the risk of posttraumatic stress disorder (PTSD) in childhood cancer survivors compared with their siblings?

A. PTSD occurs less frequently in childhood cancer survivors compared with their siblings.
B. PTSD is found in roughly the same proportion in childhood cancer survivors compared with their siblings.
C. There is roughly twice the risk of PTSD in childhood cancer survivors compared with their siblings.
D. There is roughly four times the risk of PTSD in childhood cancer survivors compared with their siblings.

The correct response is option D: There is roughly four times the risk of PTSD in childhood cancer survivors compared with their siblings.

Children with cancer, in comparison with healthy schoolchildren or children with asthma, have been found to report fewer symptoms of depression and to more often rely on repression and avoidant coping (Phipps et al. 2001). An explanation for this observation was proposed by Erickson and Steiner (2000), who found that coping styles among long-term pediatric cancer survivors were shaped by traumatic avoidance. Congruent with this finding, research now supports the conceptualization of cancer diagnosis and its treatment as being potentially traumatic, highlighting the importance of addressing these experiences early to prevent long-term psychological disturbance (Kazak et al. 2007; Mullins et al. 2014). A study of 6,542 childhood cancer survivors and 368 of their siblings found a fourfold greater risk of PTSD in the cancer survivors compared with the siblings (Stuber et al. 2010) (option D is correct; options A, B, and C are incorrect). **Chapter 32 (p. 1028)**

32.10   Which explanation is most accurate in terms of the link between asthma and panic symptoms?

A. Panic symptoms are not common in patients with asthma because the physiologic reactions to strong emotions do not trigger wheezing.
B. Panic can act like an "asphyxia alarm system" triggered by central chemoreceptors in response to changes in partial pressure of carbon dioxide.

C. Panic symptoms are uncommon because asthma medications such as steroids and beta-agonists are not associated with psychiatric side effects.
D. Periodic increases in partial pressure of carbon dioxide from asthma exacerbations are unrelated to panic attacks in patients with a genetic vulnerability to panic disorder.

The correct response is option B: Panic can act like an "asphyxia alarm system" triggered by central chemoreceptors in response to changes in partial pressure of carbon dioxide.

Panic symptoms are common, understandable given that physiological responses associated with strong emotions may trigger wheezing (option A is incorrect). One possible explanation for the association between panic and asthma is that panic acts as an asphyxia alarm system that is triggered by central chemoreceptors monitoring partial pressure of carbon dioxide in arterial blood ($PaCO_2$) (option B is correct). Children with a genetic vulnerability to panic disorder who also have periodic increases in $PaCO_2$ from asthma exacerbations may thus have panic attacks triggered by asthma attacks (option D is incorrect). Left undiagnosed and untreated, this anxiety can develop into panic disorder. Indeed, prospective epidemiological studies indicate that the primary risk factor for development of panic disorder in young adulthood is a history of childhood asthma (Goodwin et al. 2003). The heightened risk is likely also impacted by the interaction of both environmental and genetic factors. One study found that high levels of child and household stress and expressions of a susceptibility gene for PTSD and anxiety were associated with asthma morbidity (Brehm et al. 2015). Yet another reason for comorbidity is that most asthma medications (e.g., steroids, beta-agonists) are known to cause psychiatric symptoms (option C is incorrect). **Chapter 32 (p. 1030)**

References

Agorastos A, Pittman JO, Angkaw AC, et al; Marine Resiliency Study Team: The cumulative effect of different childhood trauma types on self-reported symptoms of adult male depression and PTSD, substance abuse and health-related quality of life in a large active-duty military cohort. J Psychiatr Res 58:46–54, 2014 25139009

Ahmed R, Aslani P: What is patient adherence? A terminology overview. Int J Clin Pharm 36(1):4–7, 2014 24104760

Brehm JM, Ramratnam SK, Tse SM, et al: Stress and bronchodilator response in children with asthma. Am J Respir Crit Care Med 192(1):47–56, 2015 25918834

Brosbe MS, Hoefling K, Faust J: Predicting posttraumatic stress following pediatric injury: a systematic review. J Pediatr Psychol 36(6):718–729, 2011 21262743

Bursch B, Forgey M: Psychopharmacology for medically ill adolescents. Curr Psychiatry Rep 15(10):395, 2013 23963629

Cousino MK, Hazen RA: Parenting stress among caregivers of children with chronic illness: a systematic review. J Pediatr Psychol 38(8):809–828, 2013 23843630

Davydow DS, Richardson LP, Zatzick DF, Katon WJ: Psychiatric morbidity in pediatric critical illness survivors: a comprehensive review of the literature. Arch Pediatr Adolesc Med 164(4):377–385, 2010 20368492

Duncan CL, Mentrikoski JM, Wu YP, Fredericks EM: Practice-based approach to assessing and treating non-adherence in pediatric regimens. Clin Pract Pediatr Psychol 2(3):322–336, 2014 25506046

Erickson SJ, Steiner H: Trauma spectrum adaptation: somatic symptoms in long-term pediatric cancer survivors. Psychosomatics 41(4):339–346, 2000 10906356

Gledhill J, Hodes M: The treatment of adolescents with depression. CML Psychiatry 22(3):1–7, 2011

Glenn CR, Nock MK: Improving the prediction of suicidal behavior in youth. Int J Behav Consult Ther 9(3):7–10, 2014 29924107

Goodwin RD, Pine DS, Hoven CW: Asthma and panic attacks among youth in the community. J Asthma 40(2):139–145, 2003 12765315

Hofmann SG, Asnaani A, Vonk IJ, et al: The efficacy of cognitive behavioral therapy: a review of meta-analyses. Cognit Ther Res 36(5):427–440, 2012 23459093

Horowitz LM, Bridge JA, Pao M, Boudreaux ED: Screening youth for suicide risk in medical settings: time to ask questions. Am J Prev Med 47(3)(suppl 2):S170–S175, 2014 25145735

Kazak AE, Rourke MT, Alderfer MA, et al: Evidence-based assessment, intervention and psychosocial care in pediatric oncology: a blueprint for comprehensive services across treatment. J Pediatr Psychol 32(9):1099–1110, 2007 17626069

McGrady ME, Hommel KA: Medication adherence and health care utilization in pediatric chronic illness: a systematic review. Pediatrics 132(4):730–740, 2013 23999953

Mullins LL, Gillaspy SR, Molzon ES, et al: Parent and family interventions in pediatric psychology: clinical applications. Clin Pract Pediatr Psychol 2(3):281–293, 2014

Oliva M, Singh TP, Gauvreau K, et al: Impact of medication non-adherence on survival after pediatric heart transplantation in the U.S.A. J Heart Lung Transplant 32(9):881–888, 2013 23755899

Phipps S, Steele RG, Hall K, Leigh L: Repressive adaptation in children with cancer: a replication and extension. Health Psychol 20(6):445–451, 2001 11714187

Schieveld JN, Janssen NJ: Delirium in the pediatric patient: on the growing awareness of its clinical interdisciplinary importance. JAMA Pediatr 168(7):595–596, 2014 24797545

Simon SL, Duncan CL, Horky SC, et al: Body satisfaction, nutritional adherence, and quality of life in youth with cystic fibrosis. Pediatr Pulmonol 46(11):1085–1092, 2011 21626713

Smith HA, Boyd J, Fuchs DC, et al: Diagnosing delirium in critically ill children: validity and reliability of the Pediatric Confusion Assessment Method for the Intensive Care Unit. Crit Care Med 39(1):150–157, 2011 20959783

Smith HA, Brink E, Fuchs DC, et al: Pediatric delirium: monitoring and management in the pediatric intensive care unit. Pediatr Clin North Am 60(3):741–760, 2013 23639666

Stuber ML, Meeske KA, Krull KR, et al: Prevalence and predictors of posttraumatic stress disorder in adult survivors of childhood cancer. Pediatrics 125(5):e1124–e1134, 2010 20435702

CHAPTER 33

Physical Medicine and Rehabilitation

33.1   What is expected in terms of cognitive recovery after a traumatic brain injury (TBI)?

A. TBI is associated with an acute decrement in cognitive function, which routinely improves within 2 years.
B. Individuals with severe brain injury can be expected to have made all of their cognitive gains by the first year after the injury.
C. The severity of the TBI correlates with the severity of the neurocognitive disorder (NCD).
D. In patients who have lost consciousness for 30 minutes or less, 80%–85% are expected to recover within 3–6 months without permanent deficits.

The correct response is option D: In patients who have lost consciousness for 30 minutes or less, 80%–85% are expected to recover within 3–6 months without permanent deficits.

DSM-5 specifically notes that the severity of NCD does not necessarily correspond to the severity of TBI injury, so mild TBI does not preclude more severe cognitive deficits (option C is incorrect). Although TBI is associated with an acute decrement in cognitive function that typically improves over time, recovery is very individualized, and no universally applicable description of the recovery process exists (option A is incorrect). Rao and Lyketsos (2000) offered the following general timeline: the first two periods of recovery will last from a few days to a month, the third period will last 6–12 months, and the fourth period will last beyond 12–24 months. Such guidelines are more characteristic of moderate to severe injuries. By definition, individuals with mild TBI will have loss of consciousness (LOC) of less than 30 minutes, with many having none at all (Kay et al. 1993). It is also estimated that 80%–85% of patients with uncomplicated mild TBI will recover to baseline status within 3–6 months and not enter the fourth phase of permanent deficits (Belanger and Vanderploeg 2005) (option D is correct). Among individuals with moderate to severe TBI, some recovery of cognitive function may occur 2 years or more after injury, although the gains are typically small (Millis et al. 2001) (option B is incorrect). **Chapter 33 (p. 1061)**

33.2 Which criterion for major depressive disorder does not overlap with the ICD-10 criteria for postconcussive syndrome?

    A. Insomnia.
    B. Decreased concentration.
    C. Depressed mood.
    D. Psychomotor changes.

The correct response is option D: Psychomotor changes.

Options A, B, and C are listed under diagnostic criteria for postconcussive syndrome (World Health Organization 1992). Psychomotor changes are not part of the diagnostic criteria (option D is correct). **Chapter 33 (Table 33–1, p. 1063)**

33.3 Which of the following does the research indicate as the *strongest* predictive factor for postconcussive symptoms at 6 months?

    A. Postinjury posttraumatic stress.
    B. Years of education.
    C. Anxiety.
    D. Successful outcome of litigation.

The correct response is option B: Years of education.

In the study by Cnossen et al. (2017), years of education, preinjury psychiatric disorders, and prior TBI were the strongest predictors of 6-month postconcussive symptoms (option B is correct). Postinjury disorders were not identified as predictive factors (option A is incorrect). Anxiety and litigation were identified as risk factors for persistent mild TBI symptoms in a systematic review by Carroll et al. (2004) along with depression, posttraumatic stress, negative injury perceptions, poor expectations for recovery, and emotional distress (option C is incorrect). Few individuals involved in litigation have improvement in postconcussive symptoms after settlement (King 2003) (option D is incorrect). **Chapter 33 (p. 1063)**

33.4 Which of the following defines a moderate traumatic brain injury?

    A. Loss of consciousness less than half an hour.
    B. Posttraumatic amnesia of 1–7 days.
    C. Glasgow Coma Scale of 13–15 at 30 minutes postinjury.
    D. Loss of consciousness greater than 24 hours.

The correct response is option B: Posttraumatic amnesia of 1–7 days.

DSM-5 provides thresholds for rating injury severity as *mild* (LOC less than 30 minutes and/or posttraumatic amnesia (PTA) duration of less than 24 hours, associated with Glasgow Coma Scale [GCS; Jennett and Bond 1975] scores of 13–15 at 30 minutes postinjury), *moderate* (LOC of 0.5–24 hours and/or PTA of 1–7 days, with GCS scores of 9–12 at 30 minutes postinjury), or *severe* (LOC greater than 24 hours and/or PTA greater than 7 days, with GCS scores of 3–8 at 30 minutes postinjury) (option B is correct; options A, C, and D are incorrect). **Chapter 33 (p. 1058)**

33.5   A 27-year-old man with a history of cannabis use disorder is admitted with a TBI after a motor vehicle accident. His family gets information from the internet that some people diagnosed with a TBI behave aggressively. They want to know if their loved one is likely to act aggressively once he returns home. How should this family be counseled?

   A. Approximately 95% of patients with moderate-severe TBI demonstrate aggression.
   B. Aggression in most patients with a TBI is not premeditated, does not achieve a particular goal for the individual, is triggered by an out of proportion reaction to a stimulus, does not have a prodromal buildup, and causes them distress.
   C. His preinjury history of substance abuse does not predispose him to aggression after a TBI.
   D. The most significant predictors of later aggression after TBI are worse depressive symptoms and older age.

The correct response is option B: Aggression in most patients with a TBI is not premeditated, does not achieve a particular goal for the individual, is triggered by an out of proportion reaction to a stimulus, does not have a prodromal buildup, and causes them distress.

Reported rates of aggression after moderate to severe TBI have ranged from 25% to 39% (Stéfan et al. 2016) (option A is incorrect). Although aggression may be a symptom of many disorders, aggression attributed to TBI often has certain characteristic features (Yudofsky et al. 1990). Such behavior is *nonreflective*, occurring without any premeditation or planning, and *nonpurposeful*, achieving no particular goals for the individual. It is also *reactive*, triggered by a stimulus, but often a stimulus that would not normally provoke a strong reaction (option B is correct). Aggression after TBI is *periodic*, occurring at intervals with relatively calm behavior in between, and *explosive*, occurring without a prodromal buildup. Finally, it is *ego-dystonic*, creating a great deal of distress for the patient. This classic presentation likely represents only a small proportion of aggression occurring after TBI. Risk of aggression is increased with a premorbid history of impulsive aggression, frontal lobe lesions, and preinjury history of substance abuse; evidence on cognitive function and socioeconomic status as risk factors is inconclusive (Kim et al. 2007) (option C is incorrect). Baguley et al. (2006) noted that approximately 25% of inpatient rehabilitation patients with TBI showed aggression at 6, 24, and 60 months postinjury. Greater depressive symptomatology and younger age at injury were the most significant predictors of later aggression (option D is incorrect). **Chapter 33 (pp. 1067–1068)**

33.6   When patients are depressed after spinal cord injury (SCI), which of these factors is *most* predictive of suicide?

A. Lower functional independence.
B. Poorer social integration.
C. Shame and apathy.
D. High use of paid personal care and higher medical expenses.

The correct response is option C: Shame and apathy.

Depression is a significant and disabling problem for persons with SCI. Depression is associated with longer lengths of hospital stay and fewer functional improvements (Malec and Neimeyer 1983) as well as less functional independence and mobility at discharge (Umlauf and Frank 1983) (option A is incorrect). Depression is associated with the occurrence of pressure sores and urinary tract infections (Herrick et al. 1994), poorer self-appraised health (Bombardier et al. 2004), less leisure activity (Elliott and Shewchuk 1995), poorer community mobility and social integration, and fewer meaningful social pursuits (Fuhrer et al. 1993; MacDonald et al. 1987) (option B is incorrect). Persons with SCI and significant depression spend more days in bed and fewer days outside the home, require greater use of paid personal care, and incur higher medical expenses (Tate et al. 1994) (option D is incorrect). Symptoms consistent with depression, such as documented expressions of despondency, hopelessness, shame, and apathy, are the variables most predictive of suicide 1–9 years after SCI (Charlifue and Gerhart 1991) (option C is correct). **Chapter 33 (p. 1074)**

33.7   After an SCI, a woman is told that she has suffered an incomplete lower motor neuron lesion affecting the sacral segments. How is this injury expected to impact her sexual functioning?

A. As in 25% of cases, she is expected to achieve psychogenic lubrication but will have no reflex lubrication.
B. She is likely to have vaginal lubrication from reflexive but not psychogenic mechanisms.
C. After SCI, she may, like 25% of women, achieve orgasm.
D. She will only retain psychogenic lubrication if she has intact light touch sensation in the T11–L2 thoracic and lumbar dermatomes.

The correct response is option A: As in 25% of cases, she is expected to achieve psychogenic lubrication but will have no reflex lubrication.

Vaginal lubrication and orgasm may be affected in women with SCI. Women with complete upper-motor lesions affecting the sacral segments, not lower motor neuron lesions, are likely to have vaginal lubrication from reflexive but not psychogenic mechanisms (Sipski et al. 1995) (option B is incorrect). Women with incomplete upper motor lesions affecting the sacral segments retain the capacity for reflex lubrication but will have psychogenic lubrication only if they have intact pinprick sensation in the T11–L2 thoracic and lumbar dermatomes, not light touch (option D is incorrect). Women with incomplete lower-motor lesions affecting the sacral segments are expected to achieve psychogenic lubrication in 25% of cases but will have no reflex lubrication (option A is correct). A laboratory study reported that about 50% of women with SCI were able to experience orgasm, and this ability was not significantly related to level or completeness of neurological injury (option C is incorrect). Longer stimulation, greater sexual knowledge, and higher sexual drive were associated with higher rates of orgasm (Sipski et al. 1995). **Chapter 33 (p. 1076)**

33.8   According to the Consortium for Spinal Cord Medicine (2010), what is the first-line treatment for erectile dysfunction in patients with SCI?

   A. Sildenafil.
   B. Pharmacological penile injections.
   C. Penile implants.
   D. Vacuum erection devices.

The correct response is option A: Sildenafil.

The first-line treatments for erectile dysfunction are sildenafil and other phosphodiesterase type 5 inhibitors (Lombardi et al. 2009) (option A is correct). Second-line treatments include vacuum erection devices, pharmacological penile injections, and penile implants (options B, C, and D are incorrect). **Chapter 33 (p. 1076)**

33.9   On the basis of multiple randomized controlled trials (RCTs), which of the following has been recommended by the international team of experts in cognitive rehabilitation (INCOG) to manage inattention after a traumatic brain injury?

   A. Methylphenidate.
   B. Metacognitive strategies and dual tasking.
   C. Self-cueing.
   D. Structured problem solving.

The correct response is option B: Metacognitive strategies and dual tasking.

On the basis of multiple RCTs, training in metacognitive strategies and dual tasking is recommended for attention impairments, and methylphenidate (0.3 mg/kg in divided doses) is recommended for slow speed of information processing (Ponsford et al. 2014) (option B is correct; option A is incorrect). On the basis of experimental data, the INCOG group recommended metacognitive strategies (typically, self-monitoring and incorporation of feedback into planning), structured problem-solving rubrics, and corrective feedback to manage executive dysfunction and poor awareness (Tate et al. 2014) (option D is incorrect). There is a substantial evidence base to recommend internal learning strategies (e.g., visualization, retrieval practice, self-cueing) and external compensatory techniques (e.g., memory book, electronic reminders) for memory impairment (Velikonja et al. 2014) (option C is incorrect). **Chapter 33 (p. 1088)**

33.10 A 35-year-old woman who suffered a complete SCI in a motor vehicle accident has been learning to move around with a wheelchair as well as performing self-catheterization. When discussing treatment goals with her medical team, she insists that she will be able to walk again. Psychiatry is consulted to assess the patient and to deal with her denial. On assessment, the patient does not display any signs of major depression, psychosis, or cognitive dysfunction. According to the dual-process model of grief, what would be the *most* appropriate response to this patient's insistence that she will walk again?

A. Continue to educate her on the nature of her injury.
B. Review the prognosis for recovery.
C. Discuss the limitations of current research seeking a cure for SCI.
D. Refrain from confronting her denial.

The correct response is option D: Refrain from confronting her denial.

A patient with a complete SCI who insists that he or she is going to walk again is in denial, which reflects the loss-avoidance phase of the dual-process model and his or her understandable hope or wish for neurological recovery. The consultant can express tolerance of verbal denial, especially when the patient is not engaging in behavioral denial (e.g., refusing to learn adaptive strategies such as wheelchair use or self-catheterization) (option D is correct). If verbal and behavioral denial co-occur and interfere with rehabilitation progress, more exposure-based interventions may be needed, such as education about the nature and extent of the injury (including radiographic evidence), the prognosis for recovery, and the limitations of current research seeking a cure for SCI (options A, B, and C are incorrect). **Chapter 33 (pp. 1089–1090)**

33.11 Which of the following psychological interventions is effective in improving pain and sleep in patients with a spinal cord injury?

A. Motivational interviewing plus self-management.
B. Telephone-delivered cognitive-behavioral counseling.
C. Peer-led brief action planning.
D. Telephone-delivered problem-solving therapy.

The correct response is option B: Telephone-delivered cognitive-behavioral counseling.

A meta-analysis of telephone-delivered supportive, cognitive-behavioral, and motivational counseling found evidence suggesting that these interventions can improve sleep and pain in SCI (Dorstyn et al. 2013) (option B is correct). Several RCTs have tested strategies for improving adherence to skin-care regimens. Trials of motivational interviewing alone and motivational interviewing plus self-management training in veterans with SCI failed to reduce pressure ulcer recurrence (Guihan et al. 2007, 2014) (option A is incorrect). A peer-led intervention that used brief action planning improved patient activation and resource utilization (Houlihan et al. 2017) (option C is incorrect). Telephone-based problem-solving therapy was successful in reducing emotional distress—including depression, anxiety, and PTSD symptoms—in recently deployed military service members with mild TBI (Bell et al. 2017) (option D is incorrect). **Chapter 33 (pp. 1087, 1089, 1090)**

References

Baguley IJ, Cooper J, Felmingham K: Aggressive behavior following traumatic brain injury: how common is common? J Head Trauma Rehabil 21(1):45–56, 2006 16456391

Belanger HG, Vanderploeg RD: The neuropsychological impact of sports-related concussion: a meta-analysis. J Int Neuropsychol Soc 11(4):345–357, 2005 16209414

Bell KR, Fann JR, Brockway JA, et al: Telephone problem solving for service members with mild traumatic brain injury: a randomized clinical trial. J Neurotrauma 34(2):313–321, 2017 27579992

Bombardier CH, Richards JS, Krause JS, et al: Symptoms of major depression in people with spinal cord injury: implications for screening. Arch Phys Med Rehabil 85(11):1749–1756, 2004 15520969

Carroll LJ, Cassidy JD, Peloso PM, et al; WHO Collaborating Centre Task Force on Mild Traumatic Brain Injury: Prognosis for mild traumatic brain injury: results of the WHO Collaborating Centre Task Force on Mild Traumatic Brain Injury. J Rehabil Med (43) (suppl):84–105, 2004 15083873

Charlifue SW, Gerhart KA: Behavioral and demographic predictors of suicide after traumatic spinal cord injury. Arch Phys Med Rehabil 72(7):488–492, 1991 2059121

Cnossen MC, Winkler EA, Yue JK, et al: Development of a prediction model for post-concussive symptoms following mild traumatic brain injury: a TRACK-TBI pilot study. J Neurotrauma (March):27; (Epub ahead of print), 2017 28343409

Consortium for Spinal Cord Medicine: Sexuality and reproductive health in adults with spinal cord injury: a clinical practice guideline for health-care professionals. J Spinal Cord Med 33(3):281–336, 2010 20737805

Dorstyn D, Mathias J, Denson L: Applications of telecounselling in spinal cord injury rehabilitation: a systematic review with effect sizes. Clin Rehabil 27(12):1072–1083, 2013 23823709

Elliott T, Shewchuk R: Social support and leisure activities following severe physical disability: testing the mediating effects of depression. Basic Appl Soc Psych 16(4):471–587, 1995

Fuhrer MJ, Rintala DH, Hart KA, et al: Depressive symptomatology in persons with spinal cord injury who reside in the community. Arch Phys Med Rehabil 74(3):255–260, 1993 8439251

Guihan M, Garber SL, Bombardier CH, et al: Lessons learned while conducting research on prevention of pressure ulcers in veterans with spinal cord injury. Arch Phys Med Rehabil 88(7):858–861, 2007 17601465

Guihan M, Bombardier CH, Ehde DM, et al: Comparing multicomponent interventions to improve skin care behaviors and prevent recurrence in veterans hospitalized for severe pressure ulcers. Arch Phys Med Rehabil 95(7):1246–1253.e3, 2014 24486242

Herrick S, Elliott T, Crow F: Social support and the prediction of health complications among persons with SCI. Rehabil Psychol 39:231–250, 1994

Houlihan BV, Brody M, Everhart-Skeels S, et al: Randomized trial of a peer-led, telephone-based empowerment intervention for persons with chronic spinal cord injury improves health self-management. Arch Phys Med Rehabil 98(6):1067–1076.e1, 2017 28284835

Jennett B, Bond M: Assessment of outcome after severe brain damage. Lancet 1(7905):480–484, 1975 46957

Kay T, Harrington DE, Adams R, et al: Mild Traumatic Brain Injury Committee of the Head Injury Interdisciplinary Special Interest Group of the American Congress of Rehabilitation Medicine: Definition of mild traumatic brain injury. J Head Trauma Rehabil 8(3):86–87, 1993

Kim E, Lauterbach EC, Reeve A, et al; ANPA Committee on Research: Neuropsychiatric complications of traumatic brain injury: a critical review of the literature (a report by the ANPA Committee on Research). J Neuropsychiatry Clin Neurosci 19(2):106–127, 2007 17431056

King NS: Post-concussion syndrome: clarity amid the controversy? Br J Psychiatry 183:276–278, 2003 14519601

Lombardi G, Macchiarella A, Cecconi F, Del Popolo G: Ten years of phosphodiesterase type 5 inhibitors in spinal cord injured patients. J Sex Med 6(5):1248–1258, 2009 19210710

MacDonald MR, Nielson WR, Cameron MG: Depression and activity patterns of spinal cord injured persons living in the community. Arch Phys Med Rehabil 68(6):339–343, 1987 3592945

Malec J, Neimeyer R: Psychologic prediction of duration of inpatient spinal cord injury rehabilitation and performance of self-care. Arch Phys Med Rehabil 64(8):359–363, 1983 6882174

Millis SR, Rosenthal M, Novack TA, et al: Long-term neuropsychological outcome after traumatic brain injury. J Head Trauma Rehabil 16(4):343–355, 2001 11461657

Ponsford J, Bayley M, Wiseman-Hakes C, et al; INCOG Expert Panel: INCOG recommendations for management of cognition following traumatic brain injury, part II: attention and information processing speed. J Head Trauma Rehabil 29(4):321–337, 2014 24984095

Rao V, Lyketsos C: Neuropsychiatric sequelae of traumatic brain injury. Psychosomatics 41(2):95–103, 2000 10749946

Sipski ML, Alexander CJ, Rosen RC: Orgasm in women with spinal cord injuries: a laboratory-based assessment. Arch Phys Med Rehabil 76(12):1097–1102, 1995 8540784

Stéfan A, Mathé J-F; SOFMER group: What are the disruptive symptoms of behavioral disorders after traumatic brain injury? A systematic review leading to recommendations for good practices. Ann Phys Rehabil Med 59(1):5–17, 2016 26768944

Tate DG, Stiers W, Daugherty J, et al: The effects of insurance benefits coverage on functional and psychosocial outcomes after spinal cord injury. Arch Phys Med Rehabil 75(4):407–414, 1994 8172500

Tate R, Kennedy M, Ponsford J, et al: INCOG recommendations for management of cognition following traumatic brain injury, part III: executive function and self-awareness. J Head Trauma Rehabil 29(4):338–352, 2014 24984096

Umlauf R, Frank RG: A cluster-analytic description of patient subgroups in the rehabilitation setting. Rehabil Psychol 28(3):157–167, 1983

Velikonja D, Tate R, Ponsford J, et al; INCOG Expert Panel: INCOG recommendations for management of cognition following traumatic brain injury, part V: memory. J Head Trauma Rehabil 29(4):369–386, 2014 24984098

World Health Organization: International Statistical Classification of Diseases and Related Health Problems, 10th Revision. Geneva, World Health Organization, 1992

Yudofsky SC, Silver JM, Hales RE: Pharmacologic management of aggression in the elderly. J Clin Psychiatry 51 (suppl):22–28, discussion 29–32, 1990

CHAPTER 34

Pain

34.1   What is the term for pain that results from a stimulus that does not normally pro-
        voke pain?

A. Hyperalgesia.
B. Nociception.
C. Allodynia.
D. Sensitization.

The correct response is option C: Allodynia.

Hyperalgesia is an increased response to a stimulus that is normally painful (option A is incorrect). *Nociception* is the detection of tissue damage by transducers in
skin and deeper structures and central propagation of this information via A delta
and C fibers in the peripheral nerves (option B is incorrect). *Allodynia* is pain from
a stimulus that does not normally provoke pain (option C is correct). *Sensitization*
is a lowered threshold for pain and prolonged/enhanced response to stimulation
(option D is incorrect). **Chapter 34 (Table 34–1, p. 1106)**

34.2   Which of the following statements describes the relationship between depression
        and pain?

A. Baseline depressive symptoms more accurately predict future pain and dis-
   ability than do initial ratings of the actual pain.
B. Chronic pain conditions have not been found to increase suicide risk.
C. Patients with depression have twice the prevalence of pain conditions.
D. Pain intensity is a better prediction of disability than depression.

**The correct response is option A: Baseline depressive symptoms more accurately
predict future pain and disability than do initial ratings of the actual pain.**

The relation between pain and depression is intimate and bidirectional. Baseline
depressive symptoms more accurately predict future pain and disability than do
initial ratings of the actual pain (Schieir et al. 2009) (option A is correct). Most
chronic pain conditions have been associated with an increased risk of suicide,

and patients with chronic pain complete suicide at two to three times the rate of people in the general population (option B is incorrect). It has been estimated that patients with depression have about a fourfold increase in the prevalence of pain conditions (Ohayon and Schatzberg 2003) (option C is incorrect). High levels of depression may worsen pain and pain-related disability (Lerman et al. 2015). Depression is a better predictor of disability than are pain intensity and duration (option D is incorrect). **(Chapter 34, p. 1110)**

34.3   In which of the following neuropathic conditions has lamotrigine demonstrated efficacy in treatment?

A. Fibromyalgia.
B. Postamputation phantom limb pain.
C. Central neuropathic pain.
D. HIV-related neuropathy.

The correct response is option D: HIV-related neuropathy.

Pregabalin and gabapentin are effective for the treatment of painful diabetic neuropathy, postherpetic neuralgia, fibromyalgia, postamputation phantom limb pain, and central neuropathic pain associated with spinal cord injury (Moore et al. 2014; Ogawa et al. 2016) (options A, B, and C are incorrect). Lamotrigine is effective in treating HIV-related neuropathy and central poststroke pain but has not shown efficacy in other neuropathic conditions (Wiffen and Rees 2007) (option D is correct). **(Chapter 34, p. 1121)**

34.4   A positive placebo response to a treatment would indicate which of the following?

A. The patient has not had a biological response to the treatment.
B. The patient would not benefit from active treatment.
C. Expectation has played a role in the patient's response.
D. The patient's pain is psychogenic.

The correct response is option C: Expectation has played a role in the patient's response.

Placebo analgesia is a biologically measurable phenomenon (Greene et al. 2009) (option A is incorrect). In a clinical setting, it is difficult to separate "true" improvements from placebo responses. A positive placebo response neither proves that the patient's pain is psychogenic nor shows that the patient would not benefit from an active treatment (options B and D are incorrect). The expectations and previous experiences of both patients and physicians are well-established key mediators of placebo effects (Reicherts et al. 2016) (option C is correct). **(Chapter 34, p. 1124)**

34.5   Which opioid, because of its delayed central nervous system absorption and on-set of action, has a prolonged analgesic effect relative to its plasma half-life and therefore reduced potential for accumulation and toxicity with repeated dosing?

A. Morphine.
B. Oxycodone.
C. Fentanyl.
D. Hydrocodone.

The correct response is option A: Morphine.

Morphine, because of its hydrophilicity, has poor oral bioavailability (22%–48%) as well as delayed central nervous system absorption and onset of action. This de-lay prolongs the analgesic effect of morphine relative to its plasma half-life, which reduces the potential for accumulation and toxicity with repeated dosing (option A is correct). Oxycodone has higher oral bioavailability (>60%), a faster onset of ac-tion, and more predictable plasma levels compared with morphine (option B is in-correct). Although its analgesic efficacy is similar to that of morphine, oxycodone releases less histamine and is less likely to cause hallucinations (Riley et al. 2008). Fentanyl is highly lipophilic, which allows for transdermal or transmucosal de-livery; however, it is the most potent opioid and therefore is associated with greater risk of fatal overdose (option C is incorrect). Hydrocodone is similar to oxycodone, with rapid oral absorption and onset of analgesia. Hydrocodone is metabolized by *N*-demethylation to hydromorphone, which has properties simi-lar to those of morphine but fewer side effects. **(Chapter 34, p. 1118)**

34.6   Which medication is the most effective choice for neuropathic pain?

A. Nortriptyline.
B. Fluoxetine.
C. Vortioxetine.
D. Venlafaxine.

The correct response is option A: Nortriptyline.

Meta-analyses of randomized controlled trials have concluded that tricyclic anti-depressants are the most effective agents for neuropathic pain and that they are also effective for headache syndromes (Finnerup et al. 2015) (option A is correct). Paroxetine and citalopram, but not fluoxetine, decreased the pain of diabetic pe-ripheral neuropathy in some controlled studies (Goodnick 2001) (option B is incor-rect). Duloxetine has demonstrated analgesic efficacy both in preclinical models and in clinical populations including patients with fibromyalgia (Arnold et al. 2005), painful diabetic neuropathy (Wernicke et al. 2006), or osteoarthritis (Micca et al. 2013). A Cochrane review recommends duloxetine as an effective treatment for neuropathic pain (Lunn et al. 2014). Venlafaxine is effective in migraine pro-phylaxis (Dharmshaktu et al. 2012; Ozyalcin et al. 2005) and reduces allodynia and hyperalgesia in neuropathic pain (Yucel et al. 2005) (option D is incorrect). Vortioxetine is too new to have accumulated evidence of efficacy in treating pain (option C is incorrect). **(Chapter 34, page 1119–1120)**

34.7 Which of the following is *not* an element of the fear-avoidance model of musculo-skeletal pain?

A. Pain severity.
B. Pain catastrophizing.
C. Avoidance behavior.
D. Internal locus of control.

The correct response is option D: Internal locus of control.

The fear-avoidance model of musculoskeletal pain (Leeuw et al. 2007) incorporated elements such as pain severity, pain catastrophizing, hypervigilance to pain, pain-related fear, escape or avoidance behavior, disability, disuse, and individual vulnerabilities to explain the transition from acute to chronic low back pain (options A, B, and C are incorrect). Pain-related fear and avoidance represent one of the most significant predictors of failure to return to work in patients with chronic low back pain and are also predictive of poor adjustment to chronic pain (Hasenbring et al. 2001). Patients with a variety of chronic pain syndromes who score higher on measures of self-efficacy or who have an internal locus of control report lower levels of pain, higher pain thresholds, increased exercise performance, and more positive coping efforts (option D is correct). **(Chapter 34, pp. 1111, 1123)**

References

Arnold LM, Rosen A, Pritchett YL, et al: A randomized, double-blind, placebo-controlled trial of duloxetine in the treatment of women with fibromyalgia with or without major depressive disorder. Pain 119(1-3):5–15, 2005 16298061

Dharmshaktu P, Tayal V, Kalra BS: Efficacy of antidepressants as analgesics: a review. J Clin Pharmacol 52(1):6–17, 2012 21415285

Finnerup NB, Attal N, Haroutounian S, et al: Pharmacotherapy for neuropathic pain in adults: a systematic review and meta-analysis. Lancet Neurol 14(2):162–173, 2015 25575710

Goodnick PJ: Use of antidepressants in treatment of comorbid diabetes mellitus and depression as well as in diabetic neuropathy. Ann Clin Psychiatry 13(1):31–41, 2001 11465683

Greene CS, Goddard G, Macaluso GM, Mauro G: Topical review: placebo responses and therapeutic responses. How are they related? J Orofac Pain 23(2):93–107, 2009 19492534

Hasenbring M, Hallner D, Klasen B: Psychological mechanisms in the transition from acute to chronic pain: over- or underrated? [in German]. Schmerz 15(6):442–447, 2001 11793149

Leeuw M, Goossens ME, Linton SJ, et al: The fear-avoidance model of musculoskeletal pain: current state of scientific evidence. J Behav Med 30(1):77–94, 2007 17180640

Lerman SF, Rudich Z, Brill S, et al: Longitudinal associations between depression, anxiety, pain, and pain-related disability in chronic pain patients. Psychosom Med 77(3):333–341, 2015 25849129

Lunn MP, Hughes RA, Wiffen PJ: Duloxetine for treating painful neuropathy, chronic pain or fibromyalgia. Cochrane Database Syst Rev (1):CD007115, 2014 24385423

Micca JL, Ruff D, Ahl J, Wohlreich MM: Safety and efficacy of duloxetine treatment in older and younger patients with osteoarthritis knee pain: a post hoc, subgroup analysis of two randomized, placebo-controlled trials. BMC Musculoskelet Disord 14:137, 2013 23590727

Moore RA, Wiffen PJ, Derry S, et al: Gabapentin for chronic neuropathic pain and fibromyalgia in adults. Cochrane Database Syst Rev (4):CD007938, 2014 24771480

Ogawa S, Arakawa A, Hayakawa K, Yoshiyama T: Pregabalin for neuropathic pain: why benefits could be expected for multiple conditions. Clin Drug Investig 36(11):877–888, 2016 27448285

Ohayon MM, Schatzberg AF: Using chronic pain to predict depressive morbidity in the general population. Arch Gen Psychiatry 60(1):39–47, 2003 12511171

Ozyalcin SN, Talu GK, Kiziltan E, et al: The efficacy and safety of venlafaxine in the prophylaxis of migraine. Headache 45(2):144–152, 2005 15705120

Reicherts P, Gerdes AB, Pauli P, Wieser MJ: Psychological placebo and nocebo effects on pain rely on expectation and previous experience. J Pain 17(2):203–214, 2016 26523863

Riley J, Eisenberg E, Müller-Schwefe G, et al: Oxycodone: a review of its use in the management of pain. Curr Med Res Opin 24(1):175–192, 2008 18039433

Schieir O, Thombs BD, Hudson M, et al: Symptoms of depression predict the trajectory of pain among patients with early inflammatory arthritis: a path analysis approach to assessing change. J Rheumatol 36(2):231–239, 2009 19132790

Wernicke JF, Pritchett YL, D'Souza DN, et al: A randomized controlled trial of duloxetine in diabetic peripheral neuropathic pain. Neurology 67(8):1411–1420, 2006 17060567

Wiffen PJ, Rees J: Lamotrigine for acute and chronic pain. Cochrane Database Syst Rev (2):CD006044, 2007 17443611

Yucel A, Ozyalcin S, Koknel Talu G, et al: The effect of venlafaxine on ongoing and experimentally induced pain in neuropathic pain patients: a double blind, placebo controlled study. Eur J Pain 9(4):407–416, 2005 15979021

CHAPTER 35

Medical Toxicology

35.1   What pharmacokinetic property of a drug increases the risks of toxicity?

A. Acute exposure.
B. Narrow therapeutic window.
C. Short half-life.
D. Abrupt absorption.

The correct response is option B: Narrow therapeutic window.

Effective half-life (t$_{1/2}$) defines roughly how long acute consequences will persist if a threshold of clinical effect is crossed—a longer half-life increases the duration of toxicity (option C is incorrect). In most situations involving toxicity, it will take at least two, and often three, effective half-lives for symptoms to decrease in intensity below the toxic threshold. This guiding principle of toxicokinetics outlines the necessary period of observation and expected duration of treatment, assuming no ongoing exposure and no end-organ damage has been sustained. The therapeutic window is bounded by the minimum dose necessary to produce an observable clinical effect and the maximum dose that can be tolerated without harm; a narrow window increases the probability of accidentally reaching toxicity (option B is correct). Substances that *delay* their own absorption, readily overwhelm clearance mechanisms, and/or have large volumes of distribution display abnormal toxicokinetics and make assessment more complex (option D is incorrect). Under circumstances of chronic exposure (purposeful, accidental, or iatrogenic), toxicity may persist due to high tissue burden and protracted elimination kinetics (option A is incorrect). **Chapter 35 (Figure 35–1, p. 1139)**

35.2   What is an advantage of using standard urine drug screening over other toxin assays?

A. It allows for a comprehensive detection of potentially dangerous substances.
B. It has a low rate of false negatives.
C. It is frequently updated to include novel substances of abuse.
D. It provides rapid results, which expedites intervention.

The correct response is option D: It provides rapid results, which expedites intervention.

Identifying all available toxins with a high degree of specificity and sensitivity is impossible because of limitations of time and expense. Instead, drug screening is sometimes performed. Standard urine drug screening is conducted using immunoassay techniques, offering the advantage of rapid turnaround time with detection of some commonly used and abused compounds (option D is correct). Urine screening utility is limited by relatively high false-negative and false-positive rates (option B is incorrect). Assay development for novel synthetics always lags behind use and abuse trends. Novel substances of abuse (e.g., synthetic cannabinoids, cathinones, synthetic opioids) are not detected by standard screening panels (option C is incorrect). Comprehensive toxicology screening may detect a wider range of analgesics, narcotics, psychotropics, and various other drugs but takes time to complete (option A is incorrect). Toxicology screening and/or quantitation may be more useful in the outpatient setting when chronic exposure is suspected and symptoms are less severe, rather than in the acute hospital setting, where the demand for rapid intervention does not allow time for assays (Hiemke et al. 2011; Rainey 2015; Schütze and Schwarz 2016). **Chapter 35 (pp. 1141–1142)**

35.3   What is a *main* goal in the acute phase of toxicological treatment?

A. Hastening the elimination of an absorbed toxin.
B. Rapid tranquilization with benzodiazepines or antipsychotics.
C. Preventing seizures, which can cause additional injury.
D. Use of physical restraint to prevent physical injury.

The correct response is option A: Hastening the elimination of an absorbed toxin.

The three main goals in the acute phase of toxicological treatment are preventing further drug absorption, providing antidotal therapy, and hastening the elimination of an absorbed toxin (option A is correct). Sometimes toxic effects on patients' behavior can interfere with these goals. Rapid tranquilization with benzodiazepines can protect against injury, prevent seizures, and allow vital medical interventions to proceed (option C is incorrect). Antipsychotics are effective as well (Battaglia 2005) and may be less likely to exacerbate delirium, but their greater potential for adverse effects or interactions with unknown ingestants (e.g., precipitation of seizures, induction of arrhythmias) warrants caution in their use (Martel et al. 2005; Olson 2007) (option B is incorrect). Physical restraints should be avoided but may occasionally be necessary to prevent patients from interfering with life-saving care (Rasimas and Carter 2016) (option D is incorrect). **Chapter 35 (p. 1142)**

35.4   What is the antidote to overdose with propranolol?

A. Flumazenil.
B. Glucagon.

C. *N*-acetylcysteine.

D. Physostigmine.

The correct response is option B: Glucagon.

Table 35–2 contains emergency antidotes for common toxic ingestions. The first several items are particularly common medications. Acetaminophen overdoses are treated with *N*-acetylcysteine (option C is incorrect). Anticholinergic overdose is treated with physostigmine (option D is incorrect). Benzodiazepines and some other hypnotics are reversed with flumazenil (option A is incorrect). Propranolol, a beta adrenergic, overdose is treated with glucagon (option B is correct). **Chapter 35 (Table 35–2, p. 1143)**

35.5   A patient makes a suicide attempt by overdose of lithium and presents with a high lithium level. What is the most appropriate treatment?

A. Activated charcoal.

B. Gastric lavage.

C. Chelation therapy.

D. Hemodialysis.

The correct response is option D: Hemodialysis.

Activated charcoal minimizes gastrointestinal absorption of many toxins by adsorptive binding, producing better toxin recovery and fewer complications than emesis or gastric lavage. Therefore, it should be considered as the primary means of decontamination in most overdoses (Albertson et al. 1989). Use of activated charcoal is not recommended for ingestions of agents that do not adsorb to charcoal, such as ions, solvents, alcohols, and most metals (Table 35–3) (option A is incorrect). Lithium ions and small molecules such as methanol, ethylene glycol, salicylates, and phenobarbital rapidly diffuse across synthetic membranes and are therefore removed effectively by hemodialysis (option D is correct). Activated charcoal may be beneficial when given early after an ingestion (most effective within 1 hour) and when used for an ingested drug that has delayed absorption, such as aspirin, anticholinergics, opioids, sustained-release medications, or drug packets in "body stuffers." For patients who present hours after a toxic ingestion, charcoal is usually ineffective. Furthermore, charcoal aspiration can occur, causing bronchospasm and pneumonitis (Givens et al. 1992). Gastric decontamination does not generally improve outcomes in most overdose patients (Bond 2002). Gastric lavage is rarely indicated and should be considered only when a patient is seen less than an hour after ingesting a highly toxic substance (e.g., calcium channel blocker, TCA, colchicine) or one that delays gastric emptying (e.g., opioid, anticholinergic) or forms concretions (Vale et al. 2004) (option B is incorrect). Whole-bowel irrigation (the other from of gastric decontamination) may be useful in certain cases of massive, recent ingestion of medications with sustained release and delayed absorption, including extended-release lithium. Chelation therapy (e.g., with EDTA, succimer, or DMSA) can also enhance elimination in the acute setting; it can quickly remove large amounts of lead (Goyer et al. 1995) or arsenic (Mückter et al. 1997) from the body (option C is incorrect). **Chapter 35 (pp. 1143–1145; Table 35–3, p. 1144)**

35.6   In acetaminophen overdose, what is the *most* important predictor of poor prognosis?

   A. Alcohol co-ingestion at the time of overdose.
   B. Presenting for medical care later than 24 hours after overdose.
   C. Eating disorder.
   D. Adolescent age.

The correct response is option B: Presenting for medical care later than 24 hours after overdose.

Chronic alcohol use induces cytochrome P450 (CYP) 2E1 and depletes glutathione stores, increasing the risk of a poorer outcome. Alcohol co-ingestion at the time of overdose, however, can be slightly *protective* because ethanol competes with the acetaminophen for CYP2E1, thus *decreasing* the production of the toxic *N*-acetyl-*p*-benzoquinone imine (option A is incorrect). Delay before presenting for antidotal therapy is *the most important predictor* of poor prognosis (option B is correct). Clinically, patients present with nausea, vomiting, and malaise within 24 hours of acute ingestion. Despite evolving liver injury (as reflected by elevations in hepatocellular enzymes and prolongation of prothrombin time), there can be a window of time when patients look and feel better. If they present for care at this stage and clinicians fail to consider acetaminophen overdose because of the patient's benign appearance, the consequences can be fatal. Accidental poisoning is more common in young children and in the elderly, whereas almost all adolescents and adults with acetaminophen toxicity have intentionally harmed themselves. Advanced age predisposes patients to greater toxicity (option D is incorrect), as do states of malnutrition (e.g., anorexia nervosa, option C is incorrect). **Chapter 35 (pp. 1146–1147)**

35.7   A patient was recently discharged from your hospital's addiction unit. His wife brings him into your outpatient practice visibly altered, which she cannot understand because she disposed of all of the alcohol in their house. She did notice that he had windshield wiper fluid in the bathroom. While your colleague calls 911, you quickly administer what substance to protect him from permanent damage?

   A. Ethanol.
   B. Water.
   C. 100% oxygen.
   D. Diazepam.

The correct response is option A: Ethanol.

Windshield washer fluid and fuel additives contain methanol. Methanol, ethylene glycol (in antifreeze), and isopropanol (rubbing alcohol) are rapidly absorbed after oral ingestion, and their metabolism depends on alcohol dehydrogenase. Because rapid breakdown by alcohol dehydrogenase produces organic acids from both methanol (formic acid) and ethylene glycol (glycolic and oxalic acids), metabolic acidosis with an elevated anion gap is a key finding. Isopropanol is metabolized to acetone, so the result of this ingestion is central nervous system (CNS) depression and ketosis without significant acidosis. Acidosis and the direct effects of the alcohols and their metabolites lead to end-organ damage, including nephrotoxicity with ethylene glycol and blindness with methanol. Methanol also can cause necrosis in the putamen, the result being an irreversible movement disorder resembling parkinsonism (Sefidbakht et al. 2007). The mainstay of toxic alcohol treatment is inhibition of metabolism while hastening elimination. Inhibiting alcohol dehydrogenase is a critical intervention for patients with methanol or ethylene glycol poisoning (Barceloux et al. 1999, 2002). Fomepizole is the preferred antidote (Barceloux et al. 1999, 2002), but if any delay before provision of advanced hospital treatment is anticipated, oral doses of ethanol can be temporizing and potentially lifesaving (Jacobsen and McMartin 1997) (option A is correct). Aggressive fluid hydration is part of the treatment of salicylate and nonsteroidal anti-inflammatory drug overdose (option B is incorrect). Treatment with 100% oxygen is critically important for carbon monoxide poisoning (option C is incorrect). Diazepam would be an appropriate intervention if the patient were believed to be in withdrawal instead of intoxicated with methanol (option D is incorrect). **Chapter 16 (p. 441), Chapter 35 (pp. 1147–1149)**

35.8   A patient is concerned about neurotoxicity from radiation coming from her microwave. What do you tell her?

A. Microwaves produce non-ionizing radiation, so people should not stand in front of the microwave when it's on.
B. Microwaves produce ionizing radiation, so people should not stand in front of the microwave when it's on.
C. Microwaves produce non-ionizing radiation, which does not have toxic potential.
D. Microwaves produce ionizing radiation, which does not have toxic potential.

The correct response is option C: Microwaves produce non-ionizing radiation, which does not have toxic potential.

Ionizing radiation sources include nuclear weapons and reactors, natural elements, consumer products, and diagnostic and therapeutic isotopes. Ionizing radiation preferentially harms cells with high turnover rates, including those of the skin, immune system, pulmonary epithelium, and gastrointestinal tract (options B and D are incorrect). In the CNS, radiation damage and necrosis can produce neurological dysfunction and mental status changes, including depression, sleep disturbance, fatigue, memory problems, and poor concentration. Non-ionizing radiation does not have the toxic potential outlined above, because of the low energy of electromagnetic frequencies (from radar, microwaves, television signals, mobile telephone transmission) (option C is correct; option A is incorrect). **Chapter 35 (pp. 1152–1153)**

35.9   A patient tests positive for lead level of 20 μg/dL. Which symptom would make you suspect the exposure was *chronic*?

A. Peripheral motor neuropathy.
B. Coma.
C. Convulsions.
D. Clumsiness.

The correct response is option A: Peripheral motor neuropathy.

In the United States, more than 2% of children younger than 6 years have blood lead levels greater than 10 μg/dL (Woolf et al. 2007). The major source of lead for children is old paint causing high metal content dust in their homes (Chiodo et al. 2004; Reyes et al. 2006). Lead interferes with normal development and function of the CNS. Elevated serum levels are associated with lower IQ; poor concentration; sleep problems; mood dysregulation (Bellinger et al. 1987); abnormalities in speech, language, attention, and classroom behavior; behavioral dyscontrol; antisocial personality features; reading disabilities; and decreased rates of completing high school (Needleman et al. 1990). *Acute* poisoning causes headache, emesis, clumsiness (option D is incorrect), staggering, and drowsiness and can progress to convulsions (option C is incorrect) and coma (Wiley et al. 1995) (option B is incorrect). Chronic exposure causes crampy abdominal pain, anorexia, weight loss, nausea, constipation, anemia, peripheral motor neuropathy (option A is correct), nephropathy, and adverse reproductive outcomes. **Chapter 35 (p. 1154)**

35.10 Which of the following is helpful in treating patients with "medication sensitivity"?

A. Extensive diagnostic and toxicological testing.
B. Treatment assuming the primary issue is psychiatric.
C. Using a disease model that anticipates identification of specific etiological agents.
D. Encouraging patients to seek relief from nonpharmacological therapies.

The correct response is option D: Encouraging patients to seek relief from non-pharmacological therapies.

Functional somatic presentations with external attributions when the history, examination, and laboratory testing fail to reveal a specific toxic exposure and do not suggest that an exogenous substance is responsible for the patient's suffering, such as medication sensitivity, Gulf War syndrome, idiopathic environmental sensitivity, and sick building syndrome, are collectively referred to as the "Blame-X syndromes"

(Feinstein 2001). While various toxic explanations are hypothesized, no causal role for any of the blamed compounds has been substantiated. Treatment is therefore not best accomplished using a disease model that anticipates identification of specific etiological agents (option C is incorrect). Availability of almost limitless diagnostic (including toxicological) testing contributes to medicalization of distress (option A is incorrect). Medication sensitivity syndrome, in which patients believe themselves to have multiple allergies, sensitivities, or toxicities to medications, has a high rate of psychiatric comorbidity. Assisting patients to seek relief from nonpharmacological therapies may represent the most important intervention in such cases (option D is correct). Although it is clear that psychiatric factors play a major role for many such patients, it is important to remember that the history of medicine is filled with instances of illnesses viewed as psychogenic until physiological causes were elucidated (option B is incorrect). In addition, these patients already have anticipatory anxiety and pessimistic expectations that drugs will produce unpleasant or harmful side effects (Amanzio et al. 2009), making a nonpharmacological intervention more acceptable to them. **Chapter 35 (pp. 1164–1167)**

References

Albertson TE, Derlet RW, Foulke GE, et al: Superiority of activated charcoal alone compared with ipecac and activated charcoal in the treatment of acute toxic ingestions. Ann Emerg Med 18(1):56–59, 1989 2562913

Amanzio M, Corazzini LL, Vase L, Benedetti F: A systematic review of adverse events in placebo groups of anti-migraine clinical trials. Pain 146(3):261–269, 2009 19781854

Barceloux DG, Krenzelok EP, Olson K, Watson W; Ad Hoc Committee: American Academy of Clinical Toxicology practice guidelines on the treatment of ethylene glycol poisoning. J Toxicol Clin Toxicol 37(5):537–560, 1999 10497633

Barceloux DG, Bond GR, Krenzelok EP, et al; American Academy of Clinical Toxicology Ad Hoc Committee on the Treatment Guidelines for Methanol Poisoning: American Academy of Clinical Toxicology practice guidelines on the treatment of methanol poisoning. J Toxicol Clin Toxicol 40(4):415–446, 2002 12216995

Battaglia J: Pharmacological management of acute agitation. Drugs 65(9):1207–1222, 2005 15916448

Bellinger D, Leviton A, Waternaux C, et al: Longitudinal analyses of prenatal and postnatal lead exposure and early cognitive development. N Engl J Med 316(17):1037–1043, 1987 3561456

Bond GR: The role of activated charcoal and gastric emptying in gastrointestinal decontamination: a state-of-the-art review. Ann Emerg Med 39(3):273–286, 2002 11867980

Chiodo LM, Jacobson SW, Jacobson JL: Neurodevelopmental effects of postnatal lead exposure at very low levels. Neurotoxicol Teratol 26(3):359–371, 2004 15113598

Feinstein AR: The Blame-X syndrome: problems and lessons in nosology, spectrum, and etiology. J Clin Epidemiol 54(5):433–439, 2001 11337205

Givens T, Holloway M, Wason S: Pulmonary aspiration of activated charcoal: a complication of its misuse in overdose management. Pediatr Emerg Care 8(3):137–140, 1992 1614903

Goyer RA, Cherian MG, Jones MM, Reigart JR: Role of chelating agents for prevention, intervention, and treatment of exposures to toxic metals. Environ Health Perspect 103(11):1048–1052, 1995 8605855

Hiemke C, Baumann P, Bergemann N, et al: AGNP consensus guidelines for therapeutic drug monitoring in psychiatry: update 2011. Pharmacopsychiatry 44(6):195–235, 2011

Jacobsen D, McMartin KE: Antidotes for methanol and ethylene glycol poisoning. J Toxicol Clin Toxicol 35(2):127–143, 1997 9120880

Martel M, Sterzinger A, Miner J, et al: Management of acute undifferentiated agitation in the emergency department: a randomized double-blind trial of droperidol, ziprasidone, and midazolam. Acad Emerg Med 12(12):1167–1172, 2005 16282517

Mückter H, Liebl B, Reichl FX, et al: Are we ready to replace dimercaprol (BAL) as an arsenic antidote? Hum Exp Toxicol 16(8):460–465, 1997 9292286

Needleman HL, Schell A, Bellinger D, et al: The long-term effects of exposure to low doses of lead in childhood. An 11-year follow-up report. N Engl J Med 322(2):83–88, 1990 2294437

Olson KR: Emergency evaluation and treatment, in Poisoning and Drug Overdose, 5th Edition. Edited by Olson KR, Anderson IB, Benowitz NL, et al. New York, McGraw-Hill, 2007, pp 1–57

Rainey PM: Laboratory principles, in Goldfrank's Toxicologic Emergencies, 10th Edition. Edited by Hoffman RS, Howland MA, Lewin NA, et al. New York, McGraw-Hill, 2015, pp 62–75

Rasimas JJ, Carter GL: Psychiatric issues in the critically poisoned patient, in Critical Care Toxicology: Diagnosis and Management of the Critically Poisoned Patient. Edited by Brent J, Burkhart KK, Dargan P et al. Basel, Switzerland, Springer International Publishing, 2016, pp 117–157

Reyes NL, Wong LY, MacRoy PM, et al: Identifying housing that poisons: a critical step in eliminating childhood lead poisoning. J Public Health Manag Pract 12(6):563–569, 2006 17041305

Schütze G, Schwarz MJ: Therapeutic drug monitoring for individualised risk reduction in psychopharmacotherapy. TTrAC Trends in Analytic Chemistry 84(Pt B):14–22, 2016

Sefidbakht S, Rasekhi AR, Kamali K, et al: Methanol poisoning: acute MR and CT findings in nine patients. Neuroradiology 49(5):427–435, 2007 17294234

Vale JA, Kulig K; American Academy of Clinical Toxicology; European Association of Poisons Centres and Clinical Toxicologists: Position paper: gastric lavage. J Toxicol Clin Toxicol 42(7):933–943, 2004 15641639

Wiley J, Henretig F, Foster R: Status epilepticus and severe neurologic impairment from lead encephalopathy (poster). J Toxicol Clin Toxicol 33(5):529–530, 1995

Woolf AD, Goldman R, Bellinger DC: Update on the clinical management of childhood lead poisoning. Pediatr Clin North Am 54(2):271–294, viii, 2007

CHAPTER 36

Psychopharmacology

36.1 Which of the following antidepressant side effects is long term and may not abate unless the medication is discontinued?

A. Anxiety.
B. Sexual dysfunction.
C. Vomiting.
D. Headache.

The correct response is option B: Sexual dysfunction.

Common short-term side effects with selective serotonin reuptake inhibitors (SSRIs) and serotonin-norepinephrine reuptake inhibitors (SNRIs) include nausea, vomiting (option C is incorrect), anxiety (option A is incorrect), headache (option D is incorrect), sedation, tremors, and anorexia. Common long-term side effects include sexual dysfunction (option B is correct), dry mouth, sweating, impaired sleep, and potential weight gain. **Chapter 36 (p. 1188)**

36.2 Which of the following statements most accurately describes the treatment principle for patients with comorbid mood disorder and migraine headaches?

A. Coadministration of triptans and serotonergic antidepressants is not contraindicated.
B. Coadministration of triptans and serotonergic medications is safe because there have never been case reports of serotonin syndrome.
C. All triptans should be avoided when coadministered with a monoamine oxidase inhibitor (MAOI).
D. Antidepressants have no role in the treatment of migraine headache.

The correct response is option A: Coadministration of triptans and serotonergic antidepressants is not contraindicated.

Many patients with migraine headache take triptans, which are potent $5\text{-HT}_{1B/1D}$ receptor agonists. Antidepressants are frequently prescribed for migraine prophylaxis (option D is incorrect) or comorbid depression or anxiety. Cases of serotonin syndrome from antidepressant and triptan coadministration are quite rare (option B is incorrect). Triptan use does not contraindicate use of serotonergic antidepressants (option A is correct). Triptans vary widely in their potential for pharmacokinetic interactions (Dodick and Martin 2004). Some triptans, such as sumatriptan, rizatriptan, and zolmitriptan, are metabolized by monoamine oxidase and should not be used during therapy with MAOIs (including selegeline) or within 2 weeks of MAOI discontinuation (McEvoy 2017). Other triptans are eliminated primarily through metabolism by cytochrome P450 (CYP) enzymes and/or are renally excreted and thus may be safer options in conjunction with MAOIs (option C is incorrect). **Chapter 36 (p. 1241)**

36.3   Which of the following medications requires no dosage adjustment or caution in patients with renal insufficiency?

A. Venlafaxine.
B. Pregabalin.
C. Olanzapine.
D. Gabapentin.

The correct response is option C: Olanzapine.

The following medications require no dosage adjustment in patients with renal insufficiency: asenapine, aripiprazole, clozapine, olanzapine, and quetiapine (option C is correct). Venlafaxine requires a 25%–50% dose reduction in patients with mild-to-moderate renal insufficiency and a 50%–75% dose reduction in patients with severe renal insufficiency (option A is incorrect). Gabapentin and pregabalin are both dosed based on creatinine clearance. A 50% dose reduction is recommended for patients with a creatinine clearance of 30–60 mL/min. A 75% dose reduction is recommended for patients with a creatinine clearance of 15–30 mL/min. A dose reduction of 87.5% is recommended for patients with a creatinine clearance of less than 15 mL/min (options B and D are incorrect). **Chapter 36 (Table 36–11, pp. 1235–1237)**

36.4   Which of the following natural medicines is thought to have clinically significant cytochrome interactions?

A. Ginkgo biloba.
B. Ginseng.
C. Kava.
D. Valerian.

The correct response is option C: Kava.

Kavalactones (the proposed active constituents of kava) inhibit major CYP enzymes and may cause interactions with concurrent medications (option C is correct). Ginkgo biloba has interactions with anticoagulants, nonsteroidal anti-inflammatory drugs (NSAIDs), SSRIs, and platelet inhibitors and may increase the risk of bleeding disorders. It may also reduce the efficacy of anticonvulsants (option A is incorrect). Ginseng reduces the effects of antidiabetics, antihypertensives, anxiolytics, antidepressants, mood stabilizers, anti-estrogens, and immunosuppresants. It may also have additive hypoglycemic effects with insulin and additive stimulant effects with caffeine. Similar to ginkgo biloba, it may increase the risk of bleeding disorders when combined with anticoagulants, NSAIDs, SSRIs, and platelet inhibitors (option B is incorrect). Valerian may potentiate the sedative effects of central nervous system (CNS) depressants (option D is incorrect). **Chapter 36 (Table 36–8, pp. 1224–1227)**

36.5   Which antipsychotic carries the lowest risk of affecting a patient's seizure threshold?

A. Olanzapine.
B. Clozapine.
C. Fluphenazine.
D. Quetiapine.

The correct response is option C: Fluphenazine.

Most antipsychotics lower the seizure threshold and increase seizure risk. Phenothiazines confer a dose-dependent seizure risk of 0.3%–1.2%, compared with a rate of first unprovoked seizure in the general population of about 23–61 per 100,000 person-years (Alldredge 1999; Porter and Chacko 2017). Most of the early case reports involved seizures with chlorpromazine (Alldredge 1999). Although there are no controlled comparative studies to allow an accurate assessment of relative seizure risk among the various agents, it appears that high-potency first-generation antipsychotics, aripiprazole, lurasidone, iloperidone, and risperidone (and likely paliperidone) are associated with the lowest risk of seizures (option C is correct); followed by quetiapine and then olanzapine and low-potency first-generation antipsychotics (FGAs) with an intermediate risk (options A and D are incorrect); and finally clozapine, with the highest risk (1% at 300 mg/day, increasing to 4.4% at >600 mg/day) (Alldredge 1999; Alper et al. 2007; Lertxundi et al. 2013; Williams and Park 2015) (option B is incorrect). **Chapter 36 (pp. 1201–1202)**

36.6   Which of the following psychostimulants is preferred in the treatment of patients for whom weight loss and appetite suppression are a concern?

A. Methylphenidate.
B. Dexmethylphenidate.
C. Atomoxetine.
D. Modafinil.

The correct response is option D: Modafinil.

Common adverse effects of psychostimulants (methylphenidate, dexmethylphenidate, and amphetamines) include CNS (insomnia, headache, nervousness, and social withdrawal) and GI (stomachache and anorexia) symptoms (options A and B are incorrect). Atomoxetine side effects reported in clinical trials included insomnia, nausea, dry mouth, constipation, dizziness, decreased appetite, urinary hesitancy, sexual dysfunction, and palpitations (Adler et al. 2009; Eli Lilly 2017) (option C is incorrect). Modafinil does not reduce appetite (option D is correct) (Rugino and Copley 2001). **Chapter 36 (pp. 1212–1213)**

36.7   Which of the following injectable benzodiazepines is preferred in behavioral emergencies?

A. Lorazepam, because it is readily absorbed and has no active metabolites.
B. Clonazepam, because of its onset of action.
C. Diazepam, because it is readily absorbed and has no active metabolites.
D. Diazepam, because of its onset of action.

The correct response is option A: Lorazepam, because it is readily absorbed and has no active metabolites.

Internationally, many benzodiazepines are available in intravenous, intramuscular, rectal, sublingual, and intranasal preparations. Injectable forms of diazepam, lorazepam and midazolam, and diazepam rectal gel are marketed in the United States and Canada. Intravenous benzodiazepines are commonly used to treat status epilepticus or to calm severely agitated patients. Compared with diazepam, lorazepam has more predictable pharmacokinetics after intravenous administration. For behavioral emergencies, lorazepam is the preferred agent because it is readily absorbed and has no active metabolites (option A is correct). Intramuscular diazepam is not recommended because of its erratic absorption (Rey et al. 1999) (options C and D are incorrect). Other benzodiazepines, such as clonazepam, have also been administered rectally. Although rectal benzodiazepine absorption is rapid, it is not always reliable because bioavailability is highly variable and the onset of action is delayed with rectal administration (Rey et al. 1999) (option B is incorrect). **Chapter 36 (pp. 1218–1219)**

36.8   Which medication is contraindicated in patients who have had a recent myocardial infarction?

A. Nortriptyline.
B. Ziprasidone.
C. Lorazepam.
D. Memantine.

The correct response is option B: Ziprasidone.

Ziprasidone (oral or intramuscular) is contraindicated in patients with QT prolongation or a recent myocardial infarction (option B is correct). Tricyclic antidepressants have been shown to be relatively safe for short-term treatment with stable ischemic heart disease, previous myocardial infarction, and congestive heart failure (option A is incorrect). The safety of benzodiazepines in the immediate post-myocardial infarction period has been documented (Risch et al. 1982) (option C is incorrect). Memantine is generally safe in patients with cardiovascular disease, but in rare cases, it may cause bradycardia (Gallini et al. 2008) (option D is incorrect). **Chapter 36 (pp. 1220, 1238–1240)**

36.9   Which of the following statements is true regarding psychotropic medications and syndrome of inappropriate antidiuretic hormone secretion (SIADH)?

A. Only antidepressant medications carry a risk of precipitating SIADH.
B. SSRIs and venlafaxine carry a higher risk of precipitating SIADH than other antidepressants.
C. Second-generation antipsychotics (SGAs), but not first-generation antipsychotics (FGAs), carry a risk of precipitating SIADH.
D. SIADH is not a dose-dependent phenomenon and therefore dosage adjustment has no place in the treatment of SIADH.

The correct response is option B: SSRIs and venlafaxine carry a higher risk of precipitating SIADH than other antidepressants.

In a review of the risk of SIADH in antidepressants, the risk was higher for SSRIs and venlafaxine compared with other antidepressants (De Picker et al. 2014) (option B is correct). Elderly patients, especially those with concurrent diuretic use (especially thiazides), were found to be at higher risk of hyponatremia. Other reported risk factors for SSRI-induced hyponatremia were female sex, low baseline serum sodium, and chronic illness (Varela Piñón and Adán-Manes 2017). Carbamazepine and oxcarbazepine may cause SIADH (option A is incorrect), leading to hyponatremia and water intoxication. Some studies suggest that hyponatremia can be a dose-dependent adverse effect, and, therefore, that dosage reduction can improve sodium levels (Dong et al. 2005) (option D is incorrect). SIADH can occur with FGAs as well as SGAs (option C is incorrect). **Chapter 36 (pp. 1193, 1199, 1207)**

36.10 When considering the impact of antipsychotic medication on metabolic and endocrinologic indices of glucose tolerance, lipid levels, prolactin levels, and weight gain, which of the following medications has the lowest overall risk?

A. Clozapine.
B. Risperidone.
C. Ziprasidone.
D. Quetiapine.

The correct response is option C: Ziprasidone.

Among SGAs, the relative propensity to cause weight gain (from greatest to least) is as follows: clozapine>quetiapine>risperidone>ziprasidone (Citrome 2011; Leucht et al. 2013; Murray et al. 2017) (option C is correct; options A and D are incorrect). Risperidone often elevates prolactin levels, whereas clozapine, quetiapine, and ziprasidone are regarded as prolactin-sparing (option B is incorrect). A large retrospective study suggested that the risk of new-onset diabetes is greatest for clozapine and progressively decreases for olanzapine, quetiapine, and risperidone (Miller et al. 2005). A U.S. consensus statement concluded that hyperglycemia is associated with all marketed SGAs but is less common with aripiprazole and ziprasidone (American Diabetes Association et al. 2004). **Chapter 36 (p. 1206)**

36.11   What is the definition of pharmacodynamics?

A. Determines the relationship between drug concentration and response for both therapeutic and adverse effects.
B. Characterizes the rate and extent of drug absorption, distribution, metabolism, and excretion, thus determining the rate of drug delivery to, and concentration at, its sites of action.
C. Describes the rate and extent to which the drug ingredient is absorbed from the drug product and available for drug action.
D. Is an active drug.

The correct response is option A: Determines the relationship between drug concentration and response for both therapeutic and adverse effects.

Pharmacodynamics determines the relationship between drug concentration and response for both therapeutic and adverse effects (option A is correct). *Pharmacokinetics* characterizes the rate and extent of drug absorption, distribution, metabolism, and excretion, thus determining the rate of drug delivery to, and concentration at, its sites of action (option B is incorrect). The *bioavailability* of a drug describes the rate and extent to which the drug ingredient is absorbed from the drug product and available for drug action (option C is incorrect). For example, intravenous drug delivery has 100% bioavailability. A pharmacologically active drug is, in general, unbound to plasma proteins and is therefore considered "free." Typically, acidic drugs (e.g., valproate, barbiturates) bind mostly to albumin, and more basic drugs (e.g., phenothiazines, tricyclic antidepressants, amphetamines, most benzodiazepines) bind to globulins. Decreases in protein binding increase the availability of the "free" drug for pharmacological action, metabolism, and excretion (option D is incorrect). **Chapter 36 (pp. 1181–1182)**

36.12   A patient who has been stable on aripiprazole for the alleviation of psychotic symptoms has been experiencing worsened depression. His psychiatrist starts him on fluoxetine to target his depressive symptoms. What is the possible effect of adding fluoxetine?

A. Fluoxetine will increase the activity of the metabolic enzyme, causing increased metabolism of aripiprazole.
B. Fluoxetine will increase the activity of the metabolic enzyme, causing increased metabolism of fluoxetine.

C. Fluoxetine will decrease the activity of the metabolic enzyme, causing decreased metabolism of aripiprazole.

D. Fluoxetine will decrease the activity of the metabolic enzyme, causing increased metabolism of fluoxetine.

The correct response is option C: Fluoxetine will decrease the activity of the metabolic enzyme, causing decreased metabolism of aripiprazole.

The hepatic CYP enzyme system catalyzes most phase I reactions and is involved in most metabolic drug-drug interactions. Pharmacokinetic interactions are understood in terms of the actions of an interacting drug (a metabolic inhibitor or inducer) on a substrate drug. A *substrate* is an agent or a drug that is metabolized by an enzyme. An *inducer* is an agent or a drug that increases the activity of the metabolic enzyme, allowing for an increased rate of metabolism. Induction may decrease the amount of circulating parent drug and increase the number and amounts of metabolites produced. The clinical effect may be a loss or reduction in therapeutic efficacy or an increase in toxicity from metabolites. An *inhibitor* has the opposite effect, decreasing or blocking enzyme activity needed for metabolism of other drugs. An enzyme inhibitor increases the concentration of any drug dependent on that enzyme for biotransformation, thereby prolonging the pharmacological effect or increasing toxicity (options A, B, and D are incorrect). For example, aripiprazole is primarily metabolized by both CYP2D6 and CYP3A4 isozymes. The addition of a drug that is a potent CYP2D6 inhibitor, such as fluoxetine, will inhibit aripiprazole's metabolism. Without a compensatory reduction in aripiprazole dosage, aripiprazole levels will rise (option C is correct) and increased adverse effects or toxicity may result. **Chapter 36 (pp. 1186–1187)**

36.13 Which antidepressant should be avoided in patients with comorbid depression and hypertension?

A. Fluoxetine.
B. Venlafaxine.
C. Trazodone.
D. Mirtazapine.

The correct response is option B: Venlafaxine.

Clinical trials of venlafaxine noted an average diastolic pressure increase of 7 mm Hg at dosages of more than 300 mg/day and clinically significant diastolic pressure increases ($\geq$15 mm Hg) in 5.5% of patients taking the drug at dosages of more than 200 mg/day (Feighner 1995) (option B is correct). The SSRIs and the novel/mixed-action antidepressants have a much safer cardiovascular profile than do the tricyclic antidepressants and the MAOIs. In general, the SSRIs have little effect on blood pressure or cardiac conduction (Glassman et al. 2002) (option A is incorrect). The most frequent cardiovascular adverse effect of trazodone is postural hypotension, which may be associated with syncope (option C is incorrect). Mirtazapine does not have significant effects on cardiac conduction, but because of its moderate alpha$_1$-antagonist activity, it has a 7% incidence of orthostatic hypotension (Khawaja and Feinstein 2003) (option D is incorrect). **Chapter 36 (pp. 1191–1192)**

36.14 A patient with a long history of bipolar disorder, stabilized on lithium, has a new diagnosis of diabetes insipidus. His primary doctor consults you for management recommendations. What is the treatment of choice for his patient?

A. Immediately stop his lithium as his nephrogenic diabetes insipidus will continue to progress/worsen.
B. Change his dosing from single-day to double-day dosing.
C. Increase his dose of lithium to cause his kidneys to respond to antidiuretic hormone.
D. Add amiloride to patient's medication regimen.

The correct response is option D: Add amiloride to patient's medication regimen.

Lithium reduces renal response to antidiuretic hormone, resulting in polyuria and/or polydipsia, initially in 30%–50% of patients and persisting in 10%–25% (option C is incorrect). Stopping lithium usually reverses this nephrogenic diabetes insipidus (McEvoy 2017). Apart from dry mouth, patients do not usually exhibit signs of dehydration. The long-term effects of lithium on renal function are a subject of debate, with variable findings reported in recent retrospective and cohort studies (Levenson and Owen 2017). Although long-term lithium treatment is the only well-established risk factor for lithium-induced nephropathy, other factors, such as age, previous episodes of lithium toxicity, and the presence of comorbid disorders, may also contribute. Lithium is so efficacious in bipolar disorder that the risk of renal dysfunction during long-term use is considered acceptable with appropriate monitoring of renal function. Management of polyuria may include changing to a single daily bedtime dose of lithium (option B is incorrect), decreasing the dosage, and/or administering amiloride (considered the treatment of choice) or thiazide diuretics (option D is correct). Use of amiloride does not require a reduction in lithium dosage (McEvoy 2017). Because many individuals have had their mood disorders stabilized on lithium, a consultation-liaison psychiatrist should consider all options of medication management, which include maintaining the patient on lithium despite the newly diagnosed diabetes insipidus and using other strategies (dose adjustments, changing administration times, introducing additional medications) before discontinuing a patient's lithium (option A is incorrect). **Chapter 36 (p. 1196)**

36.15 What is the correct procedure in prescribing a psychotropic drug that is primarily hepatically metabolized to a patient with impaired hepatic function?

A. Increase the initial dosage.
B. Titrate more slowly.

C. Monitor for clinical response as they would for any other patient.

D. Choose drugs with a narrow therapeutic index.

The correct response is option B: Titrate more slowly.

Psychopharmacological concerns in patients with liver disease largely center on pharmacokinetic changes brought about by the disease. Acute hepatitis usually does not require dosage alterations in psychotropics, but chronic hepatitis may require dosage adjustment, depending on the severity of liver dysfunction. In patients with cirrhosis, drug dosages will require significant modification. All plasma proteins are synthesized in the liver, so protein binding is altered in liver disease. The main clinical effect of chronic decreased protein binding is on the interpretation of blood levels. When prescribing hepatically metabolized psychotropic drugs to patients with impaired hepatic function, it is prudent to reduce the initial dosage (option A is incorrect) and titrate the drug more slowly (option B is correct), carefully monitor for clinical response and side effects (option C is incorrect), and choose drugs with a wide therapeutic index (option D is incorrect). **Chapter 36 (p. 1223)**

36.16 Which of the following medications has minimal effect on lithium levels?

A. Caffeine.

B. Nonsteroidal anti-inflammatory drugs (NSAIDs).

C. Loop diuretics.

D. Potassium-sparing diuretics.

The correct response is option D: Potassium-sparing diuretics.

Lithium is almost entirely renally excreted, and most lithium filtered by the glomeruli is reabsorbed with sodium in the proximal tubule. Serum lithium levels are increased by thiazide diuretics, NSAIDs, angiotensin-converting enzyme (ACE) inhibitors, angiotensin receptor antagonists, sodium depletion, electrolyte abnormalities, and dehydration (Finley 2016) (option B is incorrect). Symptoms of toxicity have been reported with addition of verapamil or diltiazem to lithium despite nonelevated concentrations. In patients who are elderly, medically ill, or on salt-restricted diets, loop diuretics may increase lithium; in other patient populations, loop diuretics may enhance elimination and reduce lithium levels (option C is incorrect). Carbonic anhydrase inhibitors, osmotic diuretics, methylxanthines, and caffeine reduce lithium levels (option A is incorrect), whereas potassium-sparing diuretics are considered to have no effect on lithium levels (option D is correct). In medically ill persons, it is imperative to closely monitor for toxicity whenever medication changes are made. **Chapter 36 (p. 1197)**

36.17 Among the various antipsychotic agents, which of the following medications is associated with the greatest mean QTc interval prolongation?

A. Olanzapine.
B. Aripiprazole.
C. Ziprasidone.
D. Thioridazine.

The correct response is option D: Thioridazine.

A number of antipsychotics may be associated with QTc interval prolongation and risk for torsades de pointes. Among the various antipsychotic agents, the mean QTc interval prolongation (greatest to least) is as follows: thioridazine (36 msec) (option D is correct)>ziprasidone (21 msec) (option C is incorrect)>iloperidone with metabolic inhibition (19 msec)>quetiapine (15 msec)>paliperidone (12 msec)>risperidone (10 msec)>iloperidone without metabolic inhibition (9 msec)>olanzapine (6 msec) (option A is incorrect)>oral haloperidol (5 msec)>asenapine (2–5 msec)>aripiprazole (<1 msec) (option B is incorrect)>lurasidone (negligible). Thioridazine carries a black box warning regarding dose-related QTc prolongation and risk for sudden death. Intravenous administration of haloperidol is associated with a higher risk of QTc prolongation than is oral use; risk of QTc prolongation and torsades de pointes associated with intravenous haloperidol is more similar to that of thioridazine (Beach et al. 2013). **Chapter 36 (p. 1205)**

36.18 Which SGA has been demonstrated to be *most* effective against psychosis without worsening a patient's underlying Parkinson's disease?

A. Clozapine.
B. Quetiapine.
C. Olanzapine.
D. Ziprasidone.

The correct response is option A: Clozapine.

The major concern regarding antipsychotic use in Parkinson's disease is dopamine D_2 receptor blockade, especially with high-potency FGAs, which can worsen motor symptoms. Pimavanserin (Nuplazid), a serotonin inverse agonist with no dopaminergic properties, recently received U.S. Food and Drug Administration approval for use in the treatment of Parkinson's disease psychosis (Bozymski et al. 2017) (option D is incorrect). Pimavanserin does not worsen motor symptoms or cause hypotension in patients with Parkinson's disease. Clozapine is the only SGA that has been demonstrated (in multiple controlled trials in patients with Parkinson's disease) to be effective against psychosis without aggravating the disease (for review, see Frieling et al. 2007), and it may even be beneficial in reducing tremor (Parkinson Study Group 1999) (option A is correct). As reviewed by Frieling et al. (2007), quetiapine was well tolerated but failed to demonstrate efficacy in two placebo-controlled trials (option B is incorrect), and olanzapine was ineffective in improving psychotic symptoms and caused increased extrapyramidal symptoms in two trials (option C is incorrect). **Chapter 36 (p. 1242)**

36.19 A patient with a history of chronic obstructive pulmonary disease (COPD) presents for treatment of anxiety. Which of the following best describes the approach to using benzodiazepines in this patient?

A. There is no concern about using benzodiazepines in this patient.
B. Benzodiazepines can significantly reduce the ventilatory response to hypoxia, so benzodiazepines should be used with caution.
C. Long-acting benzodiazepines are preferred over intermediate-acting benzodiazepines.
D. Benzodiazepines are contraindicated in patients with a diagnosis of COPD.

The correct response is option B: Benzodiazepines can significantly reduce the ventilatory response to hypoxia, so benzodiazepines should be used with caution.

The respiratory depressant effects of all benzodiazepines are well established (option A is incorrect); most of these agents can significantly reduce the ventilator response to hypoxia, which may precipitate respiratory failure in a patient with marginal respiratory reserve (option B is correct). Intermediate-acting agents (e.g., oxazepam, temazepam, lorazepam) have fewer respiratory depressant effects and are the benzodiazepines of first choice in patients with COPD (option C is incorrect). Patients with moderate to severe COPD are at risk of carbon dioxide retention with long-acting benzodiazepines, even at relatively low dosages. However, benzodiazepines should not automatically be avoided in patients with COPD (option D is incorrect). For patients with severe COPD, baseline assessment of blood gases and pulmonary consultation may be necessary in deciding whether benzodiazepines are appropriate for use. Oximetry is likely adequate for ongoing monitoring of the patient's clinical status during benzodiazepine use unless the patient is a known CO_2 retainer, in which case blood gases are more appropriate. Benzodiazepines are contraindicated in most individuals with sleep apnea. Benzodiazepines should not be combined with opioids in patients with respiratory compromise. **Chapter 36 (pp. 1243–1244)**

36.20 Which one of the following is a clinical feature of neuroleptic malignant syndrome (NMS)?

A. Hypothermia.
B. Generalized muscle flaccidity.
C. Autonomic instability.
D. Low white blood cell count, "leukopenia."

The correct response is option C: Autonomic instability.

NMS is a rare, potentially fatal idiosyncratic reaction to antipsychotics. NMS is also reported among patients with extrapyramidal disorders (e.g., Parkinson's disease) who have received antipsychotics or dopamine-depleting agents or who have had dopamine agonists (e.g., levodopa) abruptly withdrawn (Berman 2011). Estimates of the incidence of NMS are suggested to be 0.01%–0.02% (Berman 2011). NMS generally develops over a 1- to 3-day period and lasts for 5–10 days after a nondepot antipsychotic is discontinued (and much longer with depot agents). The main clinical features of NMS are hyperthermia (>38°C), generalized muscle rigidity, mental status changes, and autonomic instability (options A and B are incorrect; option C is correct). Temperature is greater than 38°C in the majority of cases and can exceed 40°C, predisposing patients to severe complications, including irreversible CNS and other organ damage. Muscle rigidity is often heterogeneous and can be either "lead-pipe" or cogwheeling. Signs of autonomic dysfunction include cardiac dysrhythmias, irregular blood pressure (hypertension or hypotension, orthostatic hypotension, labile blood pressure), tachycardia, urinary incontinence, and excessive sweating. Leukocytosis (not leukopenia) is common (option D is incorrect). **Chapter 36 (pp. 1202–1203)**

References

Adler LA, Spencer T, Brown TE, et al: Once-daily atomoxetine for adult attention-deficit/hyperactivity disorder: a 6-month, double-blind trial. J Clin Psychopharmacol 29(1):44–50, 2009 19142107

Alldredge BK: Seizure risk associated with psychotropic drugs: clinical and pharmacokinetic considerations. Neurology 53(5) (Suppl 2):S68–S75, 1999 10496236

Alper K, Schwartz KA, Kolts RL, Khan A: Seizure incidence in psychopharmacological clinical trials: an analysis of Food and Drug Administration (FDA) summary basis of approval reports. Biol Psychiatry 62(4):345–354, 2007 17223086

American Diabetes Association, American Psychiatric Association, American Association of Clinical Endocrinologists, et al: Consensus development conference on antipsychotics and obesity and diabetes. Diabetes Care 27:596–601, 2004

Beach SR, Celano CM, Noseworthy PA, et al: QTc prolongation, torsades de pointes, and psychotropic medications. Psychosomatics 54(1):1–13, 2013 23295003

Berman BD: Neuroleptic malignant syndrome: a review for neurohospitalists. Neurohospitalist 1(1):41–47, 2011 23983836

Bozymski KM, Lowe DK, Pasternak KM, et al: Pimavanserin: a novel antipsychotic for Parkinson's disease psychosis. Ann Pharmacother 51(6):479–487, 2017 28375643

Citrome L: Iloperidone, asenapine, and lurasidone: a brief overview of 3 new second-generation antipsychotics. Postgrad Med 123(2):153–162, 2011 21474903

De Picker L, Van Den Eede F, Dumont G, et al: Antidepressants and the risk of hyponatremia: a class-by-class review of literature. Psychosomatics 55(6):536–547, 2014 25262043

Dodick DW, Martin V: Triptans and CNS side-effects: pharmacokinetic and metabolic mechanisms. Cephalalgia 24(6):417–424, 2004 15154851

Dong X, Leppik IE, White J, Rarick J: Hyponatremia from oxcarbazepine and carbamazepine. Neurology 65(12):1976–1978, 2005 16380624

Eli Lilly: Strattera (atomoxetine) home page. 2017. Available at: http://www.strattera.com. Accessed October 17, 2017.

Feighner JP: Cardiovascular safety in depressed patients: focus on venlafaxine. J Clin Psychiatry 56(12):574–579, 1995 8530334

Finley PR: Drug interactions with lithium: an update. Clin Pharmacokinet 55(8):925–941, 2016 26936045

Frieling H, Hillemacher T, Ziegenbein M, et al: Treating dopamimetic psychosis in Parkinson's disease: structured review and meta-analysis. Eur Neuropsychopharmacol 17(3):165–171, 2007 17070675

Gallini A, Sommet A, Montastruc JL; French PharmacoVigilance Network: Does memantine induce bradycardia? A study in the French PharmacoVigilance Database. Pharmacoepidemiol Drug Saf 17(9):877–881, 2008 18500725

Glassman AH, O'Connor CM, Califf RM, et al; Sertraline Antidepressant Heart Attack Randomized Trial (SADHEART) Group: Sertraline treatment of major depression in patients with acute MI or unstable angina. JAMA 288(6):701–709, 2002 12169073

Khawaja IS, Feinstein RE: Cardiovascular effects of selective serotonin reuptake inhibitors and other novel antidepressants. Heart Dis 5(2):153–160, 2003 12713682

Lertxundi U, Hernandez R, Medrano J, et al: Antipsychotics and seizures: higher risk with atypicals? Seizure 22(2):141–143, 2013 23146619

Leucht S, Cipriani A, Spineli L, et al: Comparative efficacy and tolerability of 15 antipsychotic drugs in schizophrenia: a multiple-treatments meta-analysis. Lancet 382(9896):951–962, 2013 23810019

Levenson JL, Owen JA: Renal and urological disorders, in Clinical Manual of Psychopharmacology in the Medically Ill, 2nd Edition. Edited by Levenson JL, Ferrando SJ. Arlington, VA, American Psychiatric Publishing, 2017, pp 195–232

McEvoy GE: American Hospital Formulary Service (AHFS) Drug Information 2017. Bethesda, MD, American Society of Health-System Pharmacists, 2017

Miller EA, Leslie DL, Rosenheck RA: Incidence of new-onset diabetes mellitus among patients receiving atypical neuroleptics in the treatment of mental illness: evidence from a privately insured population. J Nerv Ment Dis 193(6):387–395, 2005 15920379

Murray R, Correll CU, Reynolds GP, Taylor D: Atypical antipsychotics: recent research findings and applications to clinical practice: Proceedings of a symposium presented at the 29th Annual European College of Neuropsychopharmacology Congress, 19 September 2016, Vienna, Austria. Ther Adv Psychopharmacol 7(1)(Suppl):1–14, 2017 28344764

Parkinson Study Group: Low-dose clozapine for the treatment of drug-induced psychosis in Parkinson's disease. N Engl J Med 340(10):757–763, 1999 10072410

Porter M, Chacko L: Antiepileptic drugs after first unprovoked seizure. Am Fam Physician 95(3):online, 2017

Rey E, Tréluyer JM, Pons G: Pharmacokinetic optimization of benzodiazepine therapy for acute seizures. Focus on delivery routes. Clin Pharmacokinet 36(6):409–424, 1999 10427466

Risch SC, Groom GP, Janowsky DS: The effects of psychotropic drugs on the cardiovascular system. J Clin Psychiatry 43(5 Pt 2):16–31, 1982 6122680

Rugino TA, Copley TC: Effects of modafinil in children with attention-deficit/hyperactivity disorder: an open-label study. J Am Acad Child Adolesc Psychiatry 40(2):230–235, 2001 11211372

Varela Piñón M, Adán-Manes J: Selective serotonin reuptake inhibitor-induced hyponatremia: clinical implications and therapeutic alternatives. Clin Neuropharmacol 40(4):177–179, 2017 28622213

Williams AM, Park SH: Seizure associated with clozapine: incidence, etiology, and management. CNS Drugs 29(2):101–111, 2015 25537107

CHAPTER 37

Psychotherapy

37.1   Hypnotherapy has the best evidence in treating which of the following conditions?

   A. Irritable bowel syndrome.
   B. Cancer.
   C. Chronic obstructive pulmonary disease (COPD).
   D. Diabetes.

The correct response is option A: Irritable bowel syndrome.

The best evidence for hypnotherapy in the field of consultation-liaison psychiatry comes from work in relation to irritable bowel syndrome (Schaefert et al. 2014) and fibromyalgia (Bernardy et al. 2011) (option A is correct). From systematic reviews (Jacobsen and Jim 2008) that evaluated psychosocial interventions for patients with cancer, some reviews reached positive conclusions, with the best evidence for behavioral therapy and counseling/psychotherapy (option B is incorrect). From a systematic review (Coventry et al. 2013) of randomized controlled trials evaluating psychological and/or lifestyle interventions for adults with COPD, multicomponent exercise training was found to be the only intervention with significant treatment effects for depression and for anxiety (option C is incorrect). A systematic review (van der Feltz-Cornelis et al. 2010) and meta-analysis of randomized controlled trials to determine the effectiveness of antidepressant therapies, including psychological treatments, in type 1 and type 2 diabetes mellitus, reported a slightly higher effect size for psychological treatments in reducing depressive symptoms than the effect size for combination treatment or for pharmacological treatment alone. There was no evidence, however, that treatments that improved depression had any impact on glycemic control (Baumeister et al. 2014; van der Feltz-Cornelis et al. 2010) (option D is incorrect). **Chapter 37 (pp. 1264, 1276–1277)**

37.2   Which of the following should be offered first in the stepped-care model to deliver psychological treatment?

   A. Guided self-help.
   B. Watchful waiting.

415

C. Cognitive-behavioral therapy (CBT).

D. Inpatient treatment.

The correct response is option B: Watchful waiting.

The stepped-care model involves five different intensities of treatment that are offered to the patient or client according to the severity or complexity of his or her problems. Most patients start at the bottom of this model and progress to the next step only if their symptoms do not improve: Step 1 involves watchful waiting, because many patients who present with symptoms will find that these resolve spontaneously without requiring any help (option B is correct). Step 2 usually involves some form of guided self-help and may include computerized CBT, psychoeducation, or help from volunteer organizations. Exercise may also be prescribed (option A is incorrect). Step 3 involves brief psychological therapy (e.g., CBT, counseling, interpersonal therapies) for six to eight sessions. Antidepressants may be prescribed if there is a previous history of moderate to severe depression (option C is incorrect). Step 4 involves depression case management, and the patient may be assigned a case manager or key worker. Medication and more intensive psychological treatments may be offered, with care coordinated by the case manager working with the patient's primary care physician. Step 5 is for patients who have not responded to the previous four steps. Step 5 may involve crisis intervention services, inpatient treatment, or even more intensive multicomponent treatment (option D is incorrect). **Chapter 37 (p. 1271)**

37.3   Homework is often assigned to patients in what type of therapy modality?

A. Supportive and problem-solving approaches.

B. Person-centered counseling.

C. Structured therapies.

D. Psychodynamic interpersonal therapy (PIT).

The correct response is option C: Structured therapies.

Participation in any form of meaningful psychotherapy requires an individual to be able to concentrate during the therapy and to recall and think about the therapy between sessions. In structured therapies, there is an explicit expectation that homework will be carried out between sessions (option C is correct). Problem-solving therapy improves individuals' abilities to cope with stressful life difficulties. It has three main steps: 1) symptoms and problems are identified, and the two are linked together; 2) the problems are defined and clarified; and 3) strategies are developed in a collaborative fashion with the patient to help solve the problems in a systematic way (option A is incorrect). Person-centered counseling, one of the most common forms of therapeutic counseling, is nondirective counseling in which emphasis is placed on the development of a personal relationship in which an individual can talk openly and freely about his or her problems (option B is incorrect). PIT combines elements of psychodynamic and interpersonal therapies. One of the central tenets of PIT is the importance of human experience and an individual's sense of self within a personal relationship. Human existence is regarded as being essentially relational, and man is regarded as a "creature of the between." This applies even to people who live a solitary existence (option D is incorrect). **Chapter 37 (pp. 1262–1266)**

37.4 On the basis of findings from systematic reviews, which of the following psychosocial interventions has the *greatest* evidence to support recommending it to cancer patients?

A. Involving families in the treatment process.
B. Pharmacotherapy.
C. Liaison activities with staff.
D. Counseling.

The correct response is option D: Counseling.

Psychosocial care is now recognized as an essential component of comprehensive cancer care. A wide range of therapies have been evaluated, including behavioral therapy, cognitive therapy, CBT, communication skills training, counseling, family therapy/counseling, guided imagery, mindfulness therapy, music therapy, problem-solving therapy, psychotherapy, stress management training, support groups, and supportive-expressive group therapy (Jacobsen and Jim 2008). A systematic review (Jacobsen and Jim 2008) of psychosocial interventions for anxiety and depression in adult cancer patients concluded that interventions involving counseling can be currently recommended for improving patients' general functional ability or quality of life, degree of depression, and interpersonal relationships (option D is correct). It is often appropriate for the therapist to involve other members of the patient's family in the therapeutic process, particularly if they have a role as a care provider, as illness affects the whole family and not just the individual with the illness. However, this is not a psychosocial intervention specific to cancer patients (option A is incorrect). Pharmacotherapy, although sometimes helpful for treating depression in cancer, is not a psychosocial intervention (option B is incorrect). For patients with cancer as well as other types of physical illness, it may also be important for the therapist to liaise with other members of the health care team and to spend time with the patient discussing relationships with nursing, medical, and other professional staff (option C is incorrect). **Chapter 37 (pp. 1263–1265, 1277)**

37.5 Women attending clinics for breast cancer were found to express which of the following preferences?

A. A more active, authoritative role in decision making by their doctors.
B. Emotional space to voice their fears and uncertainties.
C. Pharmacotherapy.
D. Hypnotherapy

The correct response is option A: A more active, authoritative role in decision making by their doctors.

There should be a collaborative approach to treatment so that patients themselves can make most of the decisions about their treatment. However, sometimes patients want doctors to play a more active, authoritative role in decision making, as was found in women attending clinics for breast cancer (Wright et al. 2004) (option A is correct). This emphasizes the need to find out what different people want and to tailor responses accordingly. If possible, patients should be given emotional space to voice their fears and uncertainties about their illness or reflect on loss and explore ways of coping (option B is incorrect). Although pharmacotherapy can be helpful for patients with depression and hypnotherapy has been shown to be helpful for certain medical conditions, these were not the expressed preferences of the women attending the breast cancer clinics (options C and D are incorrect). **Chapter 37 (pp. 1263–1264)**

37.6   Which of the following is *least* supported by findings from published studies of patients with cancer?

   A. Breast cancer patients may want doctors to play an authoritative role in decision making.
   B. Supportive group therapies reduce distress and prolong survival in cancer patients.
   C. Collaborative care models have shown benefit in depressed patients with cancer.
   D. Psychosocial treatments for cancer have positive effects on mood and well-being.

The correct response is option B: Supportive group therapies reduce distress and prolong survival in cancer patients.

Early studies of supportive group therapies involving cancer patients demonstrated emotional benefits and pain reduction, and some found apparent enhanced survival (e.g., Spiegel et al. 1989). The survival claims were controversial and were ultimately not replicated. More recent studies have not found evidence that supportive group therapies reduce distress or prolong survival (Classen et al. 2008; Ho et al. 2016) (option B is correct). Sometimes patients want doctors to play a more active, authoritative role in decision making, as was found in women attending clinics for breast cancer (Wright et al. 2004). This emphasizes the need to find out what different people want and tailor responses accordingly (option A is incorrect). Positive effects from collaborative care have been demonstrated in people with diabetes or cardiovascular disease in a U.K. population (Coventry et al. 2015), and this approach has also shown benefit in depressed patients with cancer (Dwight-Johnson et al. 2005; Ell et al. 2008) (option C is incorrect). Many systematic reviews published over the past 30 years have evaluated the evidence supporting the benefits of psychosocial treatments for anxiety and depression in patients with cancer, as well as for other outcomes, including quality of life, emotional well-being, and survival. From more recent systematic reviews of psychosocial therapies in the treatment of cancer (see Table 37–5), most, but not all, point to small but significant effects on mood or psychological well-being (option D is incorrect). **Chapter 37 (pp. 1263, 1265, 1271, 1277; Table 37–5, p. 1278)**

37.7 Which type of therapy is best described as using a treatment strategy to facilitate discussion of topics uppermost in the minds of patients with terminal illness, with an existential orientation based on the rationale that living with a terminal illness amplifies existential concerns of death, meaning, freedom, and isolation?

A. Interpersonal therapy.
B. Supportive-expressive group therapy.
C. CBT.
D. Mindfulness-based cognitive therapy (MBCT).

The correct response is option B: Supportive-expressive group therapy.

Supportive-expressive group therapy is an unstructured but quite intensive and existentially based treatment (Spiegel and Glafkides 1983). The rationale for the existential orientation presumes that living with terminal illness amplifies existential concerns of death, meaning, freedom, and isolation (option B is correct). Interpersonal therapy has been used to treat depression in HIV-positive patients (Markowitz et al. 1995) and has been adapted for PTSD and for use in hypochondriasis, focusing on the interpersonal consequences of being preoccupied with physical illness (Stuart and Noyes 2005) (option A is incorrect). The central tenet of CBT is that emotions, behavior, and cognitions are all interlinked. According to the cognitive model, distressing emotions such as anxiety or depression are linked to particular beliefs, assumptions, or thoughts. It is assumed that persistent distress is linked to underlying maladaptive beliefs and that modification of these beliefs and cognitions will result in reductions in emotional distress (option C is incorrect). MBCT has been adapted from mindfulness stress reduction approaches as a treatment for depression (Segal et al. 2002). MBCT includes basic education about depression and several exercises from cognitive therapy that show the links between thinking and feeling and demonstrate how people can look after themselves when depression threatens to overwhelm them (option D is incorrect). **Chapter 37 (pp. 1265–1267, 1270)**

37.8 For which condition does the existing evidence base show comparable effects of internet-based and face-to-face psychological treatments?

A. Diabetes.
B. Tinnitus.
C. Pain.
D. Breast cancer.

The correct response is option C: Pain.

A systematic review (Cuijpers et al. 2008) evaluated 12 studies of internet-based psychological therapies in diverse physical conditions, including headache, tinnitus, chronic pain, back pain, breast cancer, diabetes, and physical disability with accompanying loneliness. The reviewers found that the effects of the interventions that targeted pain were comparable to those of face-to-face treatments, with less robust evidence for the other conditions (option C is correct; options A, B, and D are incorrect). Other reviews (Macea et al. 2010) of internet-based therapies for chronic pain found small effects for the internet-based approaches in comparison with mainly wait-list control subjects. **Chapter 37 (pp. 1277, 1279)**

37.9 Which therapies are based on the premise that feelings, thoughts, and relationships are intimately tied up with each other?

A. Stepped care.
B. PIT.
C. Collaborative care.
D. Relational therapies.

The correct response is option D: Relational therapies.

Relational therapy refers to a broad group of therapies that have in common a model of human development and the mind in which nature and quality of human interpersonal relationships play a key role in the maintenance of "emotional homeostasis" (option D is correct). Psychological treatments can be offered as stand-alone treatments, although they are increasingly delivered as part of a package of care or part of a stepped-care model, which involves different intensities of treatment according to the severity or complexity of a patient's problems (option A is incorrect). Sometimes stepped-care programs are incorporated into collaborative care interventions, as in the Pathways Study (Katon et al. 2004), which tested a complex intervention to treat depression in patients with diabetes. The intervention involved an initial choice of two treatments, either an antidepressant or problem-solving therapy, followed by a stepped-care algorithm in which patients received different types and intensities of treatment according to their observed outcomes. PIT combines elements of psychodynamic and interpersonal therapy (option B is incorrect). Collaborative care models have five essential elements, including collaborative definition of problems, in which patient-defined problems are identified alongside medical problems diagnosed by health care professionals (option C is incorrect). **Chapter 37 (pp. 1265–1266, 1271)**

37.10 Which of the following is specific to PIT as compared with interpersonal therapy?

A. The creation of an interpersonal inventory.
B. The use of role play to modify problematic interactions.

C. The focus on strategies to prevent recurrent depression.

D. The use of the therapeutic relationship to address problems in the "here and now."

The correct response is option D: The use of the therapeutic relationship to address problems in the "here and now."

There are three stages in interpersonal therapy when it is used to treat depression. In the first phase, an interpersonal inventory of the patient's relationships is compiled, and the main interpersonal problem areas are identified, classified into four groups: grief, role transitions, role disputes, and interpersonal deficits (option A is incorrect). During the intermediate sessions of therapy, the therapist and client try to modify these problematic interactions using a variety of techniques, including role play (option B is incorrect). In the final phase, the therapist works to consolidate the client's gains and addresses the termination of therapy, with a focus on strategies that can prevent the depression from recurring (option C is incorrect). PIT combines elements of psychodynamic and interpersonal therapies. Key features of the model include 1) the assumption that the patient's problems arise from or are exacerbated by disturbances of significant personal relationship; 2) a tentative, encouraging, supportive approach from the therapist, who seeks to develop a deeper understanding with the patient through negotiation, exploration of feelings, and use of metaphor; 3) the linkage of the patient's distress to specific interpersonal problems; and 4) the use of the therapeutic relationship to address problems and test out solutions in the "here and now" (option D is correct). **Chapter 37 (pp. 1266–1267)**

References

Baumeister H, Hutter N, Bengel J: Psychological and pharmacological interventions for depression in patients with diabetes mellitus: an abridged Cochrane review. Diabet Med 31(7):773–786, 2014 24673571

Bernardy K, Füber N, Klose P, Häuser W: Efficacy of hypnosis/guided imagery in fibromyalgia syndrome--a systematic review and meta-analysis of controlled trials. BMC Musculoskelet Disord 12:133, 2011 21676255

Classen CC, Kraemer HC, Blasey C, et al: Supportive-expressive group therapy for primary breast cancer patients: a randomized prospective multicenter trial. Psychooncology 17(5):438–447, 2008 17935144

Coventry PA, Bower P, Keyworth C, et al: The effect of complex interventions on depression and anxiety in chronic obstructive pulmonary disease: systematic review and meta-analysis. PLoS One 8(4):e60532, 2013 23585837

Coventry P, Lovell K, Dickens C, et al: Integrated primary care for patients with mental and physical multimorbidity: cluster randomised controlled trial of collaborative care for patients with depression comorbid with diabetes or cardiovascular disease. BMJ 350:h638, 2015 25687344

Cuijpers P, van Straten A, Andersson G: Internet-administered cognitive behavior therapy for health problems: a systematic review. J Behav Med 31(2):169–177, 2008 18165893

Dwight-Johnson M, Ell K, Lee PJ: Can collaborative care address the needs of low-income Latinas with comorbid depression and cancer? Results from a randomized pilot study. Psychosomatics 46(3):224–232, 2005 15883143

Ell K, Xie B, Quon B, et al: Randomized controlled trial of collaborative care management of depression among low-income patients with cancer. J Clin Oncol 26(27):4488–4496, 2008 18802161

Ho RT, Fong TC, Lo PH, et al: Randomized controlled trial of supportive-expressive group therapy and body-mind-spirit intervention for Chinese non-metastatic breast cancer patients. Support Care Cancer 24(12):4929–4937, 2016 27470259

Jacobsen PB, Jim HS: Psychosocial interventions for anxiety and depression in adult cancer patients: achievements and challenges. CA Cancer J Clin 58(4):214–230, 2008 18558664

Katon WJ, Von Korff M, Lin EH, et al: The Pathways Study: a randomized trial of collaborative care in patients with diabetes and depression. Arch Gen Psychiatry 61(10):1042–1049, 2004 15466678

Macea DD, Gajos K, Daglia Calil YA, Fregni F: The efficacy of Web-based cognitive behavioral interventions for chronic pain: a systematic review and meta-analysis. J Pain 11(10):917–929, 2010 20650691

Markowitz JC, Klerman GL, Clougherty KF, et al: Individual psychotherapies for depressed HIV-positive patients. Am J Psychiatry 152(10):1504–1509, 1995 7573591

Schaefert R, Klose P, Moser G, Häuser W: Efficacy, tolerability, and safety of hypnosis in adult irritable bowel syndrome: systematic review and meta-analysis. Psychosom Med 76(5):389–398, 2014 24901382

Segal Z, Teasdale J, Williams M: Mindfulness-Based Cognitive Therapy for Depression. New York, Guilford, 2002

Spiegel D, Glafkides MC: Effects of group confrontation with death and dying. Int J Group Psychother 33(4):433–447, 1983 6642804

Spiegel D, Bloom JR, Kraemer HC, Gottheil E: Effect of psychosocial treatment on survival of patients with metastatic breast cancer. Lancet 2(8668):888–891, 1989 2571815

Stuart S, Noyes R Jr: Treating hypochondriasis with interpersonal psychotherapy. J Contemp Psychother 35(3):269–283, 2005

van der Feltz-Cornelis CM, Nuyen J, Stoop C, et al: Effect of interventions for major depressive disorder and significant depressive symptoms in patients with diabetes mellitus: a systematic review and meta-analysis. Gen Hosp Psychiatry 32(4):380–395, 2010 20633742

Wright EB, Holcombe C, Salmon P: Doctors' communication of trust, care, and respect in breast cancer: qualitative study. BMJ 328(7444):864, 2004 15054034

CHAPTER 38

Electroconvulsive Therapy and Other Brain Stimulation Therapies

38.1 Whose responsibility is it to ensure that information obtained from previous electroconvulsive therapy (ECT) treatments is passed on before starting a new course of ECT?

A. The anesthesiologist.
B. The internist.
C. Other specialist consultants.
D. The psychiatrist.

The correct response is option D: The psychiatrist.

Good communication among the primary psychiatrist, other specialist consultants, and the anesthesiologist is essential. In many ECT clinics, the anesthesiologist of the day varies from treatment to treatment (option A is incorrect), so it falls on the psychiatrist to ensure that information obtained from previous treatments is passed on (option D is correct). Also, the patient's medical status prior to treatments may change during the course of treatments, so ongoing vigilance to assess new-onset medical issues is critical, and this too usually falls on the psychiatrist rather than on the specialist consultants (option C is incorrect). Thus, it is unwise for a psychiatrist treating a patient with ECT to assume an attitude that it is the anesthesiologist's, internist's, or specialist consultant's (option B is incorrect) responsibility to deal with medical problems—good care of these patients begins with the psychiatrist. **Chapter 38 (p. 1285)**

38.2 What is the initial autonomic response to the electrical stimulus during ECT?

A. Bradycardia.
B. Tachycardia.

C. Hypotension.
D. Atrial fibrillation.

The correct response is option A: Bradycardia.

After the electrical stimulus, there is a parasympathetically mediated short-lived bradycardia (option A is correct), occasionally with an asystole of several seconds. However, a tachycardia (option B is incorrect), which is sympathetically mediated, then follows. As opposed to hypotension (option C is incorrect), there occurs a rise in blood pressure during and for a few minutes after the seizure. Myocardial work-load and cardiac output increase significantly. Transient electrocardiogram abnormalities may occur during this time, including ST segment depression and T wave changes as well as temporary echocardiographic abnormalities, mainly abnormal wall motion, but atrial fibrillation (option D is incorrect) would not be expected as a normal autonomic response to ECT. The parameters that are monitored routinely include blood pressure and electrocardiogram abnormalities, and any untoward measurements can be treated promptly by the anesthesiologist (e.g., with blood pressure medication or antiarrhythmics) to prevent serious complications. These physiological changes might predispose cardiac patients to higher-than-usual risks during ECT, but the literature does not permit precise conclusions about such risks. **Chapter 38 (p. 1286)**

38.3   What cardioprotective agent is administered during ECT for patients with congestive heart failure (CHF)?

A. An antimuscarinic is administered.
B. All cardiac medications should be held on the morning of the ECT.
C. A beta-blocker is administered.
D. CHF is an absolute contraindication to ECT.

The correct response is option C: A beta-blocker is administered.

Patients with CHF are particularly sensitive to increased myocardial demand such as occurs during ECT. The keys to maximum safety with such patients are to stabilize ventricular pump function, optimally before proceeding, and to obtain expert anesthesiological management during the sessions. There have been six case series describing 58 patients with CHF given ECT, with two deaths (Gerring and Shields 1982; Goldberg and Badger 1993; Petrides and Fink 1996; Rivera et al. 2011; Stern et al. 1997; Zielinski et al. 1993) (option D is incorrect). CHF should optimally be stabilized prior to commencing ECT. Cardiac medications should be administered in the morning before the treatments with a small amount of water, with enough time to ensure absorption (option B is incorrect). Whether to use an antimuscarinic agent in the patient with CHF must be decided on a case-by-case basis (option A is incorrect). The potential for such medication to increase myocardial workload through added tachycardia and hypertension has been established (Rasmussen et al. 1999). The attending anesthesiologist may elect to use other cardioprotective agents when ECT is being administered to the patient with CHF. For example, a beta-blocker such as esmolol or labetalol may dampen the seizure-induced sympathetic stimulation (option C is correct). Other strategies include preload reduction (e.g., nitrates), peripheral vasodilators (e.g., hydralazine), and calcium channel blockade (e.g., verapamil or diltiazem). **Chapter 38 (pp. 1286–1287)**

38.4   Which is the most common dysrhythmia among patients presenting for ECT?

A. Atrial fibrillation.
B. Sinus arrhythmia.
C. Premature ventricular contractions.
D. Premature atrial contractions.

The correct response is option A: Atrial fibrillation.

The most common dysrhythmia in ECT patients is atrial fibrillation (option A is correct). There are several reports of patients in atrial fibrillation who safely received ECT (Petrides and Fink 1996). Occasionally, such patients will convert to sinus rhythm during ECT or convert back to atrial fibrillation if already converted before ECT to sinus rhythm. Atrial fibrillation newly identified before ECT should be assessed by a cardiologist for optimal management, including the decision of whether to choose rate control or cardioversion. The patient without a history of atrial fibrillation who develops this rhythm during ECT obviously should have a cardiac evaluation before treatment is resumed. In patients taking warfarin, therapeutic anticoagulation should be continued throughout ECT (Mehta et al. 2004). Findings of premature atrial contractions (option D is incorrect) are not particularly worrisome nor are premature ventricular contractions (option C is incorrect) or sinus arrhythmias (option B is incorrect) (see Chaudhary and Rajuria 1995). **Chapter 38 (pp. 1288–1289)**

38.5   Following ECT, which of the following conditions in neurological disorders have been shown to improve?

A. Treatment-emergent dyskinesias.
B. Core motor deficits.
C. Cognitive impairment.
D. Symptoms of recent stroke.

The correct response is option B: Core motor deficits.

In the literature, ECT has been described as helping patients with Parkinson's disease with the motor (option B is correct), depressive, and psychotic components of Parkinson's disease. However, there is no evidence to demonstrate that ECT improves cognitive impairment (option C is incorrect) and treatment-emergent dyskinesias (option A is incorrect). In fact, treatment-emergent dyskinesias are common during ECT and (after consultation with a neurologist) may call for careful reduction of levodopa doses during the index ECT. Because relapse is high, maintenance ECT may help to sustain the initial benefits. Given that cognitive side effects tend to be exaggerated in this population, unilateral electrode placement is recommended. It is prudent for ECT practitioners to avoid using ECT in patients with a recent stroke (option D is incorrect). **Chapter 38 (pp. 1290–1291)**

38.6 Transcranial magnetic stimulation (TMS) is U.S. Food and Drug Administration (FDA)–approved for which of the following disorders?

A. Treatment-resistant depression.
B. Cognitive impairment.
C. Parkinson's disease.
D. Migraine.

The correct response is option A: Treatment-resistant depression.

TMS is FDA approved for treatment-resistant depression (option A is correct). TMS is being actively investigated for other neuropsychiatric conditions (e.g., conversion disorder, chronic pain, cognitive impairment [option B is incorrect], migraine [option D is incorrect], Parkinson's disease [option C is incorrect], poststroke depression). (See Chapter 7, "Depression," for a review of the evidence supporting the efficacy of TMS for depression after stroke and in Parkinson's disease.) TMS, in common with brain magnetic resonance imaging, is contraindicated in patients with ferromagnetic implants, including electronic devices in or near the head (e.g., deep brain stimulators, carotid stents, aneurysm clips or coils, cerebrospinal fluid shunts, cochlear implants) and ferromagnetic fragments. **Chapter 38 (p. 1293)**

38.7 Contraindications regarding vagal nerve stimulation (VNS) occur in which of the following situations?

A. Patients with epilepsy.
B. Patients with treatment-resistant depression.
C. Patients with left vagotomy.
D. Patients requiring diagnostic ultrasound.

The correct response is option C: Patients with left vagotomy.

VNS is FDA approved for treatment-resistant depression and epilepsy (options A and B are incorrect). VNS is contraindicated in patients who have cardiac conduction abnormalities or who have had a left vagotomy (option C is correct). VNS may aggravate sleep apnea and may affect programmable shunt valves. Patients with a VNS device cannot have shortwave diathermy, microwave diathermy, or therapeutic ultrasound diathermy because the generated heating of the VNS components can cause tissue damage. Diagnostic ultrasound is not contraindicated (option D is incorrect). **Chapter 38 (pp. 1293–1294)**

38.8   For which of the following conditions does deep brain stimulation have FDA approval?

A. Cerebrovascular disease.
B. Increased bleeding risk.
C. Treatment-resistant obsessive-compulsive disorder.
D. Immunodeficiency.

The correct response is option C: Treatment-resistant obsessive-compulsive disorder.

Deep brain stimulation is FDA approved for use in treatment-resistant obsessive-compulsive disorder (option C is correct) and for investigational use in depression. It is contraindicated in patients with increased bleeding risk (option B is incorrect), immunodeficiency (option D is incorrect), or cerebrovascular disease (option A is incorrect). Deep brain stimulation may be affected by—or may adversely affect—pacemakers and defibrillators. Diathermy, electrolysis, radiation therapy, and electrocautery should not be used directly over the implant site. Potential adverse effects include surgical and hardware complications, as well as mood disturbances and suicidality. **Chapter 38 (p. 1294)**

38.9   For which of the following conditions may ECT be lifesaving?

A. Patients with a recent stroke.
B. Intracerebral aneurysm.
C. Intracranial masses.
D. Neuroleptic-induced malignant catatonia.

The correct response is option D: Neuroleptic-induced malignant catatonia.

ECT may be lifesaving in some cases of refractory neuroleptic-induced malignant catatonia (option D is correct), which includes neuroleptic malignant syndrome. It is prudent for the ECT practitioner to avoid using ECT in patients with a recent stroke (option A is incorrect). However, occasionally such a patient is profoundly depressed, with marked decreases in psychomotor effort; has low or absent food intake; or is at high acute suicidal risk. In such cases, if ECT is judged to be necessary, risk-reduction strategies include continuing anticoagulation if it already is indicated (i.e., it should not be started just for ECT) and paying close attention to blood pressure to avoid high spikes and potentially dangerous declines. There is concern that intracerebral aneurysms may rupture during ECT because of the rapid increase in blood pressure during seizures (option B is incorrect). Some reports indicate that ECT can be safely used in patients with various types of intracranial masses (Kohler and Burock 2001; Patkar et al. 2000; Perry et al. 2007; Rasmussen and Flemming 2006; Rasmussen et al. 2007). Presence of any central nervous system tumor may lead to an increased risk for neurological complications caused by ECT. In the absence of focal neurological signs, brain edema, mass effects, or papilledema, the risks likely are relatively small. In the presence of such findings, ECT should be considered only when no other reasonable option exists, and only after consultation with a neurosurgeon or neurologist to discuss strategies to reduce the increase in intracranial pressure that accompanies seizures (option C is incorrect). **Chapter 38 (p. 1291)**

References

Chaudhary S, Rajuria SS: Effects of electroconvulsive therapy on cardiovascular system. Med J Armed Forces India 51(1):31–33, 1995 28769237

Gerring JP, Shields HM: The identification and management of patients with a high risk for cardiac arrhythmias during modified ECT. J Clin Psychiatry 43(4):140–143, 1982 7068545

Goldberg RJ, Badger JM: Major depressive disorder in patients with the implantable cardioverter defibrillator. Two cases treated with ECT. Psychosomatics 34(3):273–277, 1993 8493312

Kohler CG, Burock M: ECT for psychotic depression associated with a brain tumor (letter). Am J Psychiatry 158(12):2089, 2001 11729041

Mehta V, Mueller PS, Gonzalez-Arriaza HL, et al: Safety of electroconvulsive therapy in patients receiving long-term warfarin therapy. Mayo Clin Proc 79(11):1396–1401, 2004 15544018

Patkar AA, Hill KP, Weinstein SP, Schwartz SL: ECT in the presence of brain tumor and increased intracranial pressure: evaluation and reduction of risk. J ECT 16(2):189–197, 2000 10868329

Perry CL, Lindell EP, Rasmussen KG: ECT in patients with arachnoid cysts. J ECT 23(1):36–37, 2007 17435574

Petrides G, Fink M: Atrial fibrillation, anticoagulation, and electroconvulsive therapy. Convuls Ther 12(2):91–98, 1996 8744168

Rasmussen KG, Flemming KD: Electroconvulsive therapy in patients with cavernous hemangiomas. J ECT 22(4):272–273, 2006 17143161

Rasmussen KG, Jarvis MR, Zorumski CF, et al: Low-dose atropine in electroconvulsive therapy. J ECT 15(3):213–221, 1999 10492860

Rasmussen KG, Perry CL, Sutor B, Moore KM: ECT in patients with intracranial masses. J Neuropsychiatry Clin Neurosci 19(2):191–193, 2007 17431067

Rivera FA, Lapid MI, Sampson S, Mueller PS: Safety of electroconvulsive therapy in patients with a history of heart failure and decreased left ventricular systolic heart function. J ECT 27(3):207–213, 2011 21865957

Stern L, Hirschmann S, Grunhaus L: ECT in patients with major depressive disorder and low cardiac output. Convuls Ther 13(2):68–73, 1997 9253526

Zielinski RJ, Roose SP, Devanand DP, et al: Cardiovascular complications of ECT in depressed patients with cardiac disease. Am J Psychiatry 150(6):904–909, 1993 8494067

CHAPTER 39

Palliative Care

39.1   Which of the following statements best describes the *primary* role of the consultation-liaison psychiatrist in the palliative care setting?

A. Address bereavement issues with the patient and family.
B. Encourage discussion of end-of-life ethical issues regarding provision or
   nonprovision of treatment.
C. Assist clinicians in how to deliver bad news and discuss treatment preferences.
D. Diagnose and treat comorbid psychiatric disorders in the palliative care setting.

**The correct response is option D: Diagnose and treat comorbid psychiatric dis-
orders in the palliative care setting.**

The traditional role of the psychiatrist is broadened in several ways in the care of
the dying patient. The psychiatrist's primary role in the palliative care setting is
the diagnosis and treatment of comorbid psychiatric disorders (option D is correct). Consultation-liaison psychiatrists can provide expert care and teaching
about the management of depression, suicide, anxiety, delirium, fatigue, and pain
in terminally ill patients (Chochinov and Breitbart 2012). The role of the psychiatrist in the care of the dying extends beyond management of psychiatric symptoms and syndromes to encompass existential issues, family and caregiver
support, bereavement, doctor-patient communication, and education and training (option A is incorrect). Psychiatrists can play an important role in addressing
social, psychological, ethical, and spiritual issues that complicate the care of dying patients. Psychiatrists also have a role in encouraging discussion of end-of-life
ethical decisions regarding treatment provision or nonprovision (e.g., withhold-
ing of resuscitation, withdrawal of life support) (option B is incorrect). The capacity of the patient to make rational judgments and/or the ability of the proxy to
make appropriate decisions for the patient may require psychiatric evaluation.
The decision to withdraw life support is highly emotional and may require psychiatric consultation (Subcommittee on Psychiatric Aspects of Life-Sustaining
Technology 1996). Psychiatrists can assist in teaching providers how to deliver
bad news and discuss do-not-resuscitate orders and other treatment preferences,
ideally with the patient, or with family members when the patient is incapacitated
(Levin et al. 2008; Weissman 2004) (option C is incorrect). **Chapter 39 (p. 1300)**

39.2   A 60-year-old woman with advanced chronic obstructive pulmonary disease and current tobacco use disorder is admitted for workup and care of a newly diagnosed left lung adenocarcinoma. She and her family report that she does not drink alcohol and has been using e-cigarettes for the past year. On the third hospital day, her nurses report that she is highly anxious. The psychiatric consultant notes that she is irritable, anxious, and complains of confusion; however, she is not delirious. What is the single best first approach to patient engagement and management in this case?

A. Start citalopram 20 mg daily.
B. Offer counseling only because e-cigarette use does not cause withdrawal.
C. Initiate nicotine replacement therapy with a transdermal nicotine patch.
D. Instruct house staff to give a stat dose of intramuscular lorazepam 1 mg.

The correct response is option C: Initiate nicotine replacement therapy with a transdermal nicotine patch.

Symptoms of anxiety in the terminally ill individual may arise from a medical complication of the illness or its treatment (Breitbart et al. 1995; Roth and Massie 2009). Hypoxia, sepsis, poorly controlled pain, medication side effects such as akathisia, and withdrawal states often present as anxiety (Miovic and Block 2007). Withdrawal in terminally ill patients often manifests first as agitation or anxiety and becomes clinically evident days later than might be expected in younger, healthier patients because of impaired metabolism. Electronic cigarettes, also referred to as "e-cigarettes," consist of a battery and a heating element that vaporizes a solution ("e-liquid"), which the user inhales (known as "vaping"). E-liquids contain nicotine, flavorings, and propylene glycol or vegetable glycerin (Weaver et al. 2014). Symptoms of nicotine withdrawal are similar with all tobacco products, whether cigarettes, e-cigarettes, chewing tobacco, or snuff. Withdrawal symptoms include irritability, difficulty concentrating, restlessness, anxiety, depression, and increased appetite (Karan et al. 2003) (option B is incorrect). Symptoms of nicotine withdrawal peak around 48 hours after the last use, then gradually diminish over several weeks. Nicotine replacement therapy is used in hospitalized smokers to treat acute nicotine withdrawal symptoms (Rigotti et al. 2008) (option C is correct). Symptoms of dysphoria, anhedonia, and depression may continue for several months after cessation of nicotine; nicotine replacement products all provide similar relief from withdrawal symptoms and efficacy for smoking cessation (option A is incorrect). During the terminal phase of illness, when patients become less alert, there is a tendency to minimize the use of sedating medications. It is important to slowly taper benzodiazepines and opioids, which may have been sustained at high doses to provide extended relief of anxiety or pain, in order to prevent acute withdrawal. In anxious patients with severely compromised pulmonary function, benzodiazepines may suppress central respiratory mechanisms, making them unsafe (option D is incorrect). **Chapter 16 (pp. 452–453); Chapter 39 (pp. 1301–1302)**

39.3 You are consulting in hospital on a 66-year-old man with advanced metastatic prostate cancer. He has multiple painful bony metastases to spine and femur and is expected to live for only a few weeks. Parenteral hydromorphone is effective at controlling his pain, radiation therapy is started, and a discussion regarding home hospice is held with the patient and family. The patient becomes acutely depressed, hopeless, and feels guilty about his illness. The symptoms are distressing and persist over the next week. What is the best initial medical approach to managing depression in this patient?

A. Start fluoxetine at 20 mg daily.
B. Start methylphenidate 2.5 mg at 8 A.M. and 1 P.M.
C. Reduce hydromorphone dosage.
D. Start sertraline at 50 mg daily.

The correct response is option B: Start methylphenidate 2.5 mg at 8 A.M. and 1 P.M.

A depressed patient with only days or weeks to live is unlikely to have the time required for antidepressants to exert their desired effects; recent meta-analyses suggest that antidepressants show their clearest benefit after 6 weeks of treatment (options A and D are incorrect). In view of the time required for antidepressants to exert their effects, a depressed individual with less than 3 weeks to live may derive more benefit from a rapid-acting psychostimulant (Block et al 2000; Homsi et al. 2001). Psychostimulants are particularly helpful in the treatment of depression in the terminally ill because they have a rapid onset of action and energizing effects and typically do not cause anorexia, weight loss, or insomnia at therapeutic doses (Candy et al. 2008). Methylphenidate and dextroamphetamine are usually initiated at low dosages (2.5–5.0 mg in the morning and at noon). The benefits can be assessed during the first 1–2 days of treatment and the dose gradually titrated (usually to no greater than 30 mg/day total) (option B is correct). An additional benefit of stimulants is that they reduce sedation secondary to opioids and provide adjuvant analgesic effects (Bruera et al. 1987) (option C is incorrect). Occasionally, treatment with a selective serotonin reuptake inhibitor (SSRI) and a psychostimulant may be initiated concurrently so that depressed patients may receive the immediate benefits of the psychostimulant while waiting for the SSRI to work. When the SSRI becomes effective, the psychostimulant may be withdrawn. **Chapter 39 (pp. 1305–1306)**

39.4 Which of the following statements is *most* accurate regarding models of delivery of palliative care?

A. Palliative care is synonymous with end-of-life care.
B. Bereavement programs are carved out of traditional models of palliative care delivery.
C. Model palliative care programs are hospital based in setting.
D. Model programs typically include both research and education as core components.

The correct response is option D: Model programs typically include both re-search and education as core components.

Palliative care is not restricted to people who are dying; rather, it can be applied to the control of symptoms in and the provision of support to those living with chronic life-threatening illnesses (option A is incorrect). In recognition of the expanded role of palliative care in the United States, the Department of Health and Human Services Centers for Medicare and Medicaid Services defined palliative care as

> Patient and family-centered care that optimizes quality of life by anticipating, preventing, and treating suffering. Palliative care throughout the continuum of illness involves addressing physical, intellectual, emotional, social, and spiritual needs and [facilitating] patient autonomy, access to information and choice. (73 Federal Register 32204, June 5, 2008)

Model palliative care programs ideally include all of the following components: 1) a home care (e.g., hospice) program (option C is incorrect); 2) a hospital-based palliative care consultation service; 3) a day care program or ambulatory care clinic; 4) a palliative care inpatient unit (or dedicated palliative care beds in a hospital); 5) a bereavement program (option B is incorrect); 6) training and research programs (option D is correct); and 7) internet-based services. An updated U.S. national expert consensus process led to publication of the third edition of the *Clinical Practice Guidelines for Quality Palliative Care* (National Consensus Project for Quality Palliative Care 2013). **Chapter 39 (p. 1299)**

39.5   You are consulting in an inpatient hospice setting on an 82-year-old man with advanced lung cancer with recent progression of disease who is actively dying; he is both anxious and dyspneic. Which medicine would be the most appropriate to palliate these distressing symptoms?

A. Buspirone.
B. Morphine.
C. Trazodone.
D. Mirtazapine.

The correct response is option B: Morphine.

Sedating antidepressants such as trazodone or mirtazapine may help patients with persistent anxiety, insomnia, and anorexia (options C and D are incorrect). SSRIs are also effective in the management of anxiety disorders (Roth and Massie 2009). The utility of antidepressants and buspirone for anxiety disorders is often limited in the dying patient because they require weeks to achieve therapeutic effect (option A is incorrect). Opioids are primarily indicated for pain but are also effective in relieving dyspnea and associated anxiety (Elia and Thomas 2008) (option B is correct). Continuous intravenous infusions of morphine or other narcotic analgesics allow for careful titration and control of respiratory distress, anxiety, pain, and agitation (Portenoy and Foley 1989). **Chapter 39 (p. 1302)**

39.6 A 66-year-old woman has end-stage refractory leukemia with impaired quality of life (pain, fatigue). She begins a palliative psychotherapy intervention, which combines didactics and personal exploration with assigned writing to promote self-reflection outside of sessions. Which of the following palliative psychotherapies is consistent with this specific intervention?

A. Dignity therapy.
B. Cognitive-behavioral therapy.
C. Meaning-centered psychotherapy.
D. Life review.

The correct response is option C: Meaning-centered psychotherapy.

Psychotherapy can be challenging in the palliative care setting. Several cultures, including the culture of medicine, create a taboo around death and illness, often fostering patterns of avoidance in both patient and provider. *Dignity therapy* is a short-term care intervention for palliative care patients; an open account of life facilitated by the therapist is recorded, transcribed, edited, and the transcription is returned to the patient within 1–2 days. The immediacy of the returned transcript is intended to bolster the patient's sense of purpose, meaning, and worth, while giving the patient tangible evidence that his or her thoughts and words will continue to be valued (option A is incorrect). Several palliative psychotherapies have been derived from the principles of cognitive-behavioral therapy. These therapies use a manualized approach, and they often combine cognitive restructuring and exposure/response prevention components of traditional cognitive-behavioral therapy with ancillary measures (option B is incorrect). Meaning-centered psychotherapy utilizes a mixture of didactics, discussion, and experiential exercises that focus on particular themes related to meaning. It is designed to help individuals with advanced cancer sustain or enhance a sense of meaning, peace, and purpose in their lives even as they approach the end of life. An abbreviated form of meaning-centered psychotherapy is being developed for use in palliative care patients, with treatment delivered in three sessions to accommodate significantly shortened life expectancies (Rosenfeld et al. 2017) (option C is correct). The *life review* is a form of an existential therapy, which provides patients with the opportunity to identify and reexamine past experiences and achievements to find meaning, resolve old conflicts and make amends, or resolve unfinished business (Lichter et al. 1993). Life review has traditionally been used in the elderly as a means of conflict resolution and to facilitate a dignified acceptance of death (Butler 1963) (option D is incorrect). **Chapter 39 (pp. 1320–1324; Table 39–2, p. 1322)**

39.7 A 36-year-old woman with breast cancer is receiving cyclic systemic chemotherapy and develops severe, refractory nausea, and vomiting. First-line antiemetics have been ineffective or intolerable because of extrapyramidal side effects. Which of the following would be the most appropriate next treatment to initiate?

A. Metoclopramide.
B. Prochlorperazine.

C. Dronabinol.
D. Haloperidol.

The correct response is option C: Dronabinol.

Antiemetic drugs are the mainstay of managing chemotherapy-induced nausea and vomiting in patients with advanced disease. Several antiemetics (e.g., metoclopramide, prochlorperazine, promethazine, haloperidol, olanzapine) have dopamine-blocking properties and thus can cause acute akathisia and dystonia (options A, B, and D are incorrect). Extrapyramidal side effects are rarely a problem with newer antipsychotics (e.g., olanzapine) and newer antiemetics (e.g., serotonin 5-HT$_3$ antagonists such as ondansetron). Agents that target the cannabinoid system may be considered in treating refractory chemotherapy-induced nausea and vomiting. Dronabinol and nabilone are two cannabinoid agents approved for treating chemotherapy-induced nausea and vomiting that are refractory to standard antiemetic therapies; however, there is insufficient evidence to support use of cannabinoids or cannabis as primary treatment (Davis 2016; Smith et al. 2015) (option C is correct). **Chapter 39 (p. 1320)**

39.8   A 52-year-old man is confronting the death of his husband due to amyotrophic lateral sclerosis (ALS) 3 months earlier. He is successfully integrating this loss without significant detriment in self-care, and he has maintained social interactions. Which of the following terms *best* describes his current coping with this loss?

A. Mourning.
B. Bereavement.
C. Uncomplicated grief.
D. Complicated grief.

The correct response is option C: Uncomplicated grief.

Although words such as *grief, mourning,* and *bereavement* are commonly used interchangeably, the following definitions may be helpful:

- *Bereavement* is the state of loss resulting from death (option B is incorrect).
- *Grief* is the emotional response associated with loss.
- *Uncomplicated grief* is the process of successfully integrating the loss of a loved one without significant detriment in self-care, social interaction, or overall well-being, with significant individual variation (option C is correct).
- *Mourning* is the process of adaptation to loss, including the cultural and social rituals prescribed as accompaniments (option A is incorrect).
- *Complicated grief,* as recently proposed, presumes a normative and adaptive grief response that has been interrupted or delayed (Shear et al. 2016) (option D is incorrect).
- *Prolonged grief disorder* focuses on the intensity and length of grief itself as contributing to a pathological state (Prigerson et al. 2009).

- *Persistent complex bereavement disorder* is a clinical entity semantically synthesizing the above two terms. DSM-5 identifies it as a "condition for further study" involving intense emotional distress centered on preoccupation with the deceased and the circumstances of death (American Psychiatric Association 2013).
- *Integrated grief*, used in the context of attachment theory, refers to a stable state in which the individual maintains an emotional attachment to the lost loved one without impaired function (Shear et al. 2016).

Chapter 39 (p. 1314)

References

American Psychiatric Association: Diagnostic and Statistical Manual of Mental Disorders, 5th Edition. Arlington, VA, American Psychiatric Association, 2013

Block SD; ACP-ASIM End-of-Life Care Consensus Panel. American College of Physicians - American Society of Internal Medicine: Assessing and managing depression in the terminally ill patient. Ann Intern Med 132(3):209–218, 2000 10651602

Breitbart W, Bruera E, Chochinov H, Lynch M: Neuropsychiatric syndromes and psychological symptoms in patients with advanced cancer. J Pain Symptom Manage 10(2):131–141, 1995 7730685

Bruera E, Chadwick S, Brenneis C, et al: Methylphenidate associated with narcotics for the treatment of cancer pain. Cancer Treat Rep 71(1):67–70, 1987 3791269

Butler RN: The life review: an interpretation of reminiscence in the aged. Psychiatry 26:65–76, 1963 14017386

Candy M, Jones L, Williams R, et al: Psychostimulants for depression. Cochrane Database Syst Rev (2):CD006722, 2008 18425966

Chochinov HM, Breitbart W (eds): Handbook of Psychiatry in Palliative Medicine, 2nd Edition. New York, Oxford University Press, 2012

Davis MP: Cannabinoids for symptom management and cancer therapy: the evidence. J Natl Compr Canc Netw 14(7):915–922, 2016 27407130

Elia G, Thomas J: The symptomatic relief of dyspnea. Curr Oncol Rep 10(4):319–325, 2008 18778558

Homsi J, Nelson KA, Sarhill N, et al: A phase II study of methylphenidate for depression in advanced cancer. Am J Hosp Palliat Care 18(6):403–407, 2001 11712722

Karan LD, Dani JA, Benowitz N: The pharmacology of nicotine and tobacco, in Principles of Addiction Medicine, 3rd Edition. Edited by Graham AW, Shultz TK. Chevy Chase, MD, American Society of Addiction Medicine, 2003, pp 225–248

Levin TT, Li Y, Weiner JS, et al: How do-not-resuscitate orders are utilized in cancer patients: timing relative to death and communication-training implications. Palliat Support Care 6(4):341–348, 2008 19006588

Lichter I, Mooney J, Boyd M: Biography as therapy. Palliat Med 7(2):133–137, 1993 8261183

Miovic M, Block S: Psychiatric disorders in advanced cancer. Cancer 110(8):1665–1676, 2007 17847017

National Consensus Project for Quality Palliative Care: Clinical Practice Guidelines for Quality Palliative Care, 3rd Edition. 2013. Available at: http://www.nationalconsensusproject.org. Accessed October 20, 2017.

Portenoy R, Foley KM: Management of cancer pain, in Handbook of Psychooncology: Psychological Care of the Patient With Cancer. Edited by Holland JC, Rowland JH. New York, Oxford University Press, 1989, pp 369–382

Prigerson HG, Horowitz MJ, Jacobs SC, et al: Prolonged grief disorder: psychometric validation of criteria proposed for DSM-V and ICD-11. PLoS Med 6(8):e1000121, 2009 19652695

Rigotti NA, Munafo MR, Stead LF: Smoking cessation interventions for hospitalized smokers: a systematic review. Arch Intern Med 168(18):1950–1960, 2008 18852395

Rosenfeld B, Saracino R, Tobias K, et al: Adapting Meaning-Centered Psychotherapy for the palliative care setting: results of a pilot study. Palliat Med 31(2):140–146, 2017 27435603

Roth AJ, Massie MJ: Anxiety in palliative care, in Handbook of Psychiatry in Palliative Medicine, 2nd Edition. Edited by Chochinov HM, Breitbart W. New York, Oxford University Press, 2009, pp 69–80

Shear MK, Reynolds CF 3rd, Simon NM, et al: Optimizing treatment of complicated grief: a randomized clinical trial. JAMA Psychiatry 73(7):685–694, 2016 27276373

Smith LA, Azariah F, Lavender VT, et al: Cannabinoids for nausea and vomiting in adults with cancer receiving chemotherapy. Cochrane Database Syst Rev (11):CD009464, 2015 26561338

Subcommittee on Psychiatric Aspects of Life-Sustaining Technology: The role of the psychiatrist in end-of-life treatment decisions, in Caring for the Dying: Identification and Promotion of Physician Competency (Educational Resource Document). Philadelphia, PA, American Board of Internal Medicine, 1996, pp 61–67

Weaver M, Breland A, Spindle T, Eissenberg T: Electronic cigarettes: a review of safety and clinical issues. J Addict Med 8(4):234–240, 2014 25089953

Weissman DE: Decision making at a time of crisis near the end of life. JAMA 292(14):1738–1743, 2004 15479939